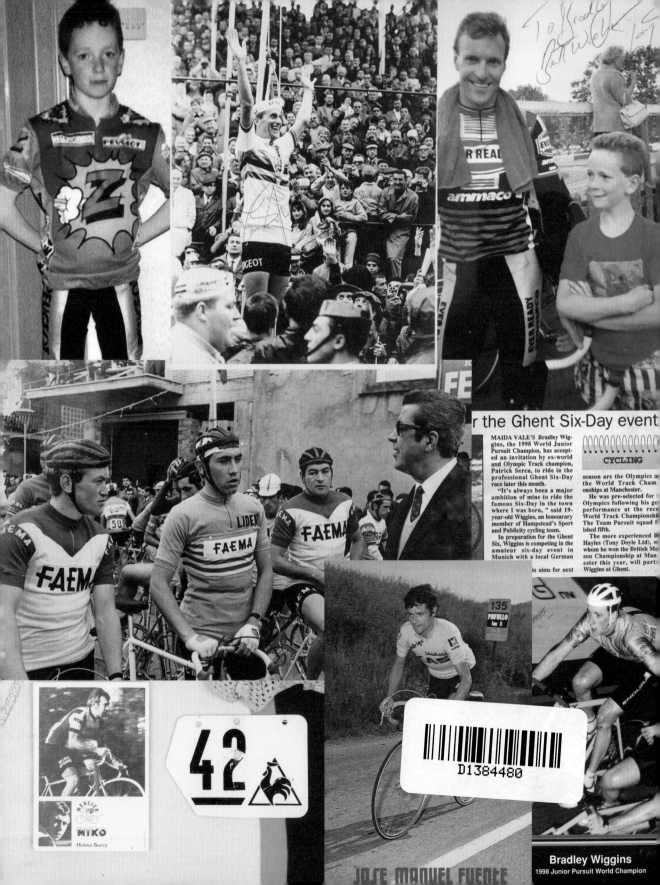

r the Ghent Six-Day event

MAIDA VALE'S Bradley Wiggins, the 1998 World Junior Pursuit Champion, has accepted an invitation by ex-world and Olympic Track champion, Patrick Sercu, to ride in the professional Ghent Six-Day race later this month.

"It's always been a major ambition of mine to ride the famous Six-Day in the town where I was born, " said 19-year-old Wiggins, an honourary member of Hampstead's Sport and Publicity cycling team.

In preparation for the Ghent Six, Wiggins is competing in the amateur six-day event in Munich with a local German

in aims for next

CYCLING

season are the Olympics a the World Track Cham onships at Manchester.

He was pre-selected for Olympics following his go performance at the rece World Track Championshi The Team Pursuit squad f ished fifth.

The more experienced R Hayles (Tony Doyle Ltd), w whom he won the British Ma son Championship at Man ester this year, will part Wiggins at Ghent.

Bradley Wiggins
1998 Junior Pursuit World Champion

JOSE MANUEL FUENTE

MIKO
Hoban Barry

42

ICONS

HarperCollins*Publishers*
1 London Bridge Street
London SE1 9GF

www.harpercollins.co.uk

First published by HarperCollins*Publishers* 2018

10 9 8 7 6 5 4 3 2 1

A catalogue record of this book is available from
the British Library

ISBN 978-0-00-830174-3

Printed and bound in China

ICONS

MY INSPIRATION. MY MOTIVATION. MY OBSESSION.

BRADLEY WIGGINS

WITH HERBIE SYKES

HarperCollins*Publishers*

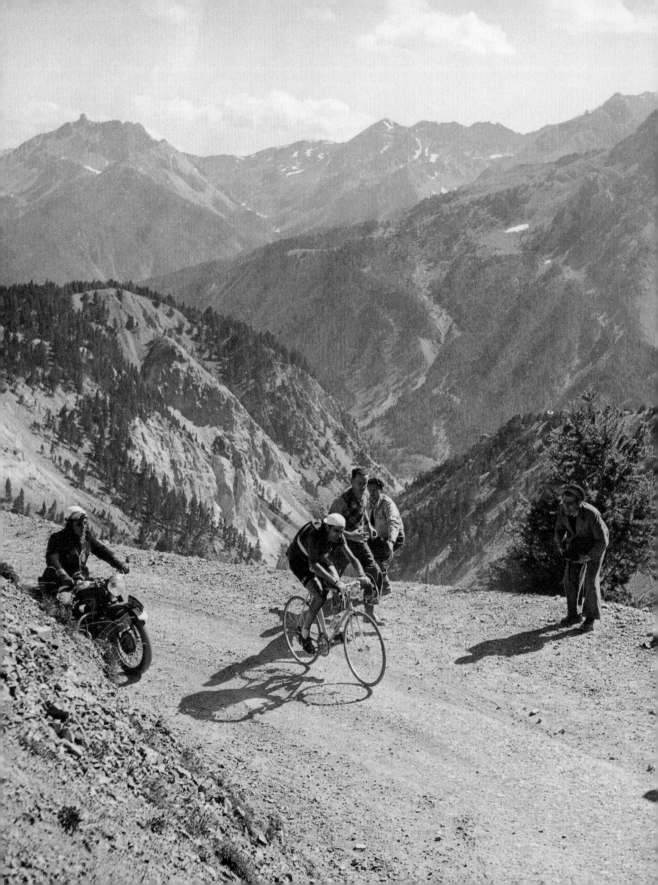

CONTENTS

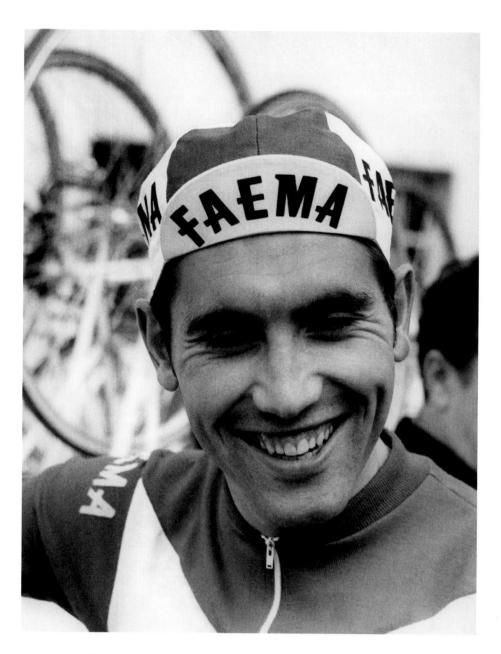

Merckx rode for the short-lived Faemino-Faema team between 1968 and 1970.
The team mostly comprised Belgian riders, with a few Italians.

FOOTBALL WAS MY FIRST LOVE, and like most kids from Brussels I was an Anderlecht fan. However, one day I discovered the great Stan Ockers, and fell in love with cycling.

Stan was a hero to me, just as he was to many Belgians. In 1955 he won the World Championships, Flèche Wallonne and Liège–Bastogne–Liège, but in general he tended to lose more races than he won. He was popular because he was a great rider, but most of all I think because he was a great sportsman. I liked to pretend I was him as I rode my bike, but then in 1956 he died following a crash on the track at Antwerp, his home town. I was only 11 at the time, but his death broke my heart.

Ultimately, Stan was the reason I started racing. I went on to win 525 professional races, so I guess you could say that he changed the course of cycling history.

The point is that we are all dreamers. We're all fans first and foremost, because if we weren't we wouldn't become sportsmen. I started out pretending to be Stan, and through him I learned about Rik Van Steenbergen, Briek Schotte and Fausto Coppi. Eventually I became a professional cyclist, and I wanted to emulate Coppi and Jacques Anquetil by winning the Tour de France and breaking the Hour Record.

Brad's story is more or less the same. He started out watching Miguel Induráin, and decided he wanted to understand cycling history for himself. That led him to me, to the Tour de France, to the Hour Record and eventually to our friendship.

We were lucky enough to be blessed with the talent to win bike races, but in reality we were no different to millions of starry-eyed kids down the years. History repeats itself in cycling, and I know for a fact that there are thousands of young British guys who took up cycling because of Brad. That's the way it rolls in cycling, and the way it always was.

Enjoy the ride . . .

Eddy Merckx

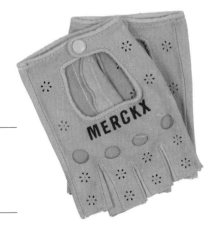

In among all the jerseys in my collection, Eddy's gloves mean a hell of a lot.

INTRODUCTION

CYCLING SEEMS TO ATTRACT A LOT OF COLLECTORS, probably because it's always been so important historically and culturally. You could say it's just a sport, but the bike itself still plays a big role in the way human civilisations think and act. You only have to look at places like Holland and China to

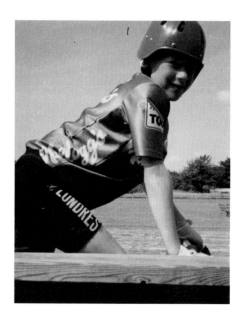

see this, and to understand that, long after fossil-fuel cars have disappeared, the humble bike will still be around. I genuinely don't think there's any one single invention that has been healthier for the human mind and body, so while it is 'just' a sport, for many people it's also a way of life and of living.

Bike racing is unique among mainstream sports because its development was totally organic. It didn't have to be 'invented' like the others, because Europeans have been learning to cycle for well over 100 years. Going fast on a pushbike is the most natural thing in the world, and organised racing is just an extension of that.

As a professional sport it has two special characteristics. The first is that it's free to watch; the second, that it goes to its public and not vice versa. What I mean by this is that there are no filters – the riders are literally within touching distance, and the public are intrinsic to the spectacle. It's much easier to watch cycling on TV, and actually being there means you're only going to see a tiny fraction of the action. The *feeling* a bike race generates, however, is electric, and I think that's one of the reasons people stand by the roadside for hours waiting for what often amounts to a few moments. The key is its sheer intimacy, and that's why the sport is so closely linked to its fans' identity. Of course, there are millions of hobby cyclists, but there are also people like me, for whom it's all-consuming.

I think all of the above – and certainly some complex anthropological stuff – explains the collecting thing. People go nuts for bidons, but also musettes, caps, race numbers, race direction signs and accreditation paraphernalia. There are guys with

Left:
Thinking I'm
Joey McLoughlin
at Herne Hill in
1988.

Opposite:
Me with 1980
and 1986 world
champion Tony
Doyle. Great
Flintstones'
shorts!

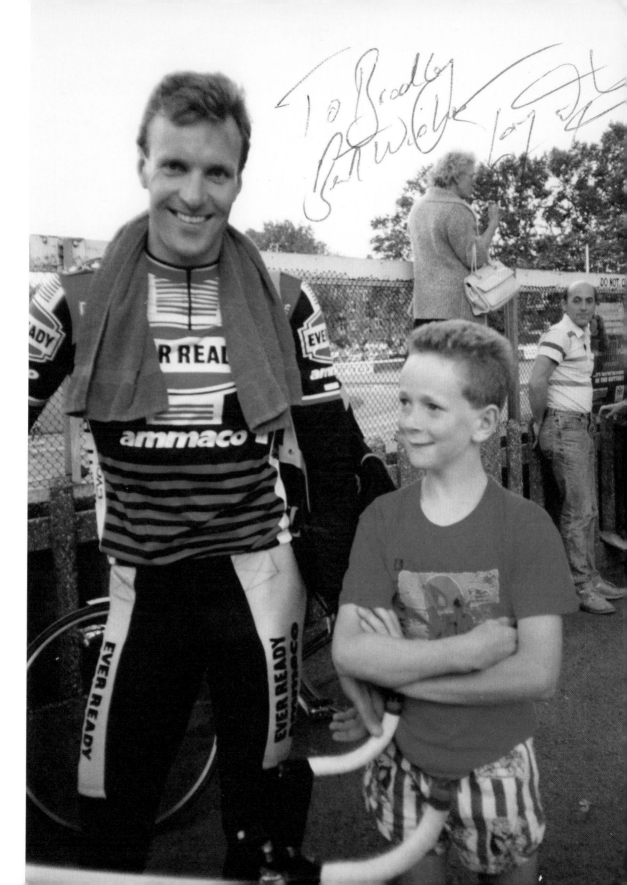

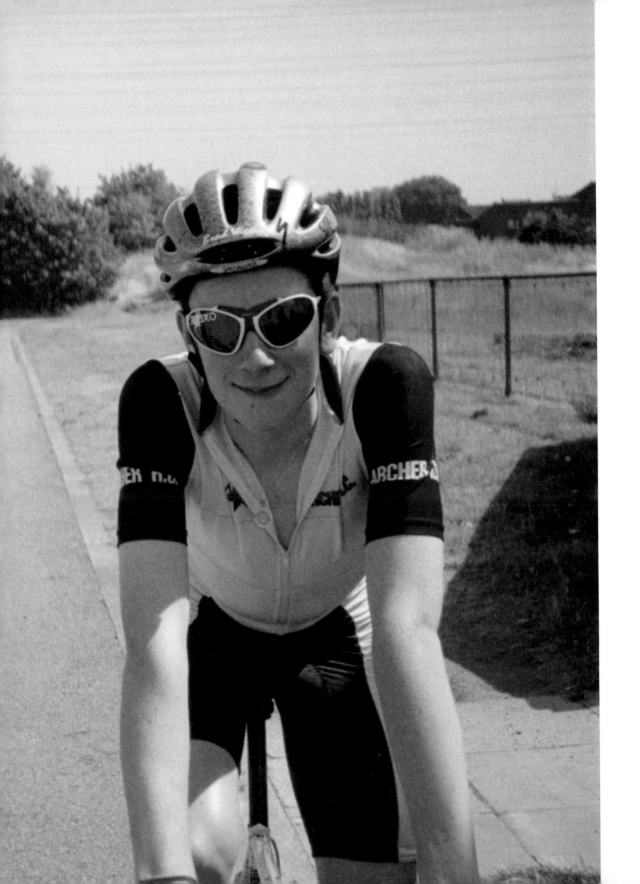

massive collections of postcards, cigarette cards, autographs, race books, photographs, miniatures, badges and magazines. There are also people who collect specific brands, especially exotic Italian ones like Campagnolo, Bianchi and Colnago. There are guys who collect stuff from specific races, typically the Giro and the Tour, and of course there are collectors of the bikes themselves. There are loads of personal museums, and I know of a chap in Italy who has over 300 perfectly restored professional racing cycles. He keeps them in a massive house he rents halfway up a mountain, and it has more security than Fort Knox. That guy also has three ex-wives, but such is life . . .

For people like me, however, it's all about the jerseys.

Football and cricket teams get a trophy if they win, or an urn full of ashes. In track and field they get a medal. In golf the winner of the Masters gets a green jacket, and in World Series baseball the champions get a ring. I'm sure they're fantastic things, but they're basically inanimate. They're not used in competition, and there's nothing used or worn in any of these sports that distinguishes the champions from the mere mortals. Diego Maradona and Michael Jordan had a number on their backs, but essentially they wore the same kit as the others, as did individual sporting greats such as Borg, Bolt and Ali.

Like all great sportsmen, champion cyclists come and go. So do their sponsors, but their jerseys remain. Over the years they accumulate value, because through them we learn the history of our sport and, as cycling people, of ourselves – they're also a mirror of the times, on our habits and our culture. First, the sponsors were the bike manufacturers and then, after the war, companies that made leisure items and consumer goods. It started with toothpaste, because as we became wealthier dental hygiene became more affordable. Next came things like aperitifs, and status symbols such as domestic appliances. They were followed by fitted kitchens, televisions, *colour* televisions, ice cream for the kids. Then cars, travel agents, video recorders, telecoms . . . As you work through the collection, it becomes apparent that the evolution of the brand logos is of as much interest and importance as that of the shirts themselves. Cycling jerseys not only tell us the story of cycling and of cyclists, but also, if we look closely, of the continent.

Then, of course, there are the leaders' jerseys and champion's jersey. They are *the* cycling icons, and there's a small army of people like me who collect them. Of course, what we're really collecting is proximity. Through the jerseys we feel closer to the champions who wore them, because they're the people who wrote the history of the thing we love.

Eastway 1995, in the exact spot on which the finish line of the velodrome now sits.

This book constitutes a thank-you note to 21 of them and, overwhelmingly, a love letter to the sport of cycling.

I hope you enjoy it.

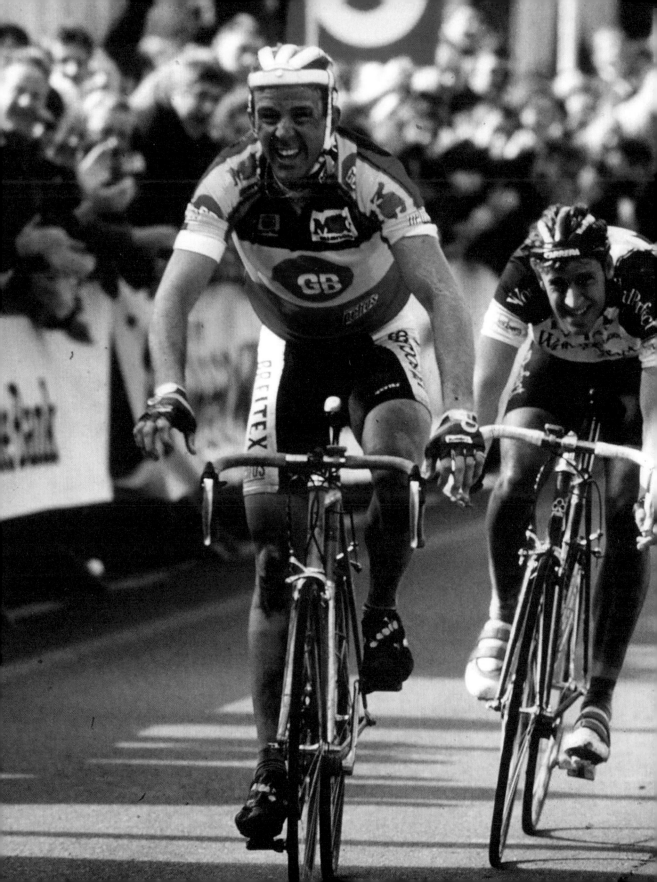

1

Johan Museeuw

1965–

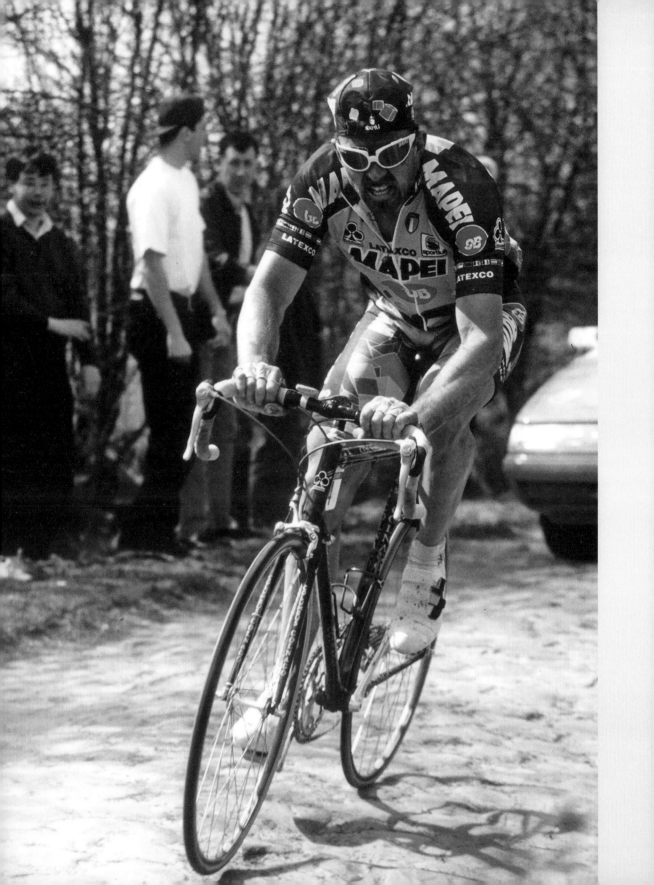

One of my first real cycling memories is the final-day time trial of the 1989 Tour de France. I was nine, we were round at my nan's house and my grandad was watching the race as usual. I wasn't much interested in Laurent Fignon and Greg LeMond – in truth I barely knew who they were – but I very well remember being struck by the visual elements. Fignon's ponytail, his yellow jersey and disc wheels, LeMond's fluorescent kit, strange handlebars and that futuristic helmet he had ... I didn't understand the magnitude of what I was witnessing, but aesthetically it was spectacular.

Like most inner-city London kids, however, I was a football fan. The sportsmen I identified with had names like Adams, Merson and Thomas, not Chioccioli, Delgado and Van Hooydonck. The Arsenal players used to drink in the local pub after the game, and most of them were Londoners. Tottenham had Gary Lineker and Paul Gascoigne in their side at the time, and Lineker lived quite close by in St John's Wood. Me and my mates saw him walking back from the shop with a pint of milk one day, and followed him to this house in Abbey Gardens. Once we knew where he lived we just knocked on the door and asked his wife if he was in, in pretty much the same way we used to ask one another's mums. She sent us on our way with an autographed publicity card each, but I've an idea the whole episode is quite illustrative. Famous sportsmen seemed more accessible, and I don't think there were so many filters between them and 'normal people' back then. Ultimately, though, it didn't matter anyway. By the summer of 1992 Lineker was playing in Japan, and my sporting world paradigm was about to be turned completely on its head.

The king of his generation.

BACK THEN GREAT BRITAIN WASN'T WINNING A GREAT DEAL at the Olympics, and it wasn't winning *at all* at Olympic cycling. As such, when Chris Boardman dominated the pursuit on his futuristic Lotus bike at the 1992 games in Barcelona, it was front-page news. Here was a British cyclist using a marvel of engineering made by a quintessentially British company – and conquering the world. The following morning I had to take the Tube across London to play football, and when I got to the station I noticed that the news stands were full of it. For better or for worse (!), British cyclists often occupy the front pages nowadays, but back then it was unheard of.

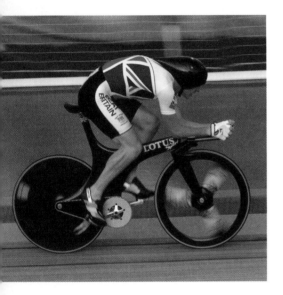

Chris had captured the public imagination, and that included me as well. I mentioned it to my mum, and she said I ought to think about giving cycling a go. I had a racing bike from Halfords, and she reasoned that I might be quite good at it. My dad had been a professional bike rider, so I had the genes if nothing else. Then if I was talented I'd have a much better chance of making it, because everyone else wanted to be a footballer. Besides, she still knew a few people in cycling and said it was a great sport. I saw no reason not to try, and so off we went to Hillingdon, where we met a guy named Stuart Benstead. He'd brought my dad over from Australia in the 1970s, and the two of them had lived together for a time. He ran the Archer Road Club, and he remembered me as a toddler. He said I ought to join the club, and before I knew it I was racing.

Truth be told it was a pretty chastening experience, at least initially. I was a 12-year-old doing under-16 races, so the others were much bigger and stronger than me. Most Friday nights I'd get an absolute pasting, then shuffle off home with my tail between my legs. Somehow, though, cycling's perverse logic started to take hold of me. The worse it got, the more I seemed to like it and the more I resolved to get better at it.

By the following spring I was half decent. I was still getting shelled out on the climbs, and the others were much more committed than I was. They used to train, where I'd pretty much just turn up and race. I'd started to look forward to the races, however, and to take an interest in the gear. By then cable TV had come to London, and Eurosport showed quite a lot of cycling.

Left:
Chris on 'that bike' at the 1992 Olympics.

Opposite:
Cornering in Bury St Edmunds in 1996.

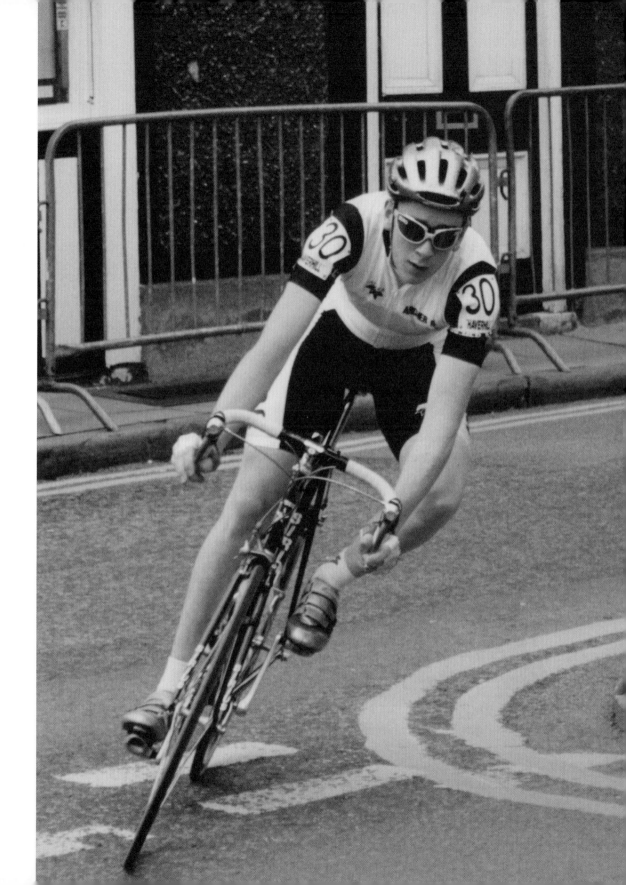

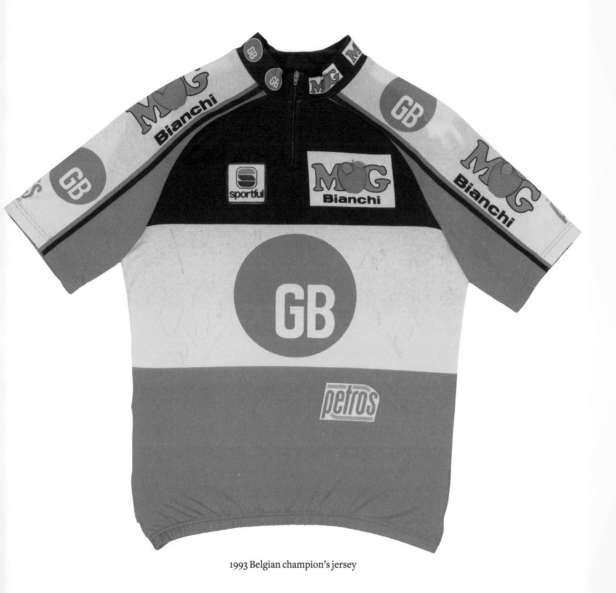

1993 Belgian champion's jersey

This was the point at which I began to understand that cycling mattered a lot in Europe, that it was very much a mainstream sport. I remember looking forward to Milan–San Remo, as well as the feeling of disappointment when I heard it wasn't going to be televised. I had to wait until the Thursday, when *Cycling Weekly* came out, to discover that an Italian named Maurizio Fondriest had won it. That waiting seems incredible now, because you can get the results of the races within seconds, but that's the way it was back then. It really was a different world.

The first live road race I watched was the Tour of Flanders. Hitherto I had really no idea that so many people would come out to watch a bike race, but there seemed to be seas of them. Nor had I any real appreciation of just how fast it all was and how ferociously the professionals raced. Johan Museeuw won it in this beautiful tricoloured jersey – red, black and yellow – and Mum told me he got to wear it because he was the Belgian national champion, which I thought was a really wicked idea. She explained some of the rituals around *De Ronde*, as the Tour of Flanders is known in Flemish. She said it was the highlight of the year for Flemish people, almost irrespective of whether or not they were cycling fans. She also told me that Museeuw would be like the king over there. He was a Flemish rider wearing the national champion's jersey to win Flanders, and nothing came close to that as regards performance or prestige. Thus Museeuw, the 'Lion of Flanders', became my first cycling hero, and so began the long and winding road that has been my journey in bike racing.

It's impossible to exaggerate how good Museeuw was, and how aggressively he rode. Almost any article you read about him at the time included words like 'warrior' or 'fighter' somewhere along the line. These were – and remain – the oldest clichés in the cycling book, but they fitted him like a glove. Other cyclists were more stylish, but nobody was ever as brave, nor looked as purposeful. The Flemish people identified with him because he was the identikit classics rider, the living embodiment of their cycling tradition. Where Boardman had been about method, science and discipline, Museeuw was an old-school blood-and-snot cyclist like no other.

A few years later, when I was 16, I went to Belgium for a week with my mum, stepdad and half-brother. We went to watch the classics, and I saw Museeuw *in the flesh*. I've italicised that for dramatic effect, but only because dramatic is precisely what it was, at least for me. My mum still has a load of photographs she took that week. Some of them are a bit bizarre, but collectively they tell an unforgettable story. Most of them are of my eight-year-old brother, standing with the champions at the start of the Tour of Flanders. Like most 16-year-olds I was too cool for school, so I'd send him up to them instead. In some ways he was acting as a sort of proxy for me, because I didn't want to come across as the smitten, star-struck teenager that I was. I feigned indifference and pretended to take it all in my stride, but in reality I was just overcome by the whole thing. Maybe I was afraid they might reject me or some such, but the long and the short of it was that metaphorically I was wetting my pants. I was at the Tour of Flanders, but I wasn't *of* the Tour of Flanders. I was trying desperately hard to pretend it was just a normal day at the races, but the reality was I was all over the place. I'd been looking forward to the moment for years, but now that it had arrived it was too much for me to compute.

During the race we went to the feed, and I remember grabbing all the musettes as they threw them away. I think I got about 20 of them from that one race – I had the others scrambling about for them as well – and the Rabobank one had a rice cake in it. I had to decide whether to eat it or keep it as a souvenir, and I can assure you that was quite a decision. I ate it in the end, and then we went to the second feed in Zottegem. We scrounged a load of caps from the *soigneurs*, watched the riders come through again, and then made for the bar to watch the last 60 kilometres on TV.

At a certain point this guy walked in with long, curly, strawberry-blond hair. I realised it was Eric Vanderaerden, and I knew all about him. By then I'd amassed the world's largest collection of cycling videotapes, and one of them showed him winning the race in 1985. Now he was getting towards the end of his career and he'd climbed off, got changed and just walked into the bar with his *soigneur*. He wasn't one of my favourites, but I was blown away all the same. I was in the same bar as Eric Vanderaerden!

Anyway, Michele Bartoli attacked on the Muur van Geraardsbergen and time-trialled to the win. He was a new star and I didn't know much about him, but after the race we went and stood around the team buses waiting for Museeuw to emerge. When he came out he didn't look happy – he'd been going for a third *Ronde* and had been undone by some sort of mechanical failure – but he had to walk 100 metres across the car park to get to his dad's car. I didn't dare speak to him, but I got close enough to be able to delude myself that I'd 'met' him. What I'd actually done was walk alongside him for a few steps, and my mum has a grainy old photo to prove it.

The first time I raced against Johan would have been the 2002 Tour of Flanders. Actually, no, strike that. Technically I was taking part in the same *race* as Johan Museeuw, but I wasn't racing against him as such. He was in a different stratosphere as a bike rider, and my abiding memory of that race is thinking, 'Hang on a minute. That's Johan Museeuw and I'm doing the same race as him!' Beyond that I just remember the size of a) his calves and b) the gear he was able to turn.

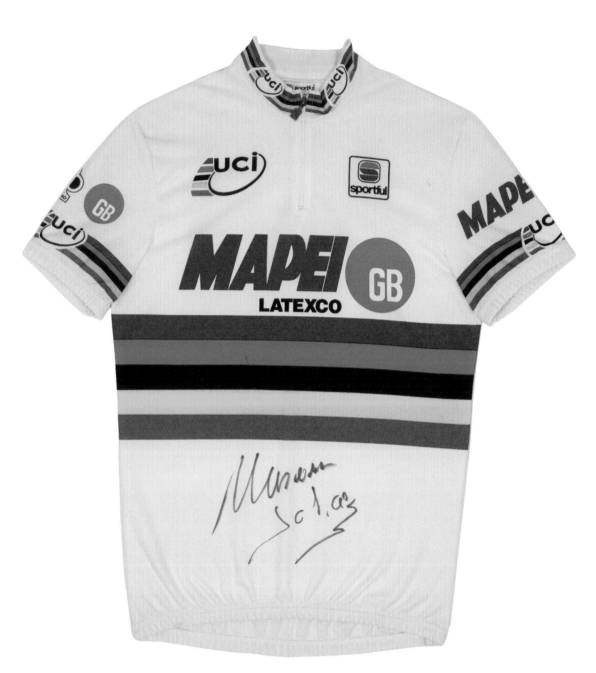

1996 world champion's jersey

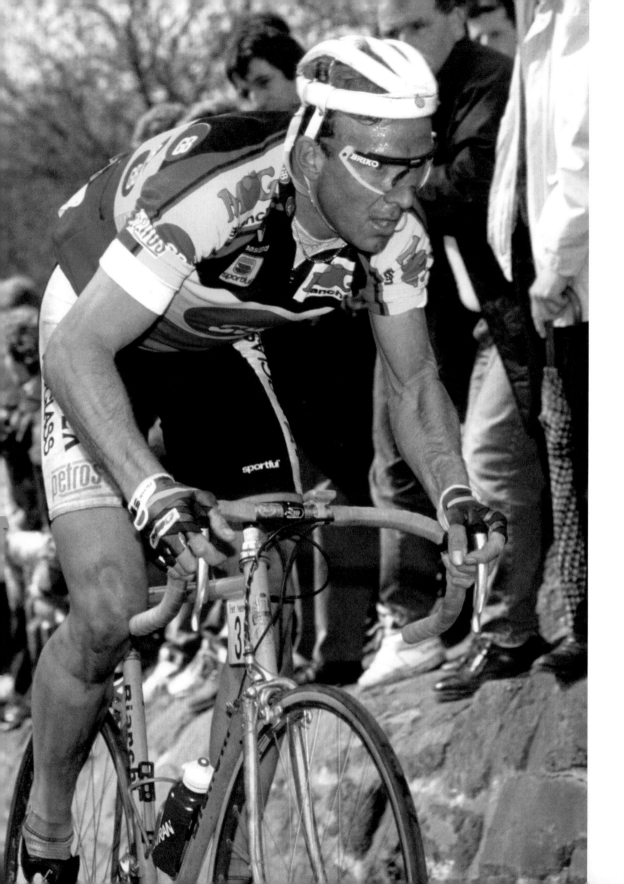

There was a big fight to get to the Molenberg in front, and I think it was there that my education as a professional road cyclist began in earnest. People were just pushing me out of their wheels all the time, and I didn't have the fight in me to do anything about it. If one of them asked me what I was doing or tried to shunt me into the gutter, I'd find myself apologising to *them*, in essence just capitulating. I was there, but I never felt like I'd earned the right to be there.

The Wednesday after Flanders it was Gent–Wevelgem. It was quite windy that day, and I decided not to allow myself to be pushed around. One of my jobs was to make sure I took my team-mates up to the front before the Kemmelberg, and I was determined I'd accomplish it. The Acqua & Sapone team were there, and their leader was Mario Cipollini, a big, macho, alpha-male Tuscan. He'd won San Remo and was favourite for the race. So I checked that my team-mates were on the wheel, and started making my way up the side of the road. Eventually I came up alongside the Italians, by now feeling quite good about myself because I felt I was doing the job that I was asked to do. The problem was that Cipollini was looking across at me with something approaching total contempt. Unbeknownst to me my colleagues had just sat up, and like a dick I'd ridden to the front of Gent–Wevelgem on my own. Cipo obviously assumed I was French – I had a Française des Jeux jersey on – and he turned to the rest of his team and said something along the lines of, 'Look at this French wanker!'

I'd thought I was being a real pro, but now these Italians were laughing at me, quite literally. I had to creep back to my place at the back of the group, and I felt like a wimpering dog. Then we hit a crosswind, then I went out the back, and then I climbed off at the first feed. It was pretty embarrassing, to say the least. Cipo could make you feel really small. I hated him for that at the time, but cycling was much more hierarchical back then. People like me didn't dare go near people like him and Museeuw, because you had to serve your apprenticeship first. The idea that I might try to converse with them never even occurred to me, and I reasoned that Museeuw wouldn't have known who I was anyway. I was a nobody, and he was far too busy trying to win the bike races I was nominally competing in. He retired in 2004, blissfully unaware of the fact that he'd been my boyhood idol. How, realistically, could it have been otherwise, given that I hadn't managed to utter a word to him?

You live and learn, and eventually I got pretty good at it. I had a long career, and towards the end of it I began a sort of sentimental journey. In the spring of 2015 I was doing an interview with the Belgian press. I was about to take part in my final Tour of Flanders, and they asked me about my cycling upbringing. I started telling them the story of how Museeuw's 1993 Flanders had been the first race I'd really watched, and it got back to him. He speaks some English, and he sent me a message on Instagram. It

Museeuw in the 1993 Tour of Flanders, his first win in the race.

was something like, 'Good luck and thanks for what you said about me.' I replied, and he told me that his 15-year-old son, Stefano, was a big fan of mine. He then asked if it would be OK for them to come and meet me before Paris–Roubaix, and I said that yes, of course it would.

Then I started to panic, because Johan Museeuw was coming to meet me.

So next thing I was having a massage after a training ride, and Servais Knaven, our DS, came up. He said, 'Johan's downstairs in the lobby waiting for you.' He was early, but I started panicking because I was keeping the great Johan Museeuw waiting. I asked Servais, 'What am I supposed to say to him?' Servais thought that was quite funny. He said, 'How should I know? Just talk to him! He's only human!'

Eventually I went down, and I was that teenager all over again. I was basically 16, but by now Johan was almost 50. He has this gentle, soft, fairly high-pitched voice anyway, and in some way he seemed almost the opposite of the ferocious rider he'd once been. When I asked him about Roubaix he gave me the usual 'Stay near the front and don't forget to eat' advice. It was exactly the same advice that cyclists have been giving one another for 100 years, because staying near the front is quite important if you want to win a bike race. The difference was that the advice came from Johan Museeuw, so it was – and is – worth its weight in gold.

I had one of my rainbow jerseys with me that day. I'd ridden De Panne a few days earlier, and there'd been a time trial. I got the jersey out, signed it and gave it to Stefano. Then Johan opened up his bag and pulled out a jersey of the same design as the one he'd worn to win the 1993 Tour of Flanders, the Belgian tricolour. He said he wanted to give it to me, which as you can imagine was pretty humbling. He also pulled out one of his famous bandanas and signed it, 'To Wiggo, Cheers. The Lion of Flanders.' Then for some reason he gave me a load of cans of beer, as you do. They're a little bit mad, the Flemish.

It had only taken me 22 years, but I'd got there in the end. I'd finally had the courage to meet Johan, and he's a mate now. However, the fact that he's a mortal, and vulnerable like the rest of us, doesn't in any way diminish the bike rider he once was. It's true that he wasn't much for talking back then, but he'd bike races to win and he was under a colossal amount of pressure. He was the torchbearer for Flemish cycling, and that's one hell of a weight to have to bear.

I keep telling him I'll go over and ride the cobblestones with him some time. I'll probably get round to it eventually, but then again maybe not. Time rolls on, but I'm still not sure I'm worthy. I may have won the Tour de France, but he's still Johan Museeuw.

Still the Lion of Flanders.

Museeuw winning the World Championships, 1996.

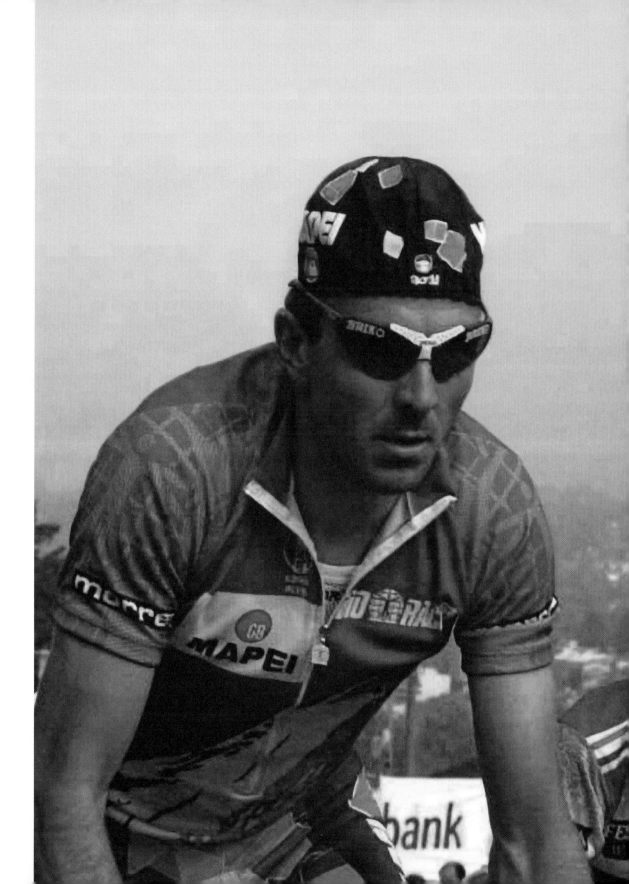

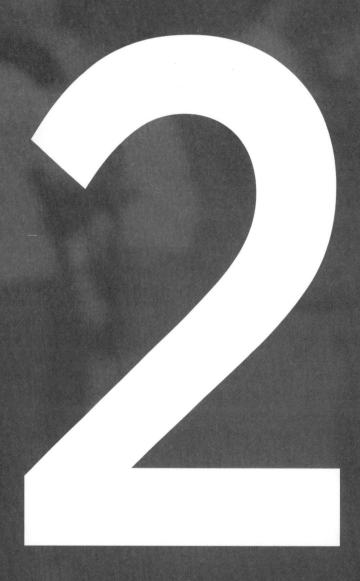

2

Franco Ballerini

1964–2010

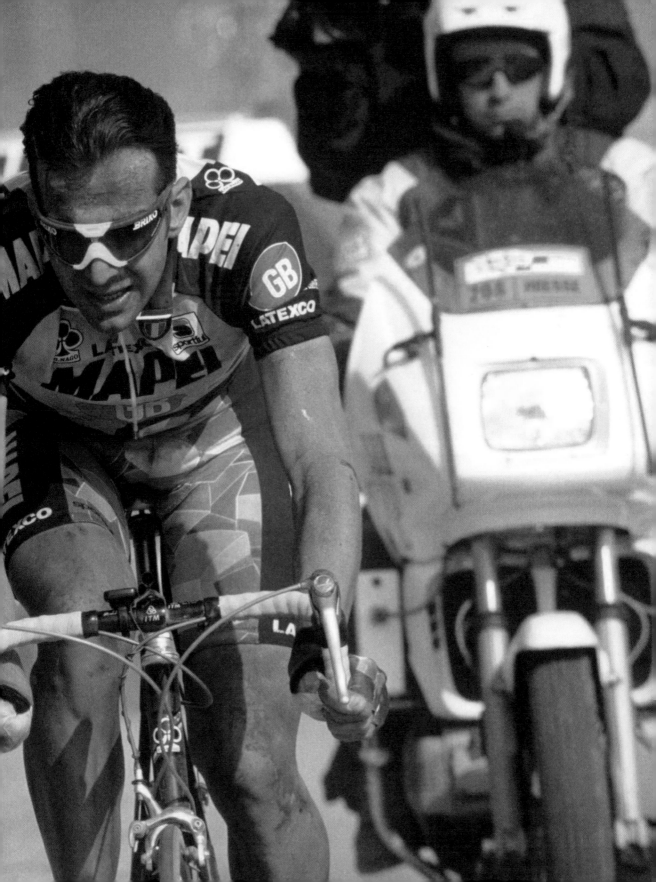

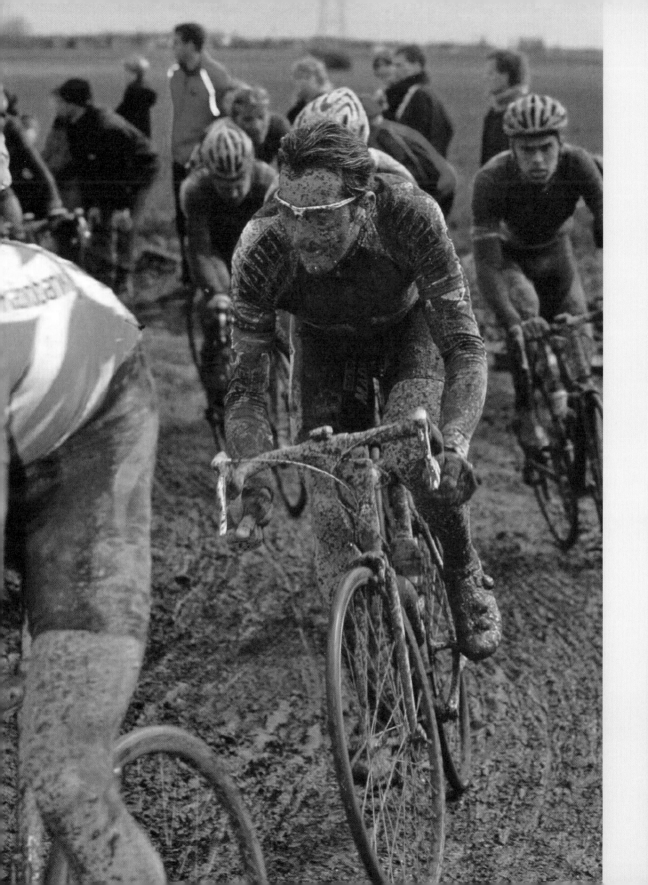

I was speaking to my mum after having watched Museeuw win Flanders, and she explained that Eurosport would be showing something called 'Paris–Roubaix' the following Sunday. She said, 'You know the mews out the back here, with the cobblestones? Well, they ride over roads like that, and the cobbled sections are called *pavé*.' I couldn't for one minute imagine how they'd be able to race their bikes over stuff like that, but I couldn't wait.

And so it was that, on 11 April 1993, I was acquainted with the wonder that is Paris–Roubaix. My first impression was just how crazy the whole thing looked. And how spectacular. I'd only ever seen sporting events that took place in hermetically sealed stadiums, but this was something else entirely. Where Boardman had gone round and round the velodrome, here they were just flaying themselves for hour after hour. You had potholes, mud and dust everywhere, and those cobbles. Then you had guys just keeling over and falling off,

Riding through the mud in his last victory at Paris–Roubaix, in 2001.

people running with their bikes or carrying them, noise and bodies everywhere. I can only really describe the scene as organised anarchy, and I loved it. It may sound dramatic, but it's no exaggeration to state that it was a life-changing moment for me.

It was an epiphany.

Two riders had broken away. One was a Frenchman named Gilbert Duclos-Lassalle, who'd won the previous year after having tried 15 times. The other was an Italian named Franco Ballerini, and he was doing all the work. He was trying to shake Duclos off, and every time he surged the electricity went straight through me. Somehow Duclos kept clinging on, and ultimately they came into the velodrome together. Then they did the sprint and literally crossed the line simultaneously.

To the naked eye it looked too close to call, but Ballerini was convinced he'd won. The race officials were looking at the photo finish, but he started riding his lap of honour anyway ...

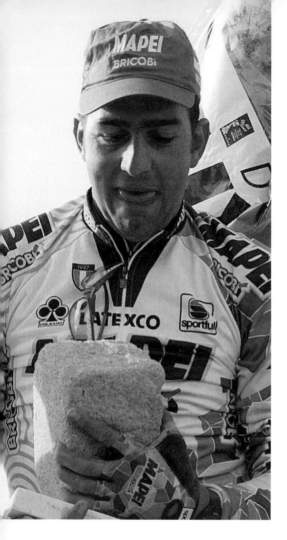

I UNDERSTAND WHAT PARIS–
ROUBAIX means to people now,
and I genuinely think he didn't dare
contemplate that he hadn't won.
I think he was actually trying to convince
himself that he hadn't *lost*. Paris–Roubaix
was who Franco Ballerini was, and
winning it was all he lived for.

In the end they gave it to Duclos,
the French guy. He'd been on Ballerini's
tail for an hour, and then stolen round
him and won by a few centimetres.
Franco had been stronger (and nobody
was in any doubt that he was the moral
victor). Duclos, though, was one stealthy,
resourceful bike rider, and he'd won by
making damned sure he didn't lose.

Ballerini had lost Paris–Roubaix,
but in the process he'd won himself a
new fan across the English Channel.
I don't suppose, in that precise instant,
he would have cared one iota, though,
because he was utterly inconsolable.

Franco Ballerini was a big, handsome
guy with a unique way of riding across the cobbles. He had this straight-armed, slightly
rocking, metronomic style that was completely different to the others. He also wore
those wonderful, fluorescent Briko glasses, and I'd often find my teenage self trying
to imitate him. Physically he was the Italian cycling archetype, but as a racer he was
made-to-measure for the northern classics. In 1994 he was second at Gent–Wevelgem,
third at Paris–Roubaix and fourth at Flanders. He was always among the strongest,
but he tended to lose because he wasn't particularly fast. In order to win he needed
to drop everyone else, and of course that's the hardest thing to do in cycling. His
greatness lay in the fact that through all the disappointments he never buckled, and
he never lost his *conviction* that one day he'd win Roubaix.

By 1995 he was riding for Mapei. They had Tony Rominger, Museeuw, Abraham
Olano, Fernando Escartín and a young Frank Vandenbroucke, and were developing
into the best team in the world, a team that would dominate cycling for almost a

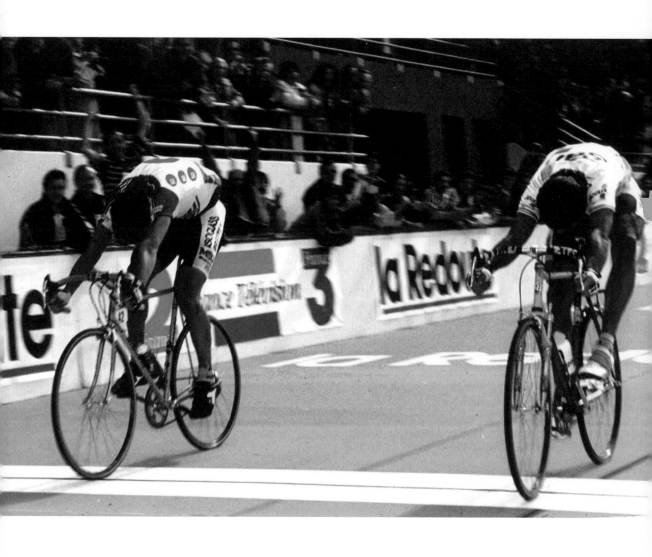

Left:
Ballerini celebrating
after winning his
second Paris–Roubaix.

Above:
The closest Paris–
Roubaix finish ever.
Ballerini (*left*) being
pipped to the line
by Duclos-Lassalle
in the Roubaix
velodrome, 1993.

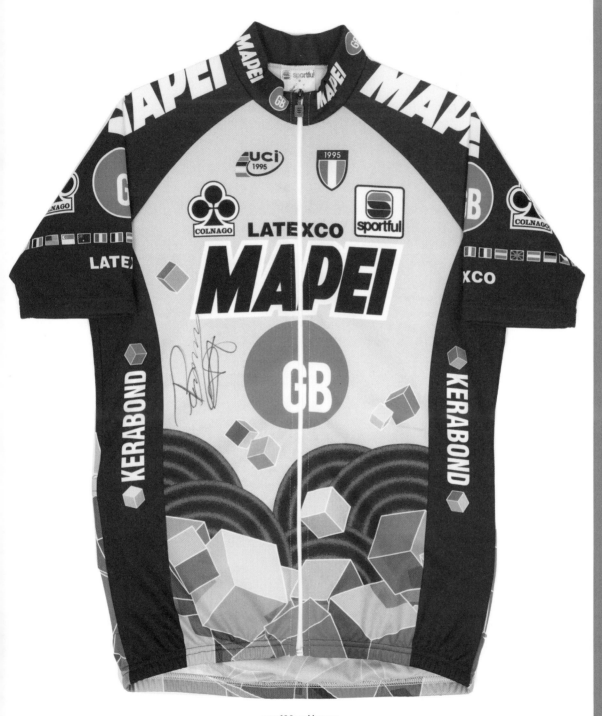

1996 Mapei jersey

decade. Talking of which, it kind of makes me smile when cycling journalists refer to Sky as the 'ruination of cycling'. In actual fact, there have always been wealthy, immensely powerful teams, and history tells us that they've generally been extremely good for the sport. The Bianchi, Peugeot, Molteni, Raleigh and Renault jerseys are iconic not because they're particularly beautiful (though to my mind some of them are), but because they are synonymous with a moment in time. Sky are just the latest iteration of the superteam.

I digress. Ballerini won Het Nieuwsblad (Het Volk, as was) in the freezing rain, and had really good form. However, three days before Roubaix he crashed at Gent–Wevelgem and dislocated his shoulder. He put the shoulder back in himself, but Ballerini's Law seemed to have struck yet again. He hung around the hotel with his arm in a sling, praying that he'd recover in time, but when he went to bed on Saturday night it was 50–50. He agreed to give it a go the following morning, but he was kidding himself. He hadn't been able to use a knife and fork for four days, let alone train for a 266-kilometre bike race over the cobblestones of northern France. The odds were stacked against him, to say the least.

But he was fresh, if nothing else, and it turned out that this was his day of grace. First one of his team-mates, a beast of a rider named Gianluca Bortolami, towed him across to the lead group. Then on Templeuve, a cobbled section 30-odd kilometres from Roubaix, Ballerini simply put on another gear and just rode away. From the best classics riders in the world.

It's often the commentary that characterises the most iconic sporting moments. Just as Sergio Agüero's title-winning goal for Manchester City has become indivisible from Martin Tyler's commentary, my abiding memory of that race is David Duffield's singalong voiceover. As Ballerini rode around the velodrome alone, old Duffers put on his very best Italian accent. It went something like, 'Fran-co-Ba-lle-rini-born-in-Fi-ren-ze . . .' Duffers's accent was rubbish, but that didn't matter at all because the moment was magical – and if I'm honest, it still is. Through all the stresses and strains of my own cycling career and post-career, that episode still brings a smile to my face. It's the unadulterated pleasure of cycling, pure and simple.

Ballerini won Roubaix again in 1998, and it's no coincidence that he chose to retire there in 2001. By then he was 36, and he rolled into the velodrome alone in 32nd place. He was caked in Paris–Roubaix mud, and that was entirely appropriate given that the race had defined his cycling career – and vice versa – for the preceding 15 years. You'll often see bike riders zip up their jersey as they approach the finish line, the better to expose their sponsor's name to the TV cameras. Ballerini, though, did the opposite. He *unzipped* his jersey, because he wanted the world to see his undervest. On it, in large blue letters, were printed two words:

MERCI ROUBAIX.

Just perfect.

By the time I turned professional I'd seen Ballerini's exploits *ad infinitum*, so when I was selected for the 2003 Paris–Roubaix it was a dream. I was 22, I'd got round Flanders the previous week, and I was about to join the Paris–Roubaix pantheon. I was with FDJ, and our protected riders were Jacky Durand, Christophe Mengin and Frédéric Guesdon, a previous winner. Our DS was Marc Madiot, whom I'd watched win it on TV, and before the race he gave us this big, dramatic, stirring team talk. He explained what it signified, the legend behind it, all the stuff I'd been daydreaming about since I watched Duclos and Ballerini slugging it out ten years earlier. To say I was excited would be an understatement.

So I knew all about it, knew every sector of the *pavé*, knew all the theories about riding it because I'd seen it on TV so many times. Nobody else really knew the first sectors because they were never televised, but I'd spent the preceding days reeling the names off to anyone who would listen. And indeed to anyone who wouldn't. I was a proper nerd.

Although Ballerini had retired, a lot of my boyhood heroes were still racing. Museeuw was there, Peter Van Petegem was there, Erik Zabel and Fabio Baldato were there . . . About 10 kilometres from the first sector I was near the front and, I have to say, doing a decent job. I was staying out of the way of the champions while simultaneously keeping Durand out of trouble. I'd have been about 20th, then suddenly there was a massive crash just behind me. It wiped everyone out, so now you'd a select group of 20. Essentially it was comprised of everyone who was anyone – and me, Bradley Wiggins, who wasn't.

I wasn't trying to mix it up at the front because I had no place there, but by the time we reached the entrance to the Arenberg I was feeling really pleased with myself. That's because the Arenberg is . . . well, *the Arenberg*, and I was in the lead group with the best of them. Then, wouldn't you just know it, 100 metres into the forest the guy in front of me, Kevin Van Impe, got his front wheel stuck in the gutter. He hopped it out, but his back wheel stayed in. He slid off in front of me, and I had no chance whatsoever. I just clattered straight into him and flew straight over the top of the bars.

I'd gone into 'The Trench' with the champions, and come out of it with a little group of back-markers. I had a buckled back wheel, and my knee and elbow hurt like hell. I couldn't hold the bars, let alone ride over the cobbles, so I had no choice but to climb into the broomwagon. Paris–Roubaix had broken me in two, but I was immediately transported back to *A Sunday in Hell*, a documentary film about the 1976 race that I'd watched fanatically as a kid. There was a shot of two riders in the wagon,

With unzipped jersey in the Roubaix velodrome at his last major professional race, in which he finished 32nd.

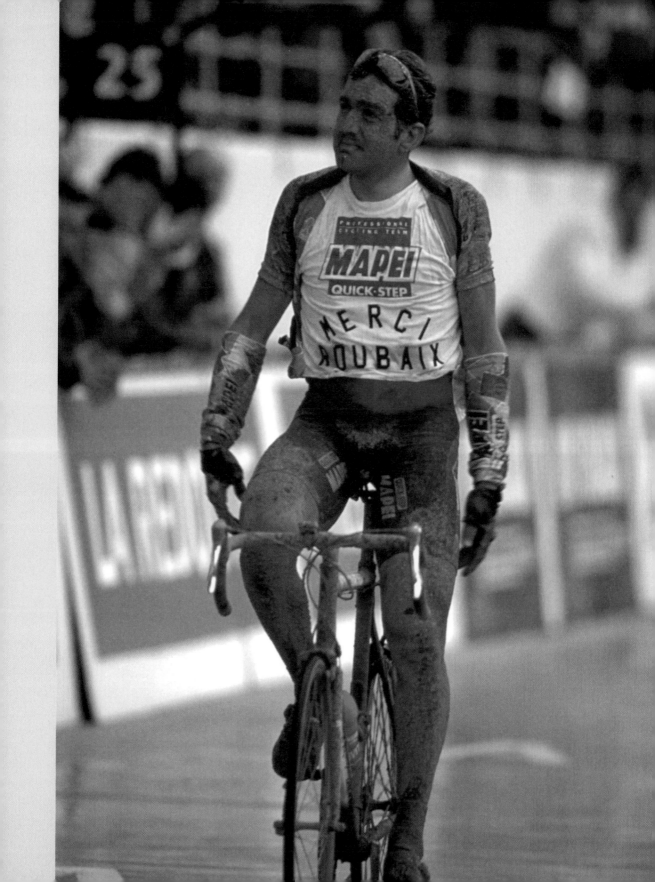

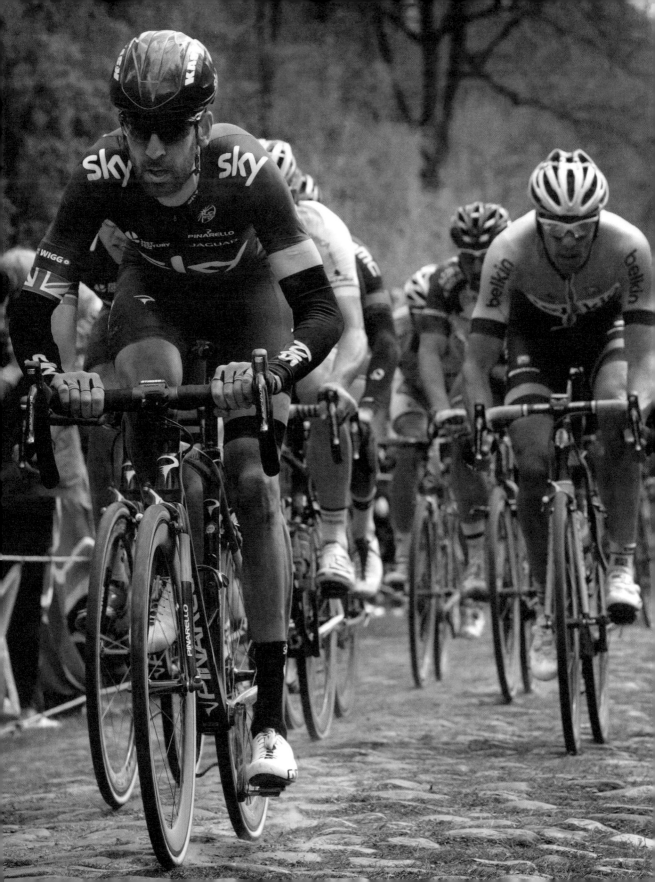

and they were telling the driver what had happened to them. Now here I was doing exactly the same thing. It sounds perverse – well, it actually *is* perverse – but I took some pleasure in that because in some way I was standing on the shoulders of giants. Giants in the sagwagon, but giants all the same.

I went back the following year, and again in 2005. I packed in both times, and by then the 'romance' of Paris–Roubaix was starting to wear thin. As a spectacle it was great, and I never failed to appreciate the grandeur of it. The problem was that actually riding it was ridiculous, a shit-fight I had not a prayer of winning. However hard I tried, something always went wrong. I couldn't figure it out. I seemed to be one of the hopeless, anonymous dozens that get sent there to make up the numbers.

And yet, I was desperate to be a factor there, and deep down I still believed I could be. I could ride, I knew how to read a race, and my bike-handling skills were good. I'd been World Madison champion, and logic suggested that if I were ever going to be competitive in a classic, it would be Roubaix. The problem was that Roubaix always did have its own twisted, indecipherable logic, and it kept making a mug of me.

In the summer of 2005 I finally got to meet Franco Ballerini, at the World Championships in Madrid. By then he was manager of the Italian national team, and he walked into the GB tent an hour and a half before the time trial. I thought, 'Bloody hell! That's Franco Ballerini!', and then Max Sciandri introduced us. Max started talking to him in Italian, telling him who I was and what I'd done. I felt ten feet tall.

I signed for Cofidis in 2006, having finally resolved to make a go of my road career. I decided to give Paris–Roubaix another shot, and found myself in a good position headed into the Arenberg. I wasn't strong enough to stay with the likes of Cancellara, Boonen and Ballan, but I settled into the main chase group of about 50 or so. Looking round I noticed that many of them were classics specialists, real class acts. I was relatively comfortable among them, and I remember being interviewed in the velodrome afterwards. I said, 'Well, even if I never do it again I'll always be able to say I finished Paris–Roubaix.' Three years later I went back, finished 25th and realised I had the ability to be competitive. I was a million miles away from winning the thing, but at least I was relevant.

Franco Ballerini died tragically in 2010, co-piloting in a rally in Tuscany. It had a profound impact on me, but also on the Italian riders who'd ridden under him. I'd idolised him as a bike rider but guys like Pippo Pozzato loved him, almost without exception, as a human being.

All of which largely explains my own efforts at the 2014 and 2015 Paris–Roubaix. In 2014 I was focused on trying to earn selection for the Tour team, so I wasn't specifically prepared for Roubaix. I was in decent form, but I was mainly

The Arenberg,
Paris–Roubaix
2014.

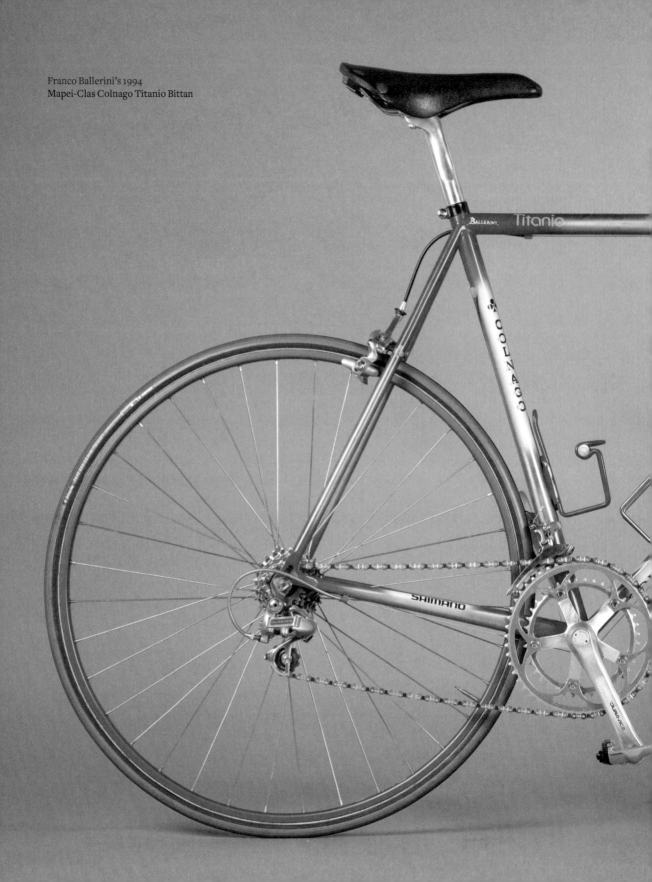

Franco Ballerini's 1994
Mapei-Clas Colnago Titanio Bittan

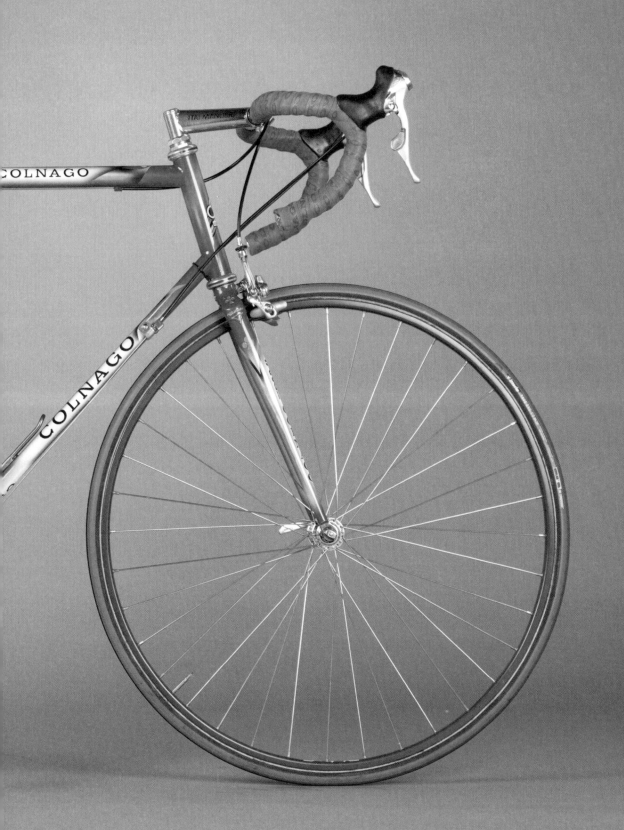

concentrating on being good for the Tour of California. Notwithstanding all of which, I was at the front all day, and I had the strength to attack in the finale. They caught me, and Niki Terpstra went clear, but I came in with Boonen, Štybar and Cancellara. I finished top ten in a race I'd never really targeted, because in my best years my career path had taken me elsewhere. Roubaix requires colossal strength and stamina, but as I'd acquired them I'd been focused, necessarily, on the Tour.

Regardless, I'd proved that I could be a player at the Hell of the North, and in 2015 I wanted to have a serious shot at it. I knew I'd need the cards to fall my way (you always need that at Roubaix, unless you're a Boonen or a Cancellara), but I was one of the elder statesmen of the peloton. The flip-side was that I was in a team containing guys like Flecha, Thomas, Stannard and Hayman, experienced riders who were more than capable of challenging for the win themselves.

The DS was Knaven, and he'd won Roubaix in 2001. When I put my hand up I knew I'd have the support of all of these people, but it was implicit that I'd need to perform. If you're asking guys like Stannard to sacrifice themselves for you, you'd better have the legs to justify it.

The rest is history. I attacked on the Templeuve, and that was no coincidence. Rather it was my way of paying tribute not only to the race itself, but also to Franco Ballerini. It was my way of honouring his memory, while simultaneously realising, as best I could, my own boyhood dream. In retrospect it probably wasn't the smartest thing to have done, but cycling's not all about watts, power meters and tactics. To me this was the very opposite of those things, and I like to think that Ballerini was of the same mind.

I didn't win Roubaix – I wasn't half the classics rider he was – but hopefully he'd have approved.

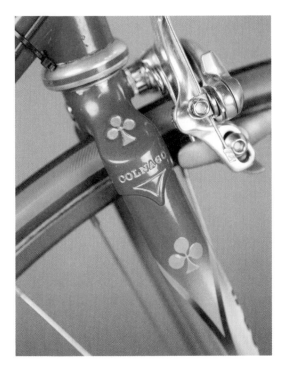

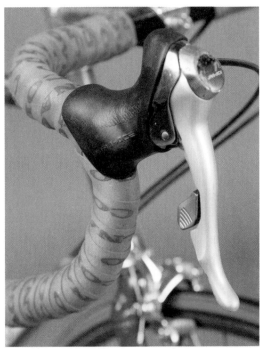

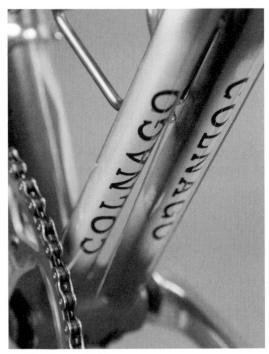

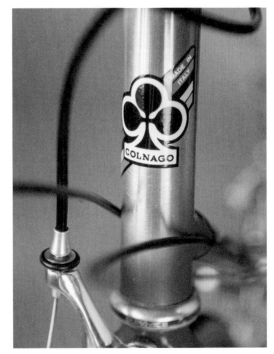

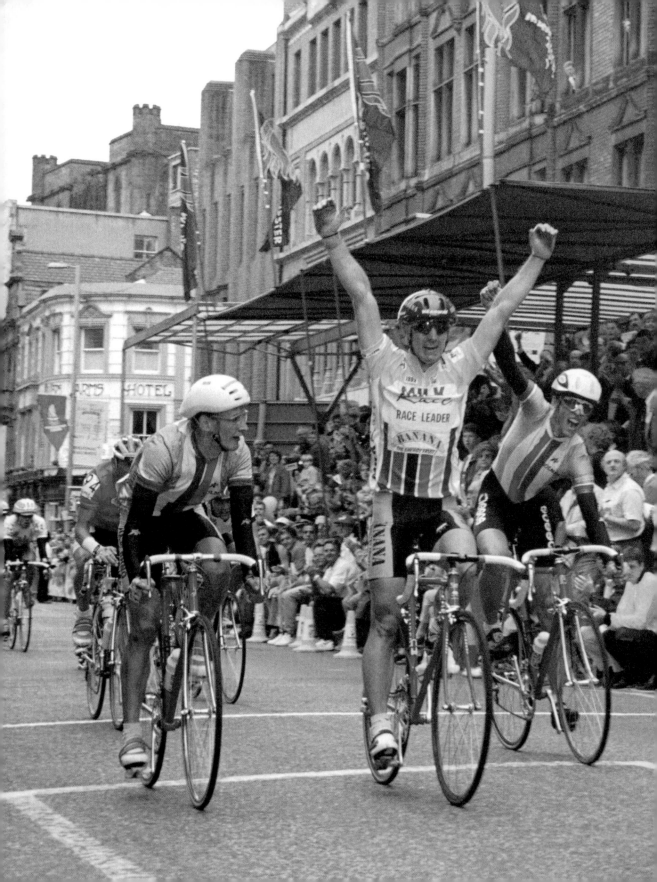

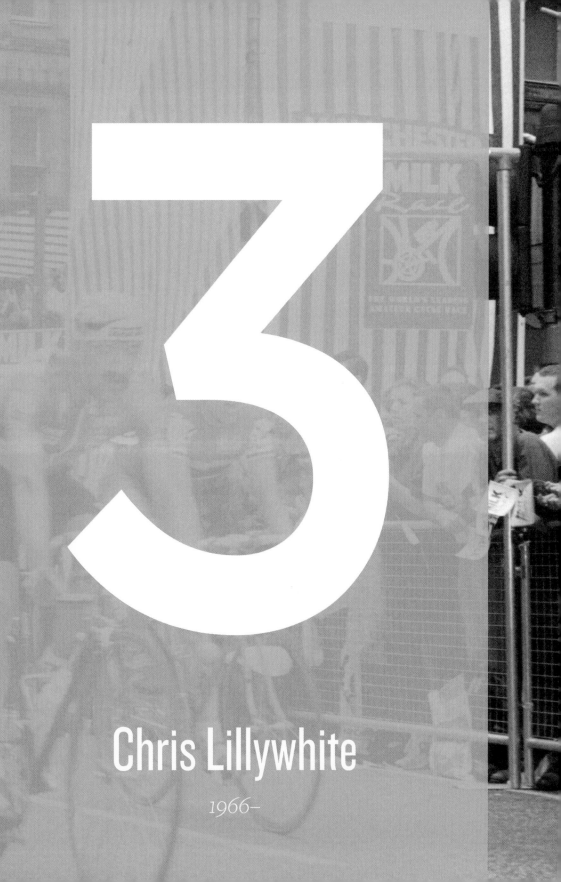

3

Chris Lillywhite

1966–

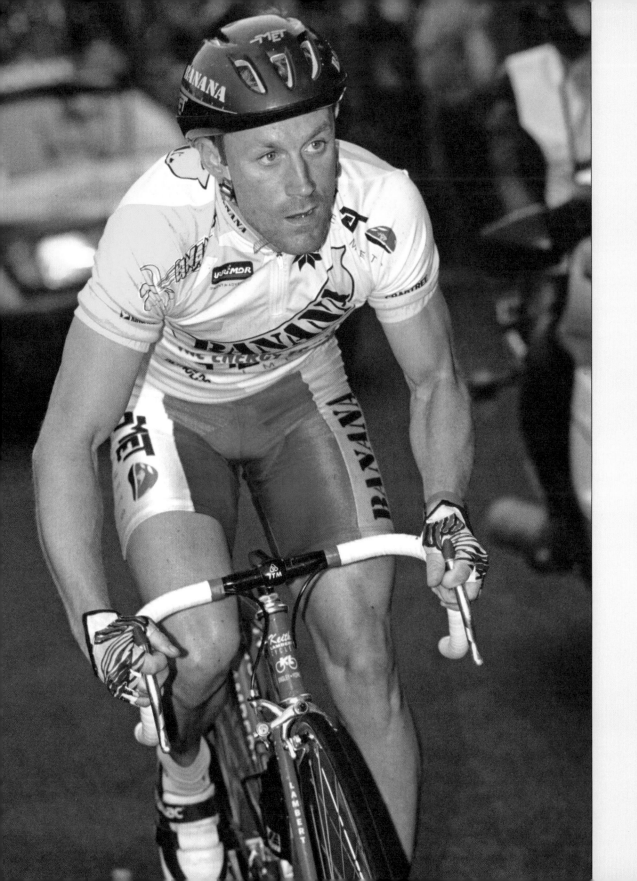

So I'd 'met' Museeuw and Ballerini, and shaken hands with Flanders and Paris–Roubaix. Next up would be a visit to the Milk Race, a pro-am Tour of Britain. I couldn't wait to see real-life riders in the flesh, but in the meantime I had my 13th birthday. Like anyone starting out in cycling, I'd quickly become obsessed by its equipment and I wanted the same gear as the champions had. I wanted to ride like them and look like them, and that meant one thing and one thing only. A date with destiny for me, and a long haul down to the cycling heartlands of deepest, darkest Croydon for my poor, put-upon mother.

It was a hell of a trip from Kilburn, and it wasn't as if we had much. She was a single mum working as a receptionist at the local school, but I wasn't interested in all that practical nonsense. Geoffrey Butler's was probably the best bike shop in the south-east in those pre-internet days, and at that age you just want stuff. The stuff I wanted was cycling stuff, and so off we set.

Before we went I made it clear that I wasn't mucking about, and that I absolutely *needed* a pair of proper cycling sunglasses in the first instance. Then there was the legwarmers issue, which I felt needed to be addressed urgently. Previously I'd worn a pair of mum's tights, and she'd elasticated the bottoms to make them seem real. I'm sure it was well meaning and all, but I wasn't prepared to put up with it any longer. As an Olympic gold medalist in the making I wasn't prepared to compromise, and I couldn't be held back by substandard equipment.

And besides, you wouldn't have seen Franco Ballerini riding around in a pair of his mum's tights ...

Racing in 1992 for the Banana-Met team.

I THINK ROOTING AROUND IN THE BARGAIN BIN AT BUTLER'S is one of my very best childhood memories. I got a pair of shorts, and I found a Carrera headband like the ones I'd seen on TV. Then a Motorola cap like Sean Yates's, a Tulip winter rain hat, a pair of Bernard Hinault cycling shoes and some Look clipless pedals. I was like a kid in a ~~sweet~~ bike shop.

It seems crazy now, but it's a classic cycling story. It's rites-of-passage stuff, and I don't suppose I was any different to thousands of other kids all over Europe. What was different was the fact that cycling was small-fry in Britain in just about every sense. Because there were so few shops you had to travel further to get kit, and I think that made it more of an event. There was a rarity value to the things you bought, and that was maybe because you had to do something and go somewhere to get them.

British cycling is unrecognisable these days from what it used to be. Back then it wasn't in the least bit 'aspirational', but rather price-sensitive. You didn't have the likes of Rapha with their huge marketing budgets, and the British cycling industry was strictly of the cottage variety. It was centred around functionality and economy as distinct from 'design' and fashion, and such marketing as existed was quite primitive. It amounted to photos of the champions on their bikes, whereas these days it's infinitely more sophisticated. Apparently it works – and whichever way you swing it, the more people out riding the better.

None of this concerned my all-new teenage self. I was far too busy strutting around the flat and preening myself in my new headband, cycling shoes and cap. I was a *racing cyclist*, and by hook or by crook I was going to assert my new identity.

The place to do that was the Archer Road Club. At first I'd been suspicious, but I was starting to feel at home there now. We had something – cycling – in common, but the collateral effects were positive as well. I was much happier, and my general demeanour was much better. Even school, which had never particularly interested me, became less of a drag. The teachers would say to my mum, 'His behaviour has improved no end. He's much more polite . . .'

I guess it was because I was going over to West London and riding with all these Oxford University types. They were all older than me, and they had ambitions to become doctors and academics, things like that. They weren't 'lads', they weren't always swearing and posturing, and they didn't go around trying to intimidate people. I'd never really been exposed to people like them before, and they were nice.

Like any impressionable adolescent I looked up to the bigger kids in my social circle, and the only thing I had to prove to them was my ability to ride a bike. Everything fitted around that – I felt like I was part of a community of equals, and people were genuinely interested in me. We rode our bikes, talked about riding them,

Bradley Wiggins – Archer R.C.

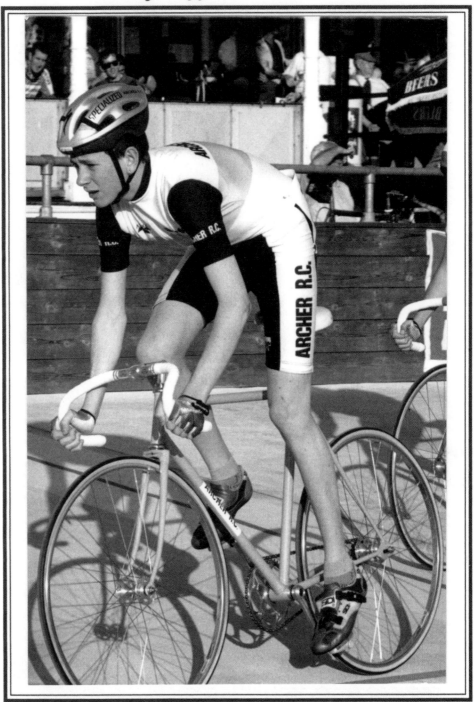

From an Archer R.C. programme. Finally kitted out and no longer wearing my mum's tights.

West London Juvenile Divisional Road Champion 1994
ESCA London & Home Counties Criterium Champion 1993/4
Herne Hill Monday Competition Juvenile Track Champion 1994

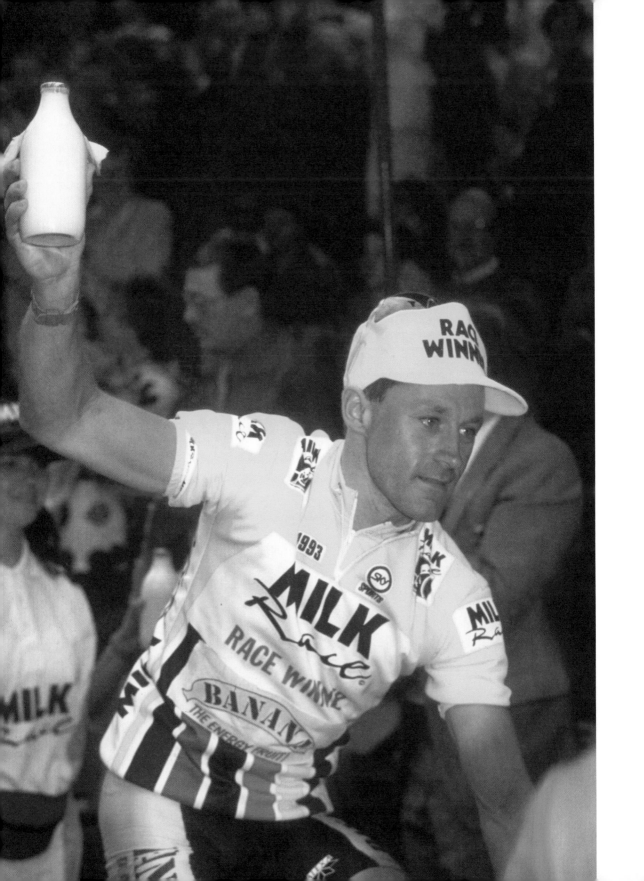

and when we weren't talking about riding them we were talking about other people riding theirs. It was a bit geeky in some ways, but I liked that aspect because, put simply, so was I. Club nights were social events, and the thing that bound us together was our love of cycling. These weren't the kind of people I'd generally run across on the estate, but I soon realised that there was nothing not to like. I'd like to pretend I made a conscious decision to change course, but it wouldn't be entirely true. I knew right from wrong, but if I'm honest it was cycling that chose me, not vice versa. I guess that's just the way of it when you fall in love, but the long and the short of it is that my football 'career' was over. As a matter of fact, so was everything else. Now it was just cycling, cycling and more cycling.

Probably just as well, because I was the beginnings of an adolescent. Everything was changing on the estate, and the innocent games of football we'd always played had started to mutate into something else. The lads I'd been knocking around with had started to ape their big brothers, which of course meant smoking, peering into car windows, that sort of thing. They were generally starting to get into a little bit of bother, and my mum could see where that might be headed. She encouraged my interest in cycling as much as possible, and I couldn't get enough of it.

And so to the Milk Race. Obviously I hadn't seen the Tour de France at this point, so this was the first time I'd been exposed to a stage race. For me the idea that there was a two-week Tour of Britain was wonderful, mystical even. In the 1950s it had been an amateur race, because there had been no British professional riders. Initially it had been sponsored by the *Daily Express*, but then the Milk Marketing Board stepped in. By now it was a bit of a hybrid – a pro-am whose peloton was made up of British domestic professionals and national amateur teams from around the world.

It started in Tunbridge Wells, and the opening stage was effectively a sort of Tour of Kent. They organised a junior criterium in Sevenoaks in advance of the race coming through, and I took part in it. After that I took my place on the side of the road with everyone else and waited for the peloton to arrive. It came through in a flash, and then we went home. That was it. Bike racing...

I remember very little – there was very little to remember! – but in my mind's eye I have a picture of Tony Doyle. He was a big star in British cycling, because he'd won the World Pursuit Championship twice. He was off the back getting a bottle or some such, and my mum said, 'That guy there used to race with your dad! You had your photograph taken with him when you were little. Do you remember?'

Sky Sports showed the highlights every night, and I spent hours studying the minutiae of the event. I was making it my business to know everything – and I mean *everything* – about the race itself, the riders and the gear they used. It was

Chris winning
the 1993 Milk
Race.

a useful geography lesson, but most of all it was a lesson in bikes, shoes, gloves, helmets, jerseys, glasses ... One of the teams was called Banana Energy. They were British, they had a really cool jersey with a big banana on it. You could buy the jersey at Yellow Jersey Cycles in London, and I went and got one in much the same way that other kids bought Arsenal or Spurs tops. A guy named Chris Lillywhite clinched the GC for them up in Manchester, and I became a fan.

Later that year I rode down to Crystal Palace to watch Lillywhite win the British Criterium Championship. That was my first real exposure to professional riding, because I saw the team cars, the presentations, all the stuff of bike racing. I also got to see professionals, albeit domestic ones, close up. They weren't perhaps as good as the top continental riders, but at 13 I wasn't making comparisons. Their kits were just as shiny, the cars just as colourful, and their bikes seemed just as beautiful.

Back then the Archer used to run the Grand Prix. It was one of the biggest races in the British calendar, and as a member you were expected to go and marshal. So each year I'd get my fluorescent bib and my flag, and watch the best of the Brits fly by.

Over time I became part of the furniture of the club, and ultimately of the national junior team. I'll never forget the first time I spent time with that generation of riders, though. It was 1998, and I'd earned a place at the Commonwealth Games in Kuala Lumpur. I was on the track team, and Lillywhite and co. were in the next door apartment. I was only 18, and they all used to laugh at me because I was this oracle of cycling knowledge. One night at dinner one of them, Matt Illingworth, said, 'Right, Bradley, tell Chris what shoes he was wearing when he won the 1993 Milk Race.' Quick as a flash I said, 'They were Carnac Podiums, and they were black and white!'

They were all dumbfounded – I probably knew more about their careers than they did themselves. I always did have an obsessive streak.

The upshot of all this is that when I set up Team Wiggins a few years back, Chris Lillywhite was the guy I wanted as sporting director. I was talking to him one day, explaining that I'd been a massive fan, and he said, 'Stop winding me up!' I think he assumed that, because I've been successful as a cyclist, I was being facetious, but he couldn't have been further from the truth. I felt a little bit aggrieved, to be honest – regardless of my own career, the relationship you have with your heroes doesn't tend to change. Guys like Chris don't see themselves as stars, but for me in some way it's still – and will forever remain – 1993. I'm still that 13-year-old kid, I'm still in awe of him and he'll always be one of my all-time cycling champions.

And that's why, for all the yellow jerseys, rainbow jerseys and champion's jerseys, I was so thrilled when he finally gave me his leader's jersey from the 1993 Milk Race.

A quintessentially 'English' scene. Fording a stream in Westerdale, Yorkshire, during Stage 12 of the 1969 Milk Race.

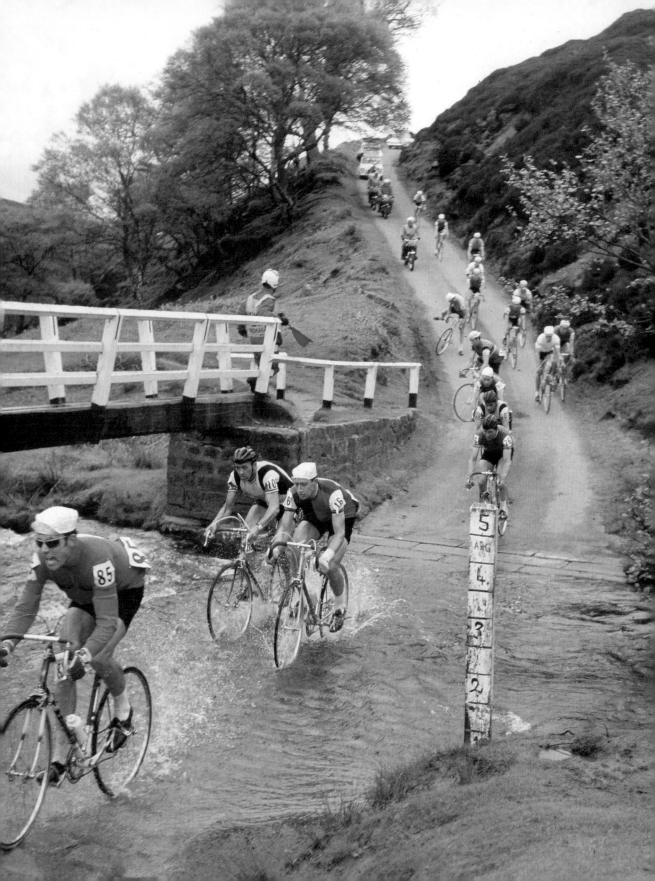

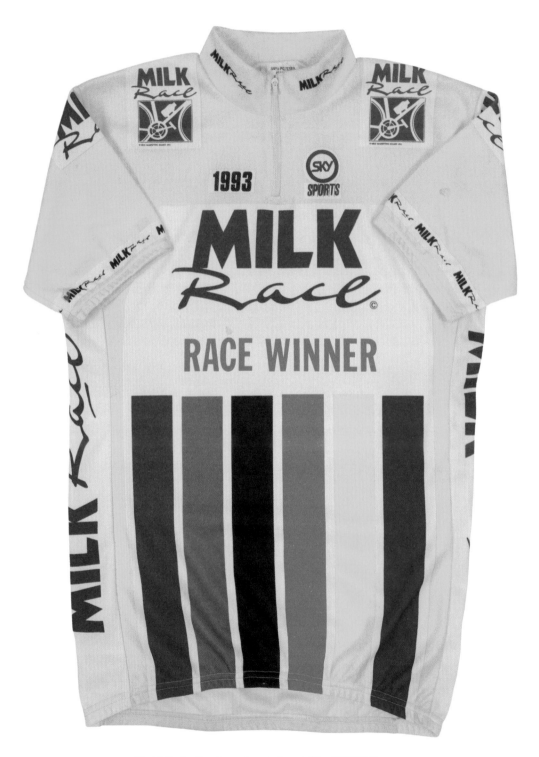

Chris's final yellow jersey as race winner of the 1993 Milk Race

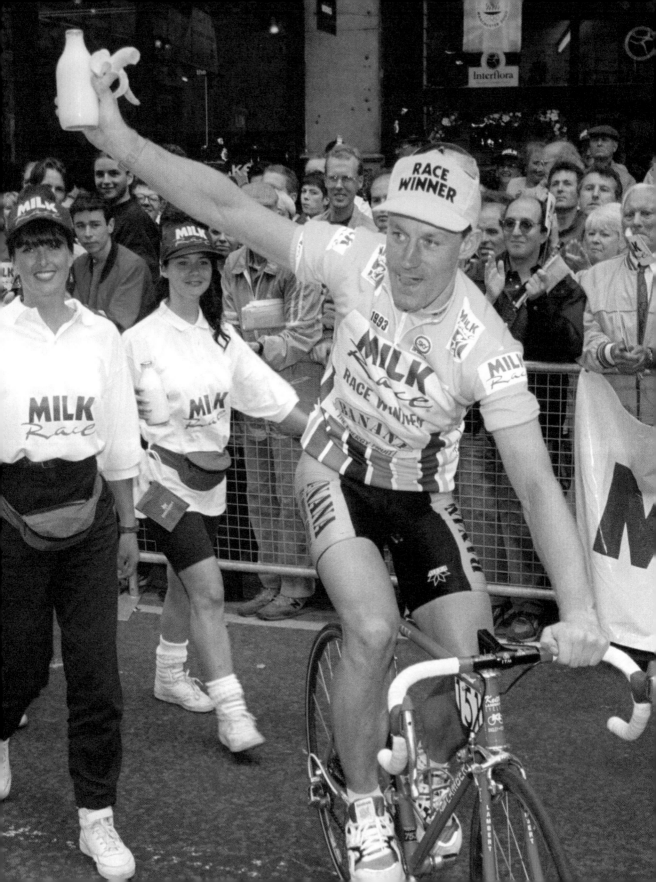

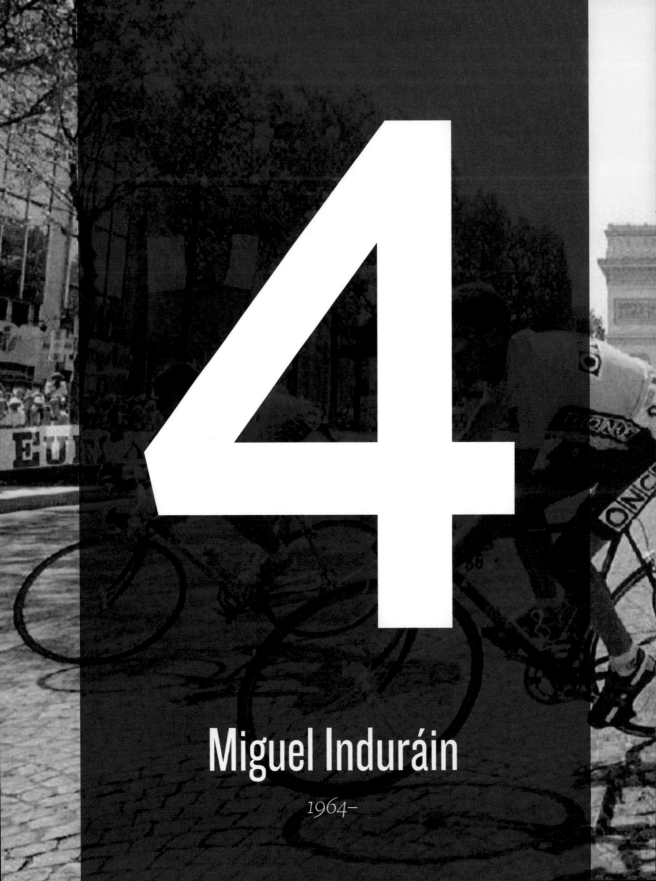

4

Miguel Induráin

1964–

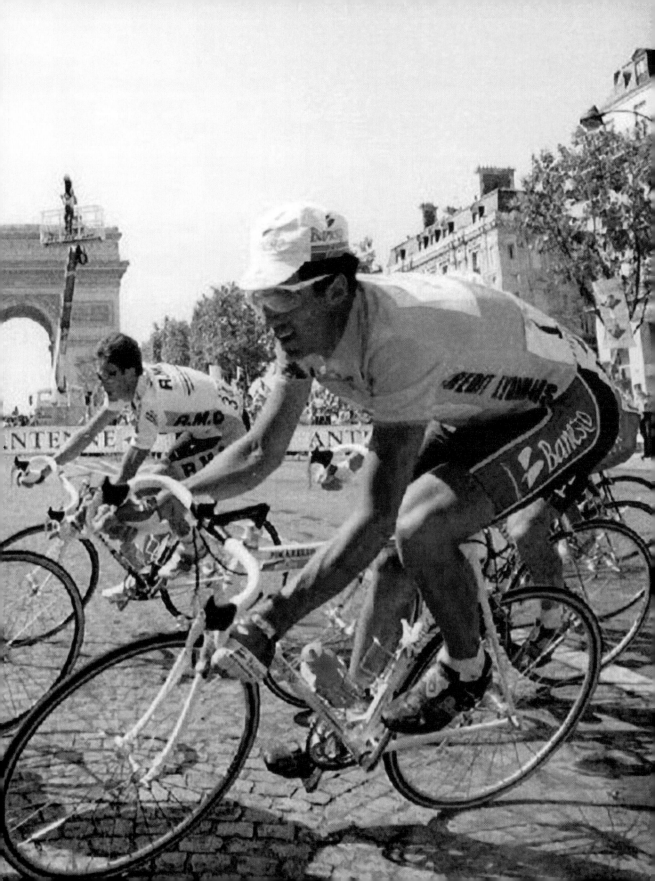

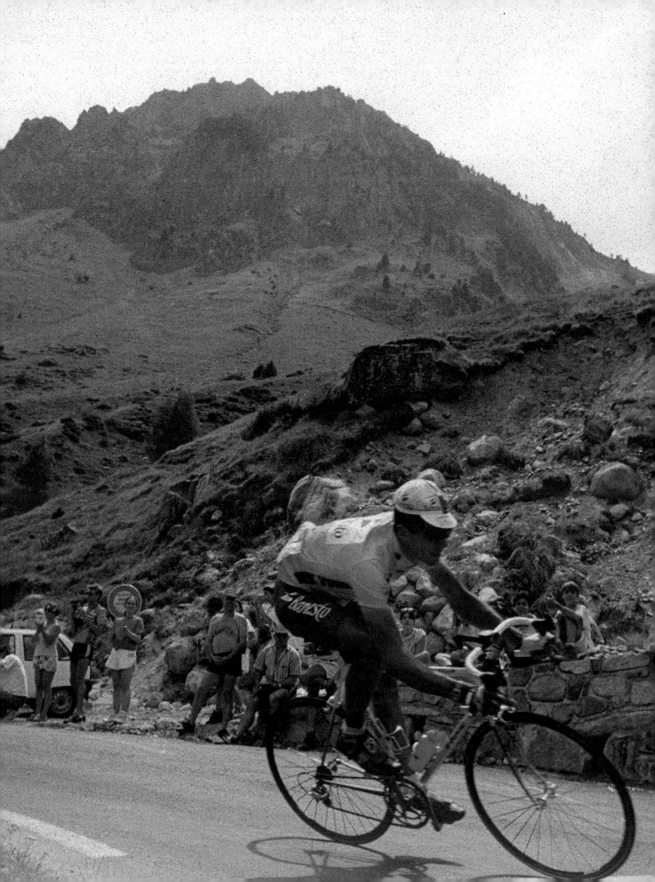

There were always copies of *Cycling Weekly* around the house. I'd never bothered with them, but after having watched Roubaix I started to devour them. I found the 1992 Tour de France editions, and started to read about the winner, this giant Spanish guy . . .

Then in June a new magazine appeared. It was a monthly called *Cycle Sport*, much glossier than *Cycling Weekly*, and much slicker. It focused almost exclusively on continental pro racing, as distinct from boring time trials in some far-flung corner of the British Isles that I'd never heard of. There was more photography, more history, more colour and more glamour, and I thought it was fantastic. I've an idea that the first issue, or at least one of the first, was a Tour de France preview. I'd never watched the Tour before, but now I couldn't wait.

If there's anything you ever want to know about the summer of 1993, I'm probably not your man. If, however, there's anything – and I mean anything – you want

Miguel in cap and sunnies at the 1996 Tour de France; he was undoubtedly one of the best descenders of his generation.

to know about the 1993 Tour de France, I'm categorically your man. I tuned in religiously, thought of nothing else, and obviously bought the compilation video when it came out. It was the first cycling film I owned, and I'm fairly sure I watched it every night that winter.

Those riders became my heroes, and to this day I can still reel them off. The sprinters were Nelissen, Cipollini, Ludwig, Moncassin and Abdoujaparov. In the GC group you had Rominger (second), Jaskuła (third), Álvaro Mejía (fourth, for Motorola). Chiappucci won a stage, Armstrong won a stage, Skibby and Bruyneel won stages. The teams had mysterious names, like Chazal, TVM, Ariostea and Telekom. I had no idea what they did or where they came from, but wherever it was I wanted to go there. Those three weeks in front of the TV were, and remain, one of the most immersive experiences of my life.

And then there was Miguel.

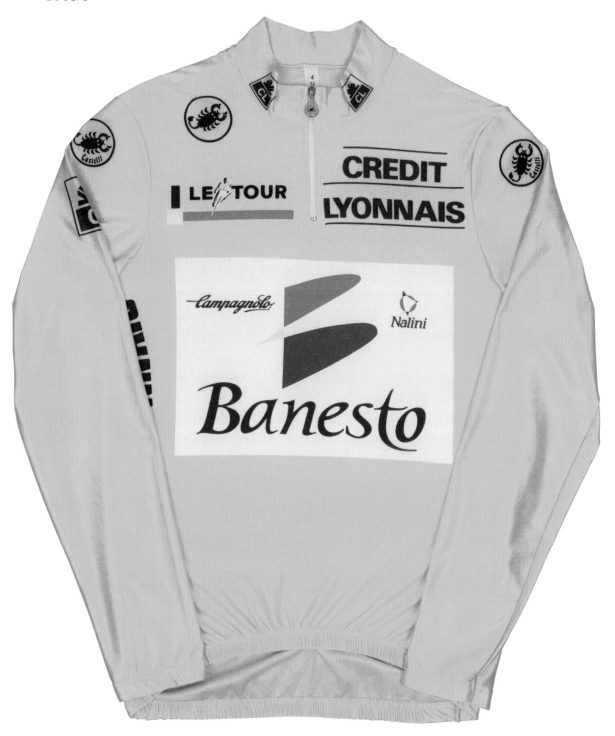

1994 Tour de France podium *maillot jaune*

CYCLING IS A VERY HARD SPORT. As often as not you're operating right at the end-stops of your physical and psychological capabilities, so it can be extremely uncomfortable. You're also competing against people whose job, essentially, is to destroy you. Any sign of weakness and they're going to bury you, because that's the business they're in. The business of suffering, and of enduring.

When I visualise guys like Marco Pantani, Tom Simpson and Luis Ocaña, I see pain etched into their features. That's maybe because they're synonymous with tragedy, but not so Museeuw, Jan Ullrich, even Eddy Merckx. They wore their suffering as well, because in cycling nobody is immune. The great champions aren't successful because they're talented per se (though talented they clearly are), but because they have the ability to hurt themselves a lot. Whatever your physical gifts, you're not going to complete the Tour, let alone win it, unless you're prepared to go really, really deep. And that's why we need to talk about *Miguelon* . . .

Miguel Induráin was the same, but completely different. He won five consecutive Tours de France because he was freakishly engineered, but also because he was a tremendous competitor. Where he was different, though, completely different, was in the *way* he won his Tours. While his opponents seemed to be wrecking themselves, he gave the impression of being out for a bike ride. They were the best climbers in the world, right at the top of their form, and yet he made beating them look easy. As a matter of fact it was anything *but* easy, and still less so given that he was much heavier than them. He was six foot three and 82 kilos, and there are mountains – big ones – to get over in France.

Imagine how soul-destroying it must have been. Whatever you tried, this great man was going to be completely unflappable. His facial expression was never going to alter for three weeks, but come what may he was going to beat you, and he was going to make beating you appear the easiest thing in the world. The horrific, brutal days in the Pyrenees were going to seem entirely routine for him, the heat and humidity only minor inconveniences. He'd hammer you in the time trial, maybe demoralise you in a couple of the mountain stages, and for the other 18 days just ride alongside you, seemingly without himself.

That sounds horrendous, but it's also entirely the point. Miguel was much, much better than the rest, but the key to the five Tours he won is that there was nothing at all gratuitous about them, or him. Where guys like Merckx and Armstrong seemed to want to crush their opponents, he killed them softly. He didn't do it painlessly – it's the Tour de France after all – but wordlessly and, in some way, mercifully. People say he was machine-like, robotic, all that stuff, and

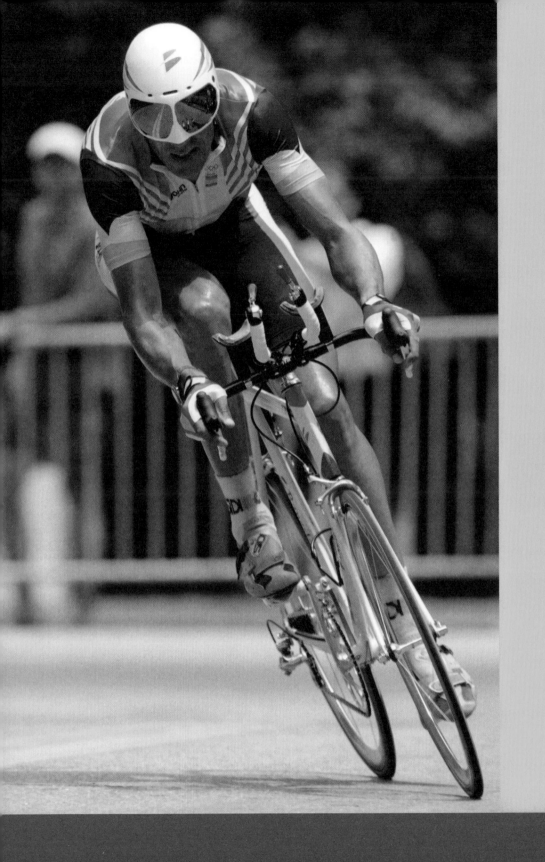

watching him race they are easy conclusions to draw. For me, though, he was the opposite of these things.

Miguel made sure he beat the guys that mattered when it mattered, but he wasn't interested in winning stages for the sake of it. In fact, he never won a single road stage in those five Tours, just time trials. That's because he had no ego, and he was more than happy for everyone to have a share of the cake. Now it could be said that they were fighting over the crumbs, but he took pains to ensure that there were plenty to go round. It's no coincidence that he always won by around five minutes, because he only ever took as much as he needed.

That, I think, is what makes him unique among the five-time Tour de France winners.

The first of them, Jacques Anquetil, understood that he needed friends in the peloton. He had a caustic rivalry with Raymond Poulidor, and the notion that Poulidor might beat him at the Tour was unthinkable. He knew that he needed as many allies as possible in the peloton, so he made it his business to ensure that the rank and file were on his side. Bernard Hinault understood this as well, but his methods were different. He was a patriarch or, in cycling parlance, a '*patron*'. His reign was built around psychology and strategy, and at times it was quite feudal. It's inarguable that his wins at the 1982 Giro and the 1985 Tour were achieved more with his head than his legs. Tommy Prim and Greg LeMond were each stronger than him, but each was brow-beaten into settling for second place. Everything Hinault did was calculated and calibrated, and nothing happened by accident.

Miguel was much less calculating than either Anquetil or Hinault, though contrary to popular misconception he was anything but naïve. He understood that it paid to have friends in high places, but he was the polar opposite of someone like Hinault. He raced hard, but he wasn't one of those who turned into an animal when he pinned a number on. The context changed, but he didn't, and his innate kindness didn't ever desert him. He didn't generally do many interviews, but when he did he was humble, respectful and courteous. The other riders liked him because it was impossible not to.

I don't ever remember him punching the air or shaking his fists when he won the Tour. The one and only time I recall him being demonstrative was at a race he didn't win, the 1995 World Championships in Colombia. He'd won the time trial, and now he was away on the final lap with the Italians, Pantani and Gianetti, and with Abraham Olano, the 'Baby Induráin'. When Olano attacked, the Italians didn't respond, so Miguel was able to sit on as his countryman disappeared up the road.

On his way to gold in the 1996 Atlanta Olympics time trial – his last big win.

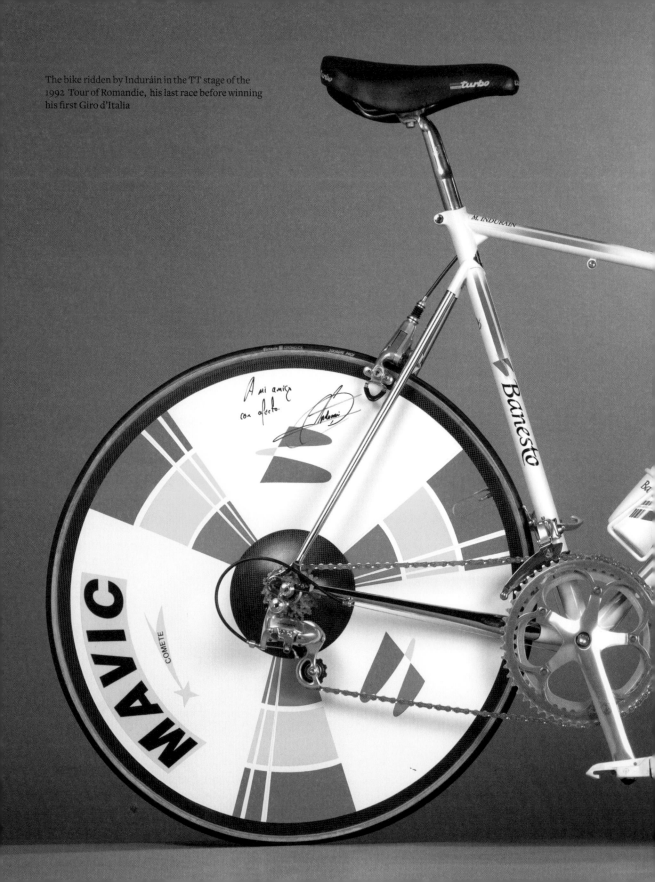

The bike ridden by Induráin in the TT stage of the 1992 Tour of Romandie, his last race before winning his first Giro d'Italia

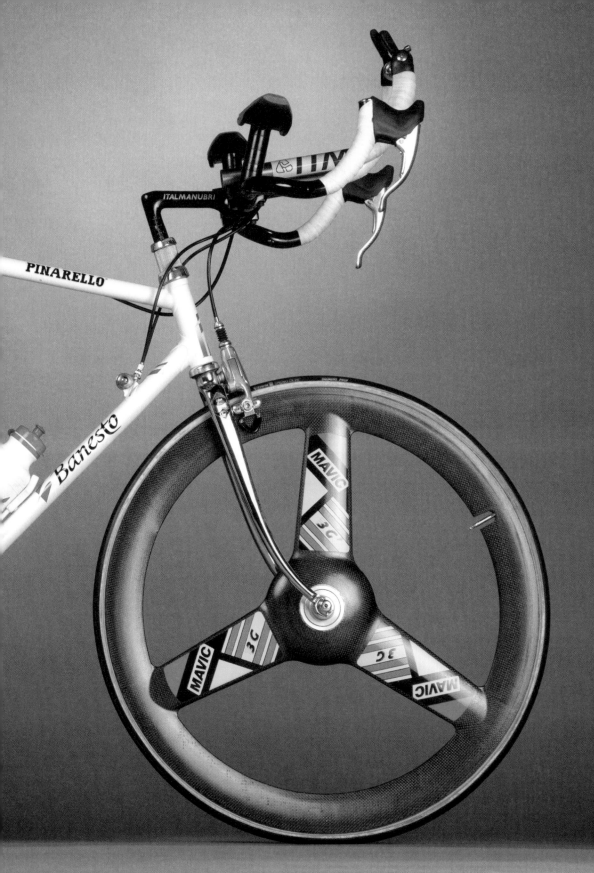

Olano subsequently punctured, but famously managed to roll over the line on his rim. That left Miguel contesting a sprint for second with the two Italians, and when he won he celebrated as if he'd won the rainbow jersey himself. Of course he hadn't, but that's entirely the point. He was delighted for Olano in the first instance, and for his country in the second. Spain had been failing to win the Worlds for 62 years, and finally his friend had achieved it.

Stories about Miguel are legion, but I think his character is best summed up by a couple that Juan Antonio Flecha told me while we were training together. One of Miguel's sponsors was Sidi, the Italian shoe manufacturer. They had a rider-liaison person there, and if the riders wanted something she was their point of contact. She told Flecha about her dealings with Induráin, and he passed the story on to me.

The first story goes that Miguel, who had won maybe four Tours de France by that point, would ring the girl and ask, extremely politely, whether it might be possible for him to have another pair of shoes, on account of the others being worn out, or broken, or whatever. The girl would say, 'Well, yes! Of course it is! You can have as many as you like! You're Miguel Induráin!,' but she said she never really felt as if she'd convinced him. Very obviously he knew he was Miguel Induráin, but he seemed to not have the faintest idea of what that meant.

When he finished he rang the girl again. It was 1996, he'd finally lost the Tour, and then they'd pretty much obliged him to do the Vuelta. He really hadn't wanted to do it, but in the end he'd succumbed to pressure from the Spanish public, the team and the sponsors. He'd only just turned 32, but he was spent psychologically as much as physically. Alex Zülle beat him in the time trial, then dropped him on Monte Naranco, and the following day Miguel famously climbed off on the road to Covadonga and walked into a bar. He said not a word to anyone, and in truth he didn't need to. He didn't want to be a cyclist anymore, so he stopped. (The extraordinary thing is that the other riders stopped as well, to see what was wrong. This was a guy who had been hammering them for five years, and yet they were worried about his well-being.) Anyway, that was that. Career over.

Now this took place on 21 September. It was the fag end of the season, and in retiring he probably missed ten days' racing, no more. Keep in mind that over the previous five years he'd delivered five Tours de France, two Giri d'Italia and goodness knows how many others, so sponsors like Sidi had gotten more than their money's worth. Miguel being Miguel, however, picked up the phone and rang the girl again. He said, 'I think I'm in breach of contract, so you need to tell me how much money I owe you, and I need to send the shoes I have back.'

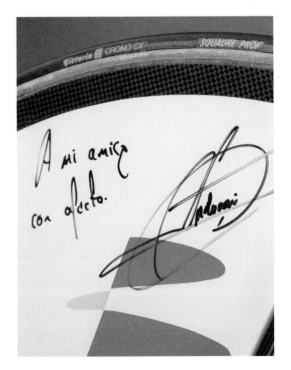

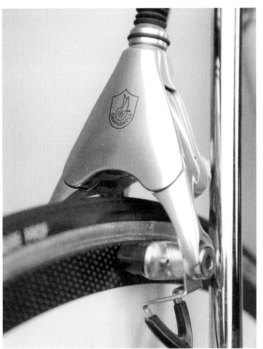

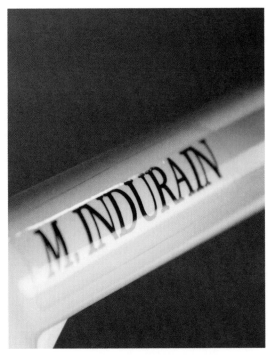

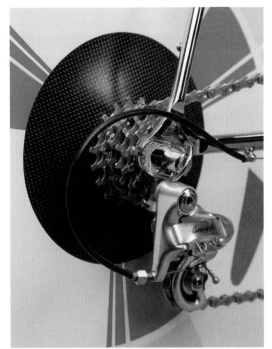

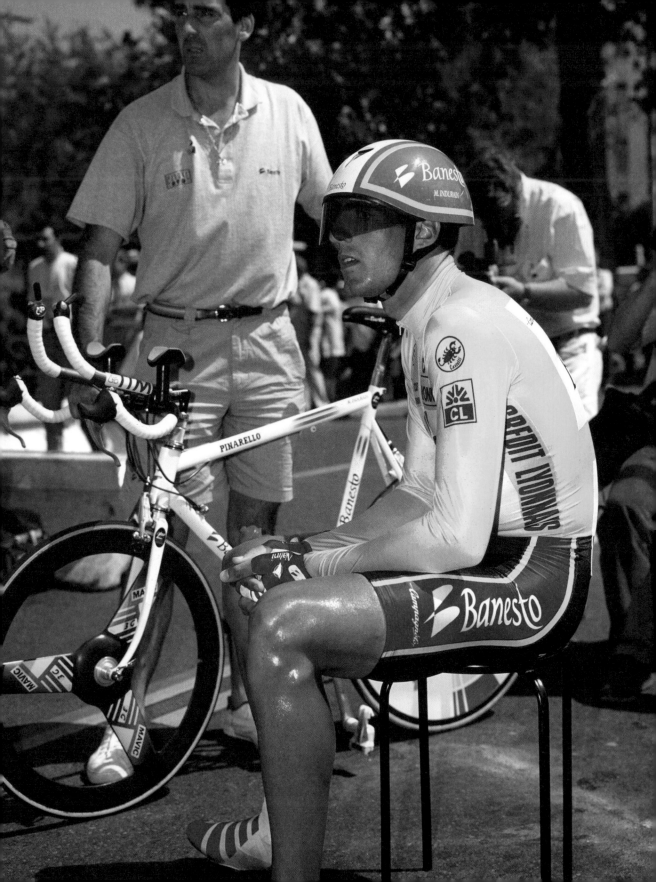

The other story that springs to mind came from Txema González. He was a lovely guy, a Team Sky *soigneur*, who died during the 2010 Vuelta. He said it was one of those horrible wet days at the Tour of the Basque Country, and the staff were all sitting on the team bus waiting for the stage finish. It was belting down with rain, and the poor spectators were standing behind the barriers waiting by the finish. One of the guys on the bus looked out of the window and said, 'There's a guy over there in a green cape, and I'm sure it's Induráin. He's the spitting image!' So Txema got off the bus and went over, and lo and behold it was – it was Miguel. He said, 'Miguel, what are you doing standing here? Come in the bus and get dry!'

The issue here is that Miguel wouldn't have dreamed of getting onto a team bus, for two reasons. First, he wouldn't have wanted to intrude, and second, the last thing he'd have wanted was to be treated differently to the other people standing there. It was raining, so as he saw it that would have been rude.

We're talking about a cyclist here, but he didn't exist in a vacuum. Spain was in turmoil while he was winning the Tour, and ETA was waging a war. Miguel is from Pamplona, on the doorstep of the Basque Country, and yet in some way he was a unifying force. They may have tried to exploit him or appropriate him, but there was a sense that, even in conflict, he represented a line that couldn't be crossed. It was as if everyone in Spain decided, subconsciously, that in some way he transcended the war. As if he were a deity.

Likewise the fallout from the doping scandals. It's a matter of public record that he rode during the EPO years, and yet he's the Tour winner that nobody – journalist, judiciary, former rider – has ever gone after. They've gone after Riis, Ullrich, Pantani and Armstrong, and history tells us they've been going after Tour winners (myself included) since Jan Janssen in 1968. There has to be a reason why only Miguel has been left alone, and to me it's pretty clear what that reason is. Whatever the context and whatever was happening in cycling, Induráin's morality is bomb-proof.

When I won the time trial at the 2012 Tour I did an interview for Spanish TV. I mentioned having grown up watching him smash them, and the journalists went to see him. Evidently he said nice things about me, and TVE said they wanted to revisit me on the second rest day, to show me the film. I said that would be fine, and when they came they had something for me.

They gave me this claret-coloured neckerchief with the Induráin family crest on it. To be perfectly honest I didn't really understand what it was, but then they explained that it was from San Fermín, the summer festival in Pamplona where they run the bulls. Afterwards I showed it to the Spanish guys on the team and they were taken aback. They explained that for someone from a Navarro family to make

With the Pinarello bike at the Tour de France, where his time-trialling ability did much to secure him his five victories.

a gift of something like that was *extremely* rare. It signified my being an extended part of the Induráin family, so it was just about the highest honour Miguel could have bestowed on me. As you can imagine, I was really touched.

Two years later I went to the Gran Fondo Pinarello in Treviso, and Fausto Pinarello told me Miguel was coming. He'd always ridden Pinarello bikes, including the legendary Espada on which he broke the Hour Record after the 1994 Tour. He'd ridden it when becoming the first man to ride over 53 kilometres in an hour, and he'd remained a friend of the Pinarello family. So it was not unlike that Museeuw moment, me panicking about meeting one of my boyhood favourites and fretting about what I would say to him.

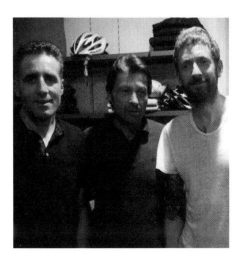

The day before the event we were wandering around the square looking at the sponsor's stands, and Fausto spotted Miguel. He said, 'It's Miguel! Come on – let's go and see him,' but I wasn't ready. I'd been building myself up for the moment, but the moment wasn't supposed to be until the following morning. I said to Fausto, 'Can't we leave it until tomorrow?' because I went into full panic mode. It sounds like a stupid cliché, but growing up on a council estate in Kilburn I couldn't have imagined something like that. He was this perfectly calibrated cycling machine from Pamplona, and I hadn't even known where Pamplona *was*!

Anyway, he was everything that everybody had said he was, just a lovely man. He and I sat together at dinner that evening, having one of those European conversations. He spoke no English but a little bit of French, I spoke good French but no Spanish, and Fausto helped us because being Italian (and very smart) he understood a bit of everything.

I mentioned the fact that I was minded to attempt the Hour, and he asked me some questions about it. When I asked him how he'd trained for it he said that he hadn't really, at least not specifically. That says it all, because he'd just ridden a time trial. He didn't expand on that, because he much preferred listening to talking about his own achievements.

Then again, his achievements speak for themselves. Volumes. He's Miguel Induráin.

Left:
The moment Fausto Pinarello introduced me to Miguel – one of my favourite riders as a boy. Hopefully not looking totally overwhelmed.

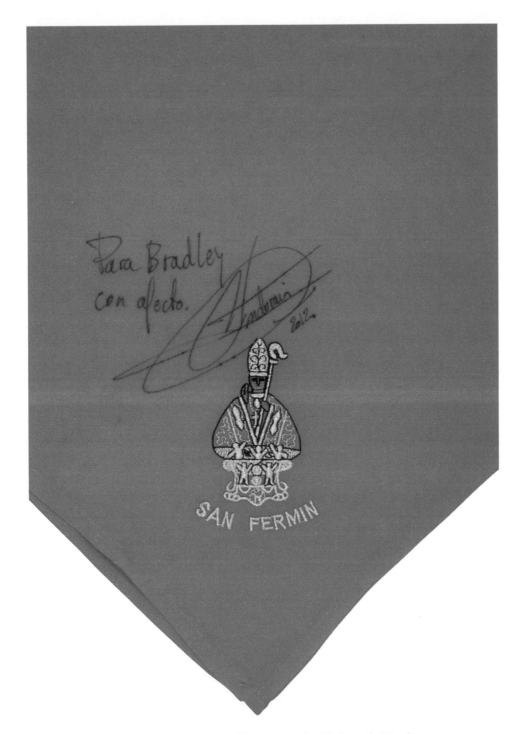

The Induráin family neckerchief from San Fermín, gifted to me by Miguel

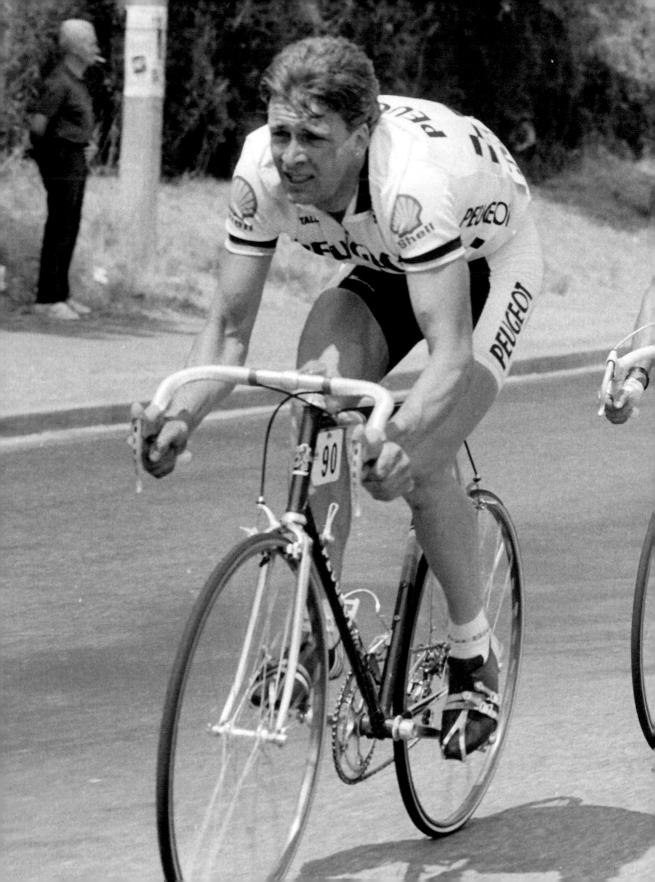

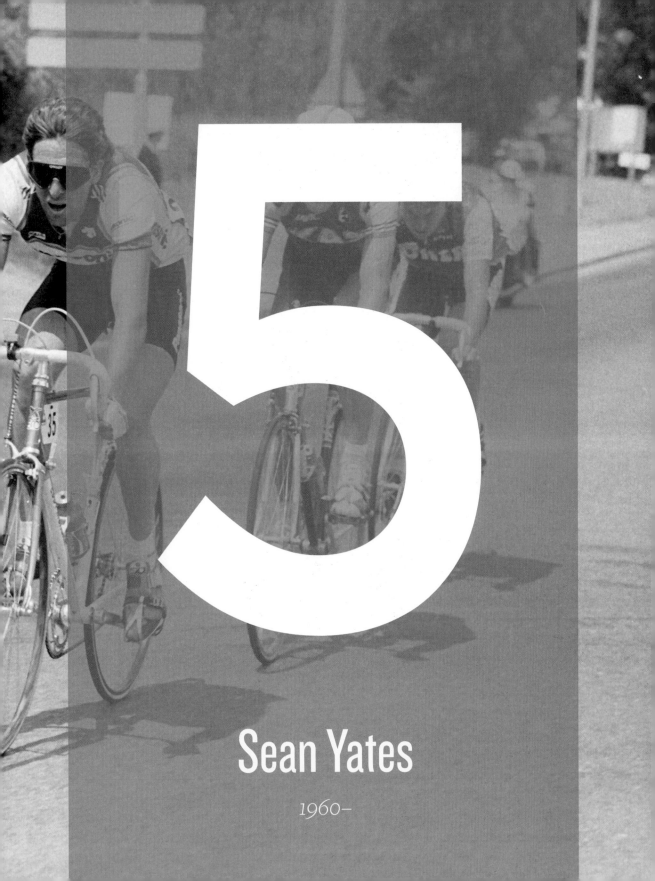

5

Sean Yates

1960–

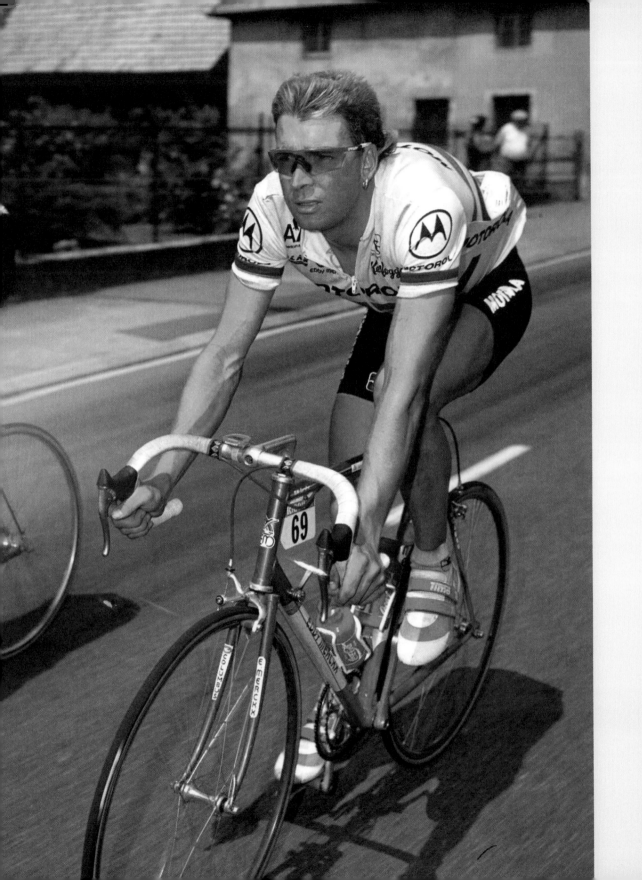

As I became a rider in my own right, so my list of cycling idols began to take shape. Museeuw was a warrior, Gianni Bugno some sort of a magician, Induráin this serene, beautiful winning machine. Top of the list, however, was a guy who wasn't a great champion. I'd never seen him win a single race, and yet somehow he was the very embodiment of everything I loved about bike racing.

When Duclos and Ballerini slipped away at the previous year's Paris–Roubaix, there was a chase group of seven or eight. Museeuw and Olaf Ludwig were in it, and so too were the classics specialists Edwig Van Hooydonck and Adri van der Poel. Then there was this other guy. He was wearing a white jersey with two horizontal stripes across the chest, a red one and a blue one. My mum explained that he was the British champion and that his name was Sean Yates. She also said he'd ridden for the Archer, just like me.

'The Animal' looking achingly cool in the British champion's jersey and gold earring.

My mum still loved cycling. She'd met my dad through it and had never really stopped following it. In the past I'd never given the sport a second thought, but this all changed after that Paris–Roubaix. Back then *Cycling Weekly* used to put a poster on the back cover, and on 15 April 1993 it was of this guy Yates. He was rounding a corner, that beautiful jersey covered in dust. Unlike the rest of them he had no gloves and no helmet, and his shorts seemed to be shorter than anyone else's. He was wearing an earring, and I thought that was impossibly cool. I cut the poster out and put it up on my bedroom wall.

It's also true to say that I spent far more time than was probably healthy staring at it.

My guilty little secret?

Not really. Not at all, in fact.

Thing is, I just really, really wanted to be like Sean Yates.

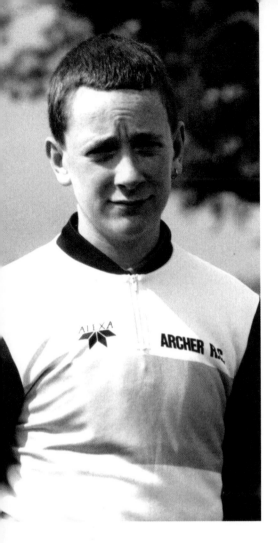

IN THE MID-NINETIES, top-end British road cyclists were few and far between on the international circuit. There were dozens of Italians, Frenchmen, Belgians and Spaniards, and quite a lot of Dutchmen and Germans. There were a few talented Swiss, some Colombian climbing specialists, and beyond that a bit of a mishmash. You had the odd American, Scandinavian and former Soviet, with a few stragglers from elsewhere thrown in here and there. The Brits were very much in the latter category, which was a bit of a double-edged sword. It meant that while the chances of one of them winning any given race were pretty slim, as a fan it wasn't hard to choose your favourites.

Boardman was immense, but essentially a time-trial specialist. He and Graeme Obree were engaged in a titanic struggle for the Hour Record, but I wasn't yet dialled into that, and Obree was a complete enigma. Chris was his total opposite, and I found him a bit methodical. Over the years I've learned to appreciate him, and there's no question he was a phenomenal athlete. He's gone on to become a really important advocate for cycling as a whole, but back then it was all a bit clinical for me. I was a romantic, idealistic teenager, and his approach seemed rather too scientific.

Robert Millar's winning days were behind him, and beyond that there was hardly anybody. Harry Lodge was holding down a job with an Italian team, Malcolm Elliott had gone to race in America, and I seem to think that Brian Smith had a contract at Motorola. Max Sciandri had been *born* in Britain, and that would come in handy when the Olympics came around. In reality, though, he'd been raised in Tuscany, and to all intents and purposes he was Italian. I knew about Sean Kelly and Stephen Roche, but they were coming to the end by then. Of course, they are Irish, not British. It was not about nationality either – at 13 I admired them all the same.

Thank God, then, for Yates.

Left:
Complete with earring and thinking that I'm Sean Yates, in 1994.

Opposite:
Hanging in there to win Stage 6 of the 1988 Tour de France – with a record average speed at the time.

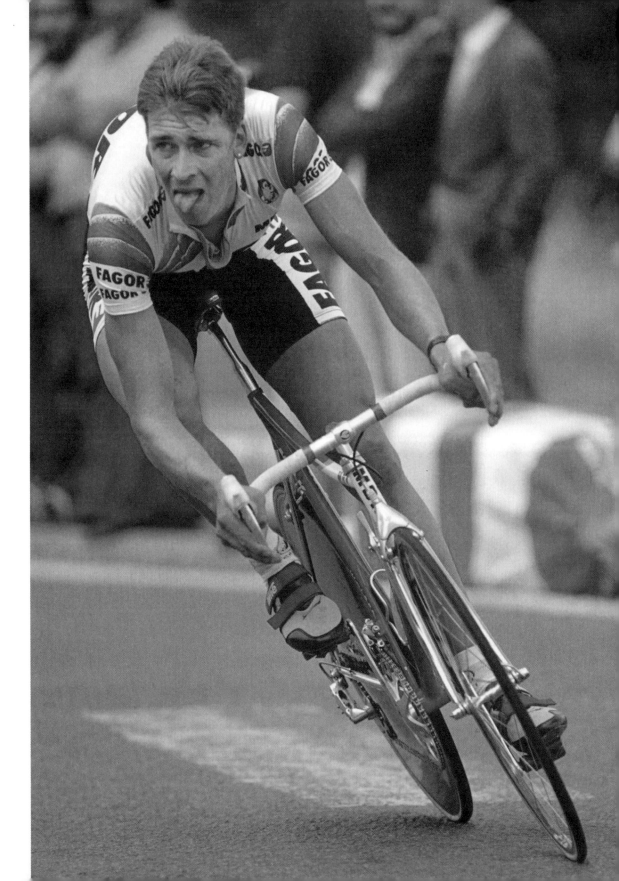

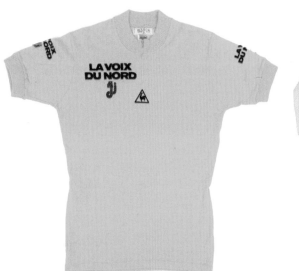

1983 Four Days of Dunkirk leader's jersey

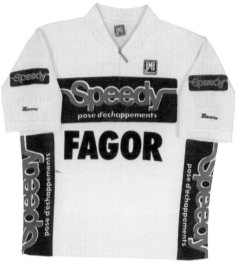

1988 Paris–Nice leader's jersey

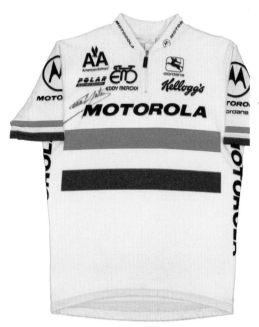

1992 Leeds Classic, national champion's jersey

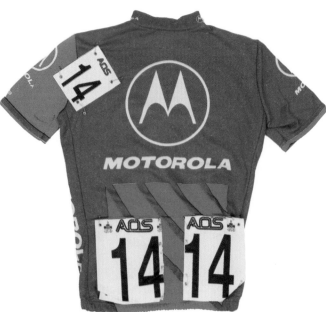

1992 National Championship jersey

Britain was far from a 'traditional' cycling country – road racing had been outlawed here before the Second World War – but contrary to popular belief it wasn't a complete desert as regards pro racing. The Milk Race was essentially for British domestic riders and foreign amateurs, but we had the Kellogg's Tour of Britain to look forward to in August. That was followed two days later by the Leeds Classic, which had been founded by Alan Rushton in 1989. It was part of the new World Cup series, and all the big teams raced there.

The UCI were trying to globalise cycling, but the race was typically British in the sense that, with the best will in the world, there was no money in it. The first edition had been in Newcastle, then it had moved to Brighton, and now it was up in Yorkshire. Everyone said they loved racing it, and the crowds were great. In retrospect, though, Britain just didn't have the critical mass for a race like that to succeed. The Leeds (or Rochester, or Wincanton . . .) would fold the following year, and Hamburg would take its place in the World Cup. That's just the way it was, I'm afraid. The sporting landscape was different back then, totally dominated by football, cricket, rugby and golf. Oh, and snooker.

Whatever. First and foremost, the 1994 Tour de France was coming back to England. I say 'coming back', because I'd learned that there had been a stage in Plymouth twenty years earlier, though seemingly it had been a bit of a dog's dinner. They hadn't managed to get it televised live – I assume it would have interfered with the wrestling on *World of Sport* – but evidently that was no bad thing because the 'racing' had been hopeless. They'd literally just ridden up the new bypass to the roundabout, and then ridden back down it again. Thirty times.

This time there would be two real stages, on days four and five. Everybody at the club was talking about them, not least because Boardman might be in yellow. He was the best prologue rider in the world, and if he could get the jersey and survive the team time trial we'd have one of our own in the *maillot jaune* when the race crossed the Channel. I learned that no Brit had worn the yellow jersey since 1962, when a certain Tom Simpson had kept it for a single day.

Chris duly won the jersey but his team, GAN, couldn't defend it in the time trial. Museeuw took it from him and wore it on the stage from Dover to Brighton, but the next day one of his team-mates, an Italian guy named Flavio Vanzella, got it in the break. He wore it into Portsmouth, and that was that for the British stages. As ever with the Tour, the fun seemed to be over before it had really begun. That's the nature of cycling, I suppose, and I was starting to understand that part of its beauty is the fact that it's so ephemeral, so fleeting.

Yates hadn't particularly extended himself in the prologue. He'd shipped almost a minute because he wasn't a GC rider, but also because he was a serious professional with a job to do. Motorola had made the team time trial one of their main objectives, and Sean

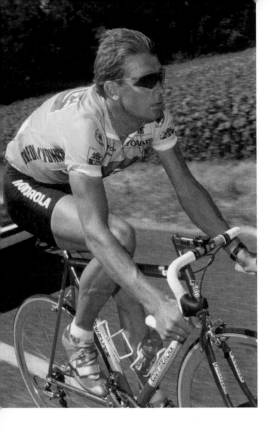

would need to preserve every ounce of energy he could for that. Motorola also had the likes of Steve Bauer and Phil Anderson, really powerful *rouleurs* with big engines, but you'd be hard-pushed to find any team time triallists better than Yates over 65 kilometres. In the event they finished second in the TTT, but as a consequence Sean found himself in seventh place overall when they got back to France.

The first French stage was Cherbourg to Rennes, 270 kilometres. A break went, Sean and one of his team-mates got in it, and then one of the escapees, Bortolami, jumped off the front. Now all hell broke loose because you had Bortolami trying to win both the stage and the jersey, Sean and co. desperately trying to bring him back, and Vanzella's team turning themselves inside out to bring *them* back. There were effectively three races in one, which is typical of the frantic, dramatic, desperate stuff you often see during the opening week of the Tour. Bortolami held on for the stage, but Sean was a monster. When the dust settled he'd taken the jersey by a single second, with Bortolami second and Museeuw third.

Now it could be argued that he fell on his feet that day, because I am not sure that he'd set out with the objective of claiming the jersey. That wasn't his job, but by the same token you don't get to wear it by accident. That's the key to it, because Sean's day in yellow was fundamentally a consequence of both his physical strength and, paradoxically, his altruism. He'd shipped some time initially, and then buried himself for his team. That had left him there or thereabouts on GC, but not so close to the race leader that they weren't prepared to cut him a little bit of slack. He grabbed it with both hands, and there was nobody better equipped to keep hold of it on that kind of terrain. It was his first yellow jersey in his 11th Tour de France, and nobody was ever more deserving. It was breathtaking, heroic stuff, the stuff of the Tour . . .

Meanwhile, back in down-at-heel Kilburn, I had no interest in anything but cycling. I was extremely ambitious, and my mind was set on winning Olympic gold on the track and wearing the yellow jersey on the road. Boardman had won the pursuit and now, in him and Sean, Britain had claimed two yellows in under a week! For me that was

Left:
Yates wearing the *maillot jaune* in 1994 for a single day, before losing it to Museeuw on Stage 7.

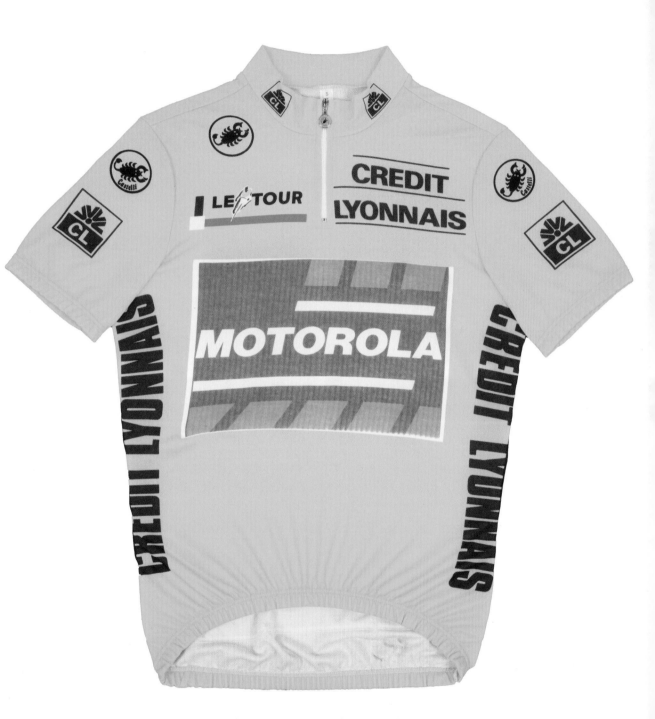

My prized possession – 1994 Tour de France *maillot jaune*

confirmation that it was possible, because I figured that if they could do it there was no reason why I couldn't. My mind was made up, and by the end of 1995 I was up and running. I was winning quite often, and I too had a British champion's jersey. It was only the junior points race, but it presaged another big moment in my cycling life.

There was a prize-giving dinner, and of course everyone who'd won a title was invited. Robert Millar was present because he'd won the road race championship, but I seem to recall that Boardman was absent because he'd had a big off at the Tour and was convalescing. Sean was presenting the prizes, though, and what with me being at the bottom of the undercard I was first up onto the stage. I asked him to autograph the programme, and suffice to say this was the highlight not only of my cycling year but also of my fledgling career.

Over the years Sean has variously been my friend, my mentor, my DS and my inspiration. Our time together at Sky is well documented elsewhere, but in essence he's been a mainstay throughout my cycling life. Whatever anyone says about cycling and cyclists, it's an irrefutable fact that Sean is a man of character and integrity.

Our sport is filled top to bottom with arcane rituals, methods and legends, which of course largely explains why its history is so absorbing for people like me. That said, it's no secret that Yates, Millar, Obree and Boardman – the handful of Brits abroad when I was starting out – were all somewhat *other*. The two Scots were pure mavericks, and still are to this day. Everyone knows about Obree's 'home-made' bikes and his revolutionary 'Superman' position. Chris was possessed of a unique intellect, but also the ability to take his body to places most sportsmen can't begin to imagine. Sean was probably the least celebrated among the wider public, but probably the most admired within the sport itself.

They were different bike riders, they came from different backgrounds and they had radically different characters. On the surface, then, there is very little connecting them beyond the fact that they all hailed from this lump of rock on the edge of the Atlantic Ocean. There *is* a common thread, however, and it's fundamental to understanding what they achieved. All of them were free thinkers, and each had the courage to challenge traditional cycling methodology and convention. As Anglo-Saxons in a resolutely European sport that's by no means easy, but it speaks volumes about them both as men and as athletes.

Sean couldn't climb like Millar nor ride a prologue like Boardman, and he certainly couldn't sprint like Johan Museeuw. He didn't win many races, but you'll be hard pushed to find anyone in cycling who doesn't hold him in the very highest regard. As a cyclist he was very much his own man, but he was also an exemplary team man. He was an excellent classics rider in his own right, but more importantly there was nobody who delighted in the hard yards more than he did. I've ridden with some sensational *domestiques*, but I'm struggling to think of a better, more reliable one.

I have to say at this point that I'm the guardian of – among other things – his yellow jersey and his British champion's jersey. I think that they're beautiful, priceless artefacts, and I feel immensely privileged to have them in my care. That said, of all the objects I hold dear, the programme from the British Cycling Annual Prize-giving Dinner is right up there with the best of them. At first glance it appears perfectly innocuous, but in reality it represents a pivotal moment for me and, if I may be so bold, for British cycling.

It's one of the reasons I won all those races and amassed all this stuff, and the reason you're reading this book.

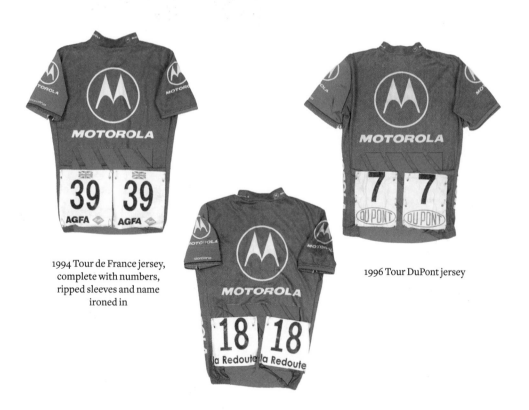

1994 Tour de France jersey, complete with numbers, ripped sleeves and name ironed in

1996 Tour DuPont jersey

1992 Paris–Roubaix jersey, with ripped sleeves, mud and dust. Sean finished 13th that day

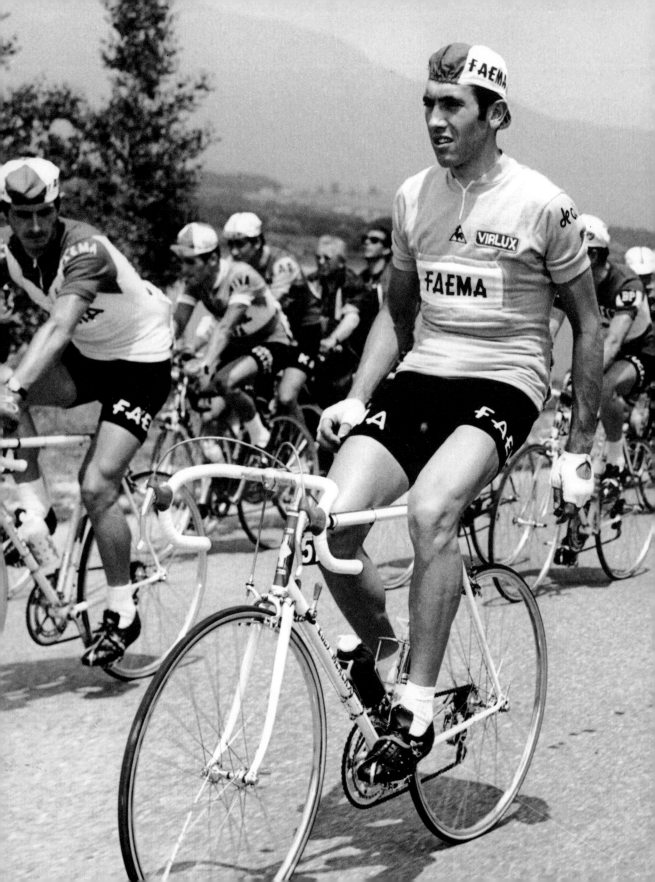

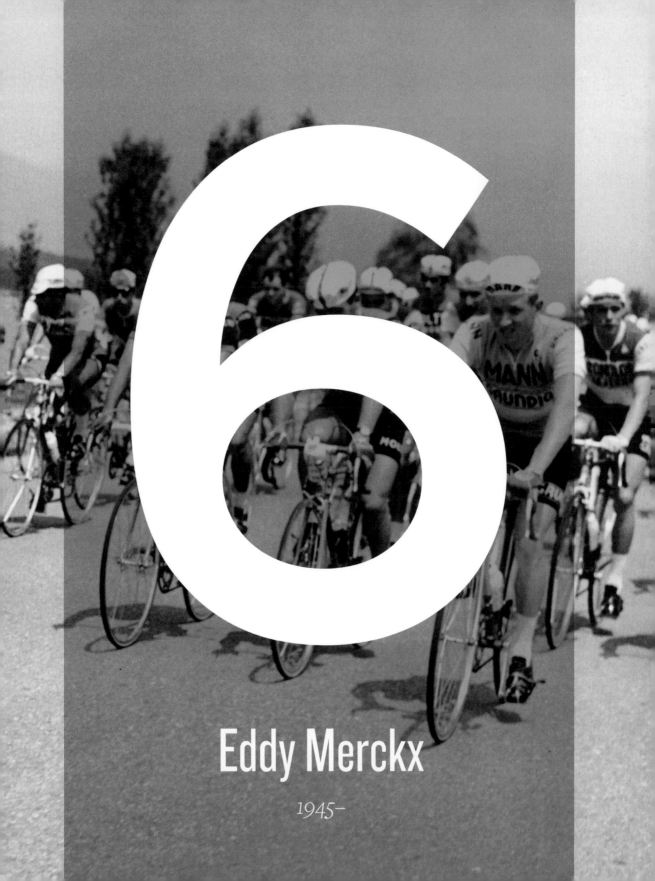

6

Eddy Merckx

1945–

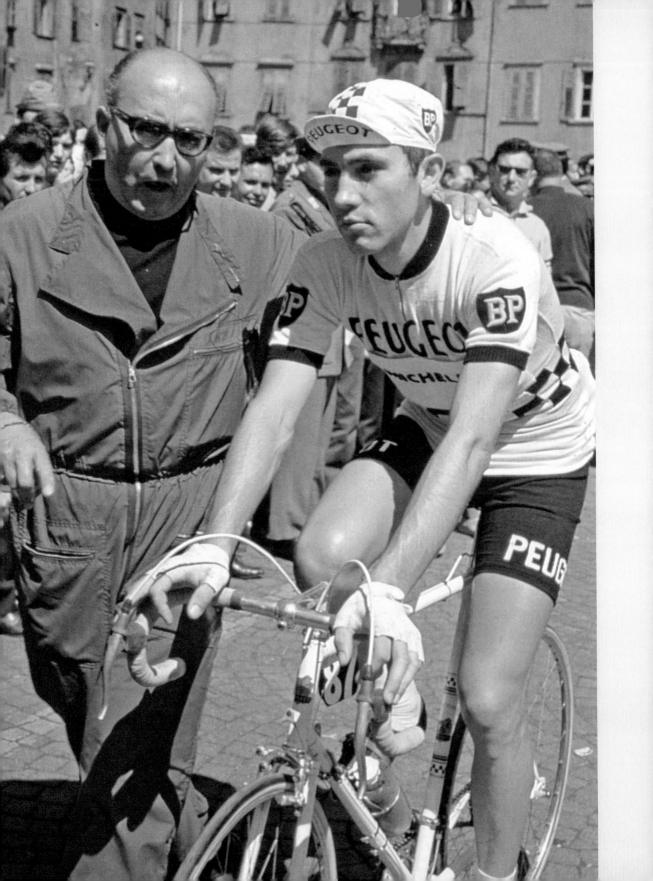

By the time I was 18, cycling had started to earn me a little money via sponsorship. As a teenager living at my mum's I was doing OK.

One night I was scanning the classified ads in *Cycling Weekly* and I saw an advert for an 'Eddy Merckx race-worn Peugeot jersey'. I rang the number and it was a guy up on the Wirral. It transpired that a 21-year-old Eddy had come over to Britain and had raced at New Brighton. Seemingly he'd given his jersey and mitts to a very good British rider named Tony Bell, and he'd passed them on to this guy. So I went up there and paid something like £500 for the lot. That was an astronomical amount of money at the time, but I didn't mind. It was my first 'real' cycling jersey, and it had belonged to Eddy.

I don't have that jersey anymore. By 2005 I was Olympic champion, I'd been awarded an OBE and I was totally skint. I was a well-known athlete, but I was much, much worse off than I'd been when I was 18. I was earning a pittance at Crédit Agricole because I hadn't yet done anything on the road, I'd become a father, and Cath and I needed a pram much more than I needed an Eddy Merckx jersey. I wouldn't say that I ever regretted selling it – needs must and all that – but I never quite managed to scratch the itch.

I never stopped wanting another one ...

Looking full of confidence at the start of Stage 22 of the 1967 Giro d'Italia. Merckx finished 9th overall that year.

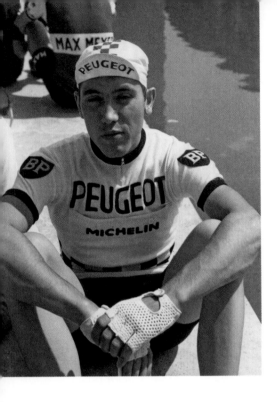

I SUPPOSE I BECAME AWARE OF EDDY MERCKX in much the same way as everyone else of my generation did. He had long been retired, but if someone did something really exceptional, as often as not it would be referenced back to his exploits. He won 525 professional races, so there's no point in my trying to list the most important ones here. Suffice to say that, between 1967 and 1975, he ruled cycling in a way nobody had before, no one has since and no one can ever hope to again. Come to think of it, I can't think of anyone in any endurance sport who has so been so utterly dominant for so long. He truly is unique.

When I was a kid there were magazines, but very few English-language cycling books. There was no internet either, so the only way to see actual footage of Merckx racing was to buy it on video. One film in particular had me spellbound. It was called *Stars and Watercarriers*, and a lot of the objects in the collection constitute a celebration of it, and of that era of racing.

The film was made by a Danish guy named Jørgen Leth. He was a fan of Ole Ritter, the brilliant Dane who rode for Bianchi, and he'd become obsessed by bike racing. He decided to make a film about the sport, with Ritter as one of the protagonists. He settled on the 1973 Giro, and the rest is history.

Stars and Watercarriers is a seminal film for anybody who loves cycling. The soundtrack and cinematography are perfect, and it does a wonderful job of evoking the race, the landscape and the Italian peloton. There's a moment in it where Bianchi roll out of their hotel, and through these tiny Italian streets towards the start in the main piazza. When they get there there's a little scaffold, and the speaker guy is booming out the names of the riders as they sign on. The crowd is quite small by today's standards, but there's a real intimacy. Leth manages to portray the sense of community both within the peloton and among the spectators, and to me that's what cycling is. The film

Left:
Young Eddy in La Spezia before the start of Stage 3 of the 1967 Giro d'Italia.

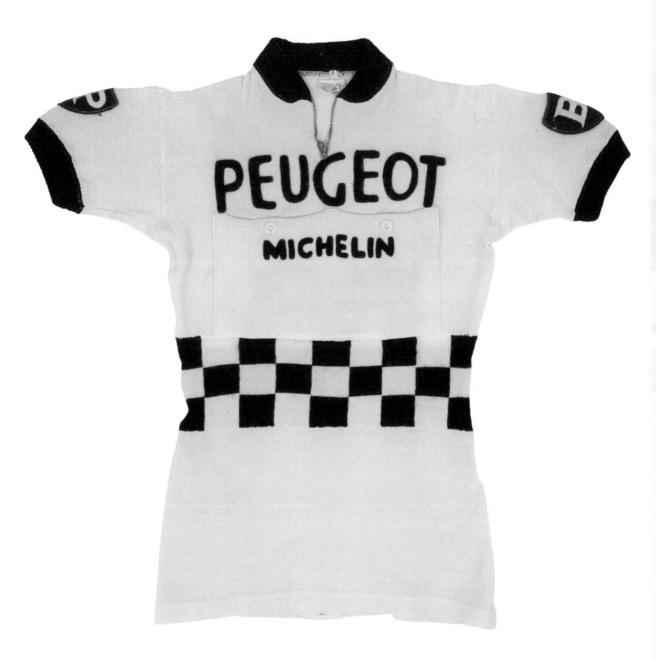

1967 Giro d'Italia, Stage 22a. Very distinctive 'G' in the Peugeot lettering,
which is chain-stitched across the zip

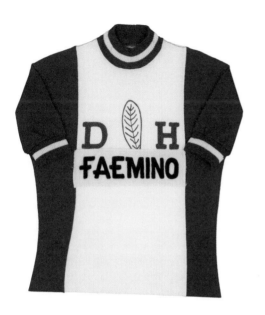

1970 Tour of Belgium leader's jersey

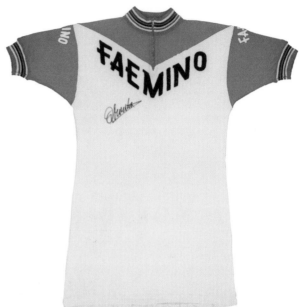

1970 Milan six-day jersey

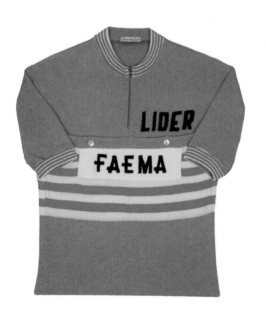

1969 Tour of Valencia leader's jersey

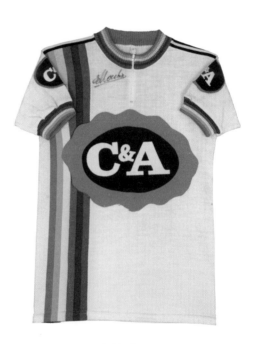

1978 C&A jersey

isn't particularly stylised, nor does it try to be too clever. It doesn't need to be to make bike racing appear the most beautiful sport in the world, because it just is.

All of which brings me, somewhat circuitously, to one of the undisputed highlights of my own cycling career. It took place neither at the Olympics nor the Tour. It wasn't a race I won, and in reality I didn't even perform that well. Ladies and gentlemen, I give you . . . the 2013 Tour of Trentino.

Trentino is a small, provincial Italian stage race. It's a preparatory event for the Giro, and as such the result didn't really matter in the big picture. That's just as well, because I didn't make the podium. I think I finished fifth, and for most people the most memorable thing about the race was a mechanical I had. I threw my bike away in disgust, but miraculously it rolled to a perfect stop against the side of the mountain. You can see the footage of it on YouTube, but it was pure fluke. However, that's not to say I didn't have a moment of divine intervention, because I did.

At a certain point I found myself on a climb I'd never ridden before. It was called the Paganella and it suddenly dawned on me that it had been there, vicariously, that I'd discovered what it was that made Eddy Merckx unique in the history of sport.

By Stage 18 of Leth's 1973 Giro, Merckx was out of sight. He'd won six stages, had led from the very first stage, and his domination was total. The others were riding for the stage win and the minor placings, and of course for money. The film shows a lead group of nine on the Paganella, and five of them are from KAS, the Spanish team famous for its climbers. Merckx is the only one from his team, and then there are three GC guys. Now in the normal course of events you'd expect for the race leader to ride defensively, and for KAS to keep sending their non-GC guys up the road until, eventually, the contenders let them go. That tends to be the way cycling works, and still more so because apparently Merckx had been on the attack all day. Instead, what we see is Merckx pounding away on the front, and the rest clinging on for dear life. The narrator of the films lists them one by one, and then one by one they crack.

So when I realised I was climbing the Paganella, I was transported back 20 years, to my mum's flat and my burgeoning collection of cycling videos. I must have watched *Stars and Watercarriers* 100 times, and the commentary was hard-wired into my memory; 'Battaglin, Lazcano, Fuente, Zilioli, Galdós, Aja, Pesarrodona . . . Merckx churns on and on – that's his way of dealing with the climbs. He has a tough, uniform, march rhythm that has the effect of slowly torturing the others. Gimondi keeps glued onto his rear wheel, but it's a murderous pace. The leading group is at breaking point. To increase the pace now is surely impossible, *inhuman* . . . For any other than Eddy Merckx.'

By the stage finish he'd ridden them all off his wheel. I can't think of anything that better encapsulates what Merckx was about.

You could argue, quite legitimately, that it's a romanticised version of cycling, and in all honesty there can't have been very much that was romantic about being bludgeoned day in, day out by Eddy Merckx. My answer to that is quite simple, though, because whether we like it or not, romance is the soul of cycling. As you go through life – and certainly as you go through a cycling career like the one I had – it's easy to lose sight of that, and of the joy of riding a bike. Cycling, however, remains the great sporting metaphor for life's journey.

I can't really remember a time in my career when Eddy wasn't present. He'd be race director at the Tour of Qatar, guest of honour at the Tour of Flanders, the Gent Six, whatever. Then he'd come to the Dave Rayner Fund dinner, which in the context of Planet Cycling is a very small thing. So it was a bit like seeing your uncle, because he was always bumbling around, doing that walk of his, just being a really nice, innocuous, middle-aged man. I don't recall the shock of the first time I met him at all, because he'd always be popping up here and there. He was just part of the furniture, and in reality I was more in awe of Axel, his son. He was a very good rider, but by no means a great one. Somehow, though, I'd be riding alongside him thinking, 'How cool must it be to have Eddy Merckx as your dad?', and I think that's because there were always two distinct Eddys. There was the one on the films, smashing it to bits, and the self-effacing bloke milling around and shaking hands with anybody and everybody.

On a personal level that tells you a great deal about him. He wouldn't make any particular distinction between the Tour of Flanders and the Dave Rayner because he's one of the least affected people I know. He's an authentic sporting icon, and yet he'd just be there, enjoying being out and about. Of course, those two things – his humility and his popularity – are two sides of the same coin. One begets the other.

You can be a great cyclist and only be *respected*, and I can think of quite a lot of those. Rik Van Looy would probably be the best example. Conversely, I don't think I've ever met anyone who actively disliked Eddy. In fact, people love him because he characterised an era, but also because he was everything you could possibly want in a sportsman. I don't think he *set out* to be an example, because he wouldn't be so presumptuous.

That became apparent to me at the Olympics in Athens. Having won my event, I decided to go to watch the road race. Eddy was there watching as well, and Axel got bronze. Eddy said Axel had done something he never had, because he'd finished 12th when he'd ridden them in 1964. He was overcome with pride in Axel, as I guess most normal dads would be, and I just found that fantastic.

Fast forward 11 years to the 2015 Tour of Qatar, the first race of my last full season as a pro. I arrived very late one night, and the following morning when I went down for

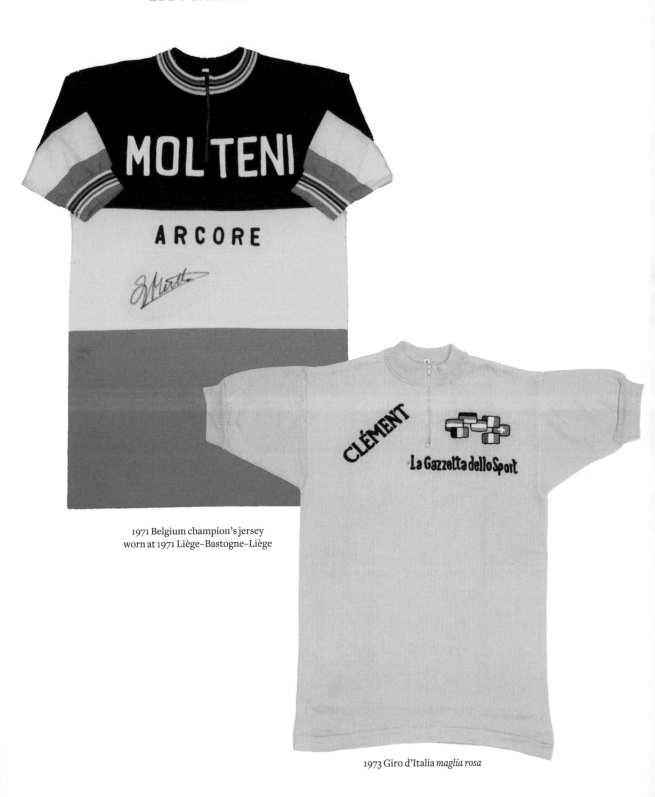

1971 Belgium champion's jersey
worn at 1971 Liège–Bastogne–Liège

1973 Giro d'Italia *maglia rosa*

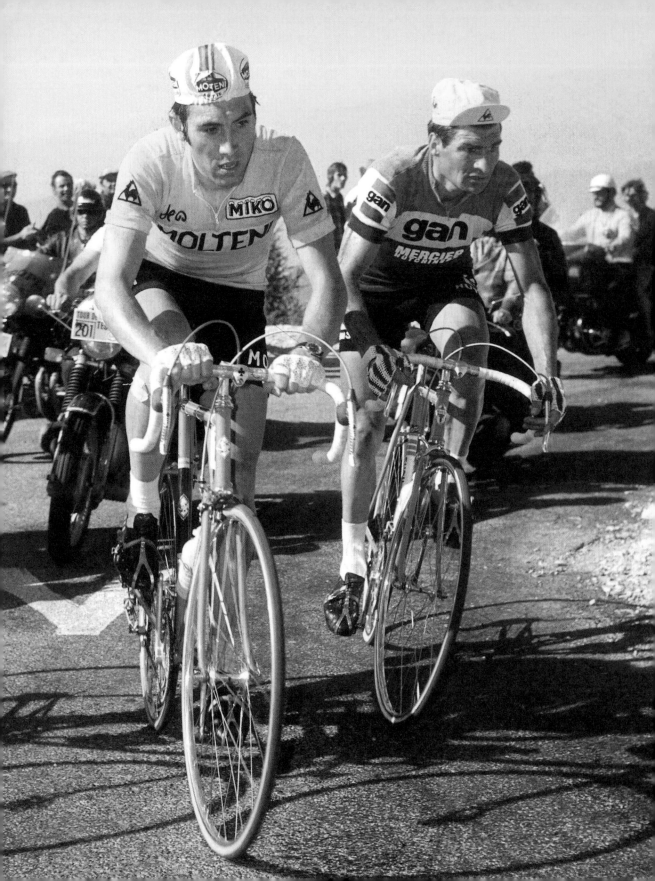

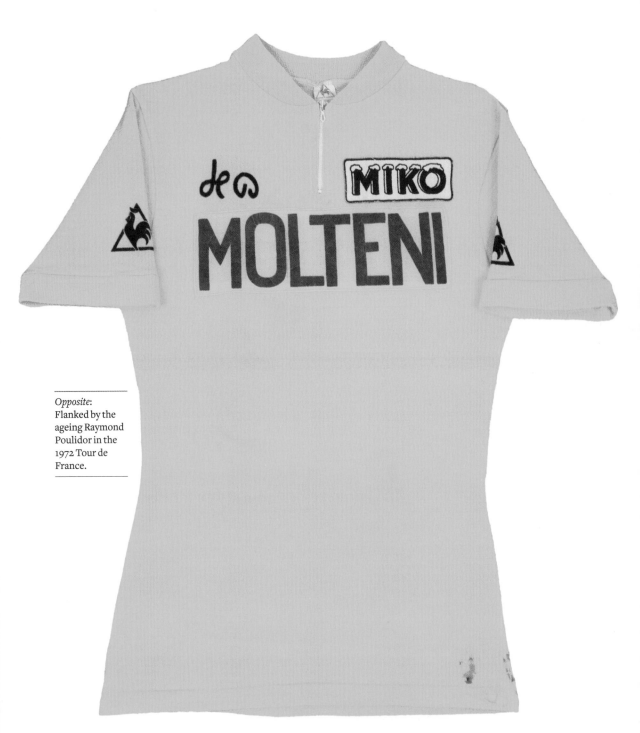

Opposite:
Flanked by the
ageing Raymond
Poulidor in the
1972 Tour de
France.

1972 . . . yellow and Merckx are synonymous with each other

breakfast there were two people sitting there, Eddy and Axel. I went over to say hello and Eddy said, 'Oh, so it's the last kilometre for you.' I'd never really had a meaningful discussion with him before, but then I bumped into him again in the corridor. He started talking to me about the Hour Record, and said he thought I should go to Stuttgart instead of London because it had longer bankings, all that stuff. So there I was talking to Eddy about the Hour Record, and he was genuinely interested. He said, 'With your position you could eat dinner on your back,' and afterwards, when I got thinking about it, the enormity of it hit me. On the one hand I'd been talking to this guy I often saw at the races. Previously he'd just been Eddy, but now in some way he was Eddy *Merckx*, and *he* was paying *me* a compliment.

When I retired I started to work on building up the collection, and it goes without saying that something from him was top of the list of priorities. So I sent him an email and arranged to go and see him after Cancellara's farewell race in Gent. It was a Sunday morning, and I was supposed to go for a ride with him and all his mates. A load of them go out, and it's essentially his old *domestiques* and the people he's been riding with all his life.

In the event the weather was atrocious and nobody wanted to go out, so I found myself sitting around the breakfast table with Eddy and Claudine, his wife. At a certain point he said, 'Oh yes, I need to get you those jerseys,' and off he shuffled. He came back with a carrier bag, and there were three in there. He said, 'I don't have a yellow jersey to give you, but you can have these.' There was a lovely silk Molteni time-trial jersey, a leader's jersey from the Tour of Valencia and another from the 1970 Tour of Belgium.

Now you might say that the Tour of Belgium's not the Tour de France. You'd be right, but that would be to miss the point, because as an athlete Eddy didn't make any distinction. He understood that some races are more prestigious than others, but his approach didn't alter. He rode each and every one of them to win, because as he saw it to do otherwise would have been dishonest. He was being paid good money to compete, and so compete he would. It's basic decency, and it largely explains the admiration that his peers had for him. They didn't necessarily *like* losing all the time, but they appreciated the fact that he treated them, and the races, with total respect. He demanded a lot of his *domestiques*, but he gave a hell of a lot more, and he was never, ever less than correct.

It turned out that the 1970 Tour of Belgium was a mythical race all the same. It began on 5 April, the day after Eddy had finished third in the Tour of Flanders. He'd been the strongest as usual, but Walter Godefroot and Eric Leman had managed to cling to his wheel. There was a three-up sprint in Meerbeke, and Leman had come round him for the win.

It's no secret that Eddy hated losing. What's more, he'd never won the Tour of Belgium, and Roger De Vlaeminck was emerging as a new challenger to his dominion.

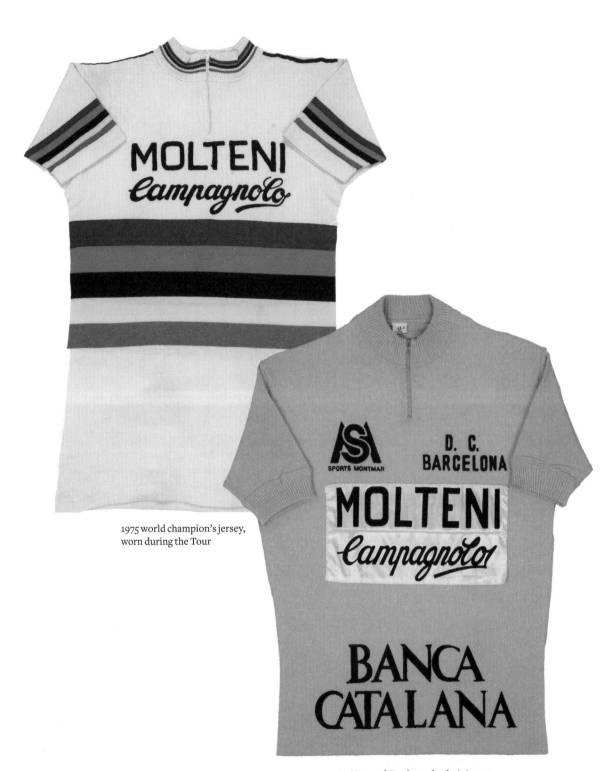

1975 world champion's jersey,
worn during the Tour

1976 Tour of Catalunya leader's jersey

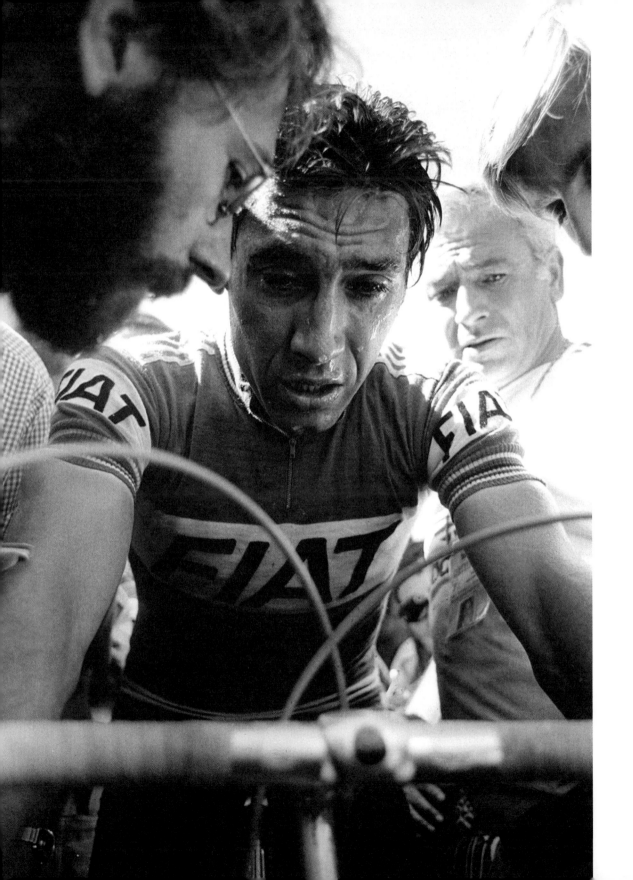

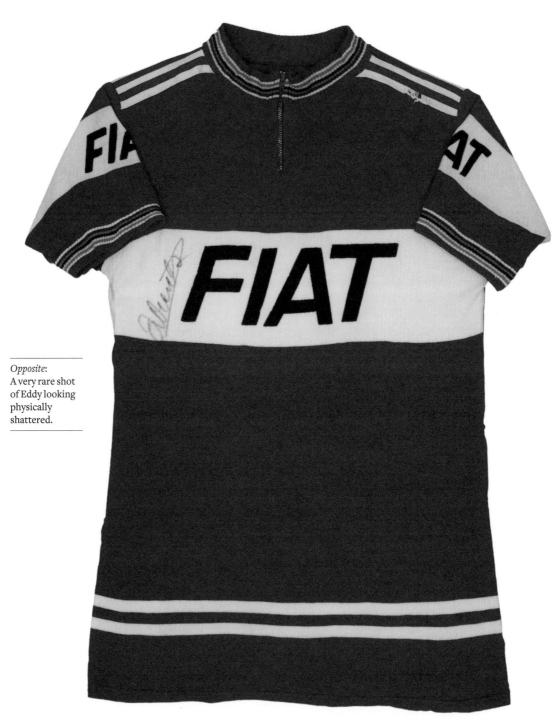

Opposite:
A very rare shot
of Eddy looking
physically
shattered.

1977 Fiat jersey, worn during the Alpe d'Huez stage of the Tour de France

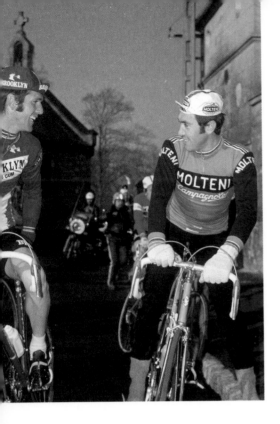

He was determined to have his pound of flesh, and the chance came on Stage 3. There was a blizzard, and while half the field abandoned, Eddy carried on being Eddy. He just rode straight into it and through it, and annihilated the field. De Vlaeminck lost 13 minutes, and started to realise what he was up against. It was pure Merckx, and the fact that the man himself gave me the jersey makes it priceless.

There are quite a lot of cycling collectors in Belgium, as you can probably imagine. Following my visit to *chez* Merckx, I called in on another of them and swapped my Hour Record skinsuit for Eddy's 1976 Catalan Week leader's jersey. Catalan Week hasn't been run since 2005, and again it wasn't a particularly big race. The Hour Record, on the other hand, is a huge event, but there are two issues there. The first is that for some reason my own jerseys aren't really important to me. I've kept some for the kids, but in some way I place more value on the bits and pieces I collected as a teenager starting out. The other is that Eddy is simply the greatest. I had a very good career, but what he did was incomparable.

I don't mean just to me, but to everyone else as well.

As of now I've accumulated about 15 of his race-worn jerseys. There are *maglie rosa* from the Giro, *maillots jaunes* from the Tour, rainbow jerseys from the 1971 and 1974 Worlds. Then I have Belgian champion's jerseys, time-trial jerseys, leader's jerseys from smaller-stage races. I even managed to track down a replacement for my Peugeot. I found a guy in Milan who had one from the 1967 Giro, worn on the penultimate stage to Ghisallo.

The thing they have in common, aside from being Eddy's, is that they all tell a unique story. That's because every race he did, big or small, was a major sporting event.

And that's the greatness of Eddy Merckx.

Left:
One of the great cycling rivalries: De Vlaeminck and Merckx at the 1976 Paris–Roubaix.

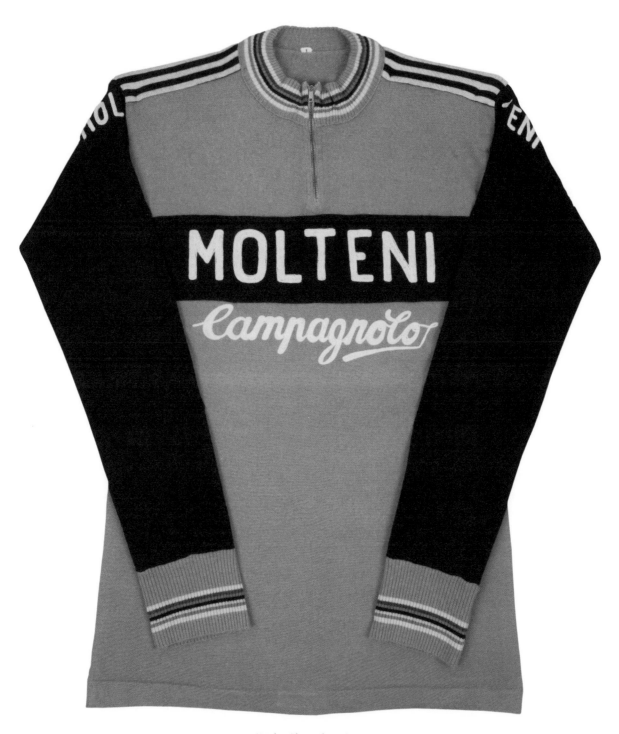

1976 Molteni long-sleeve jersey

7

Patrick Sercu

1944–

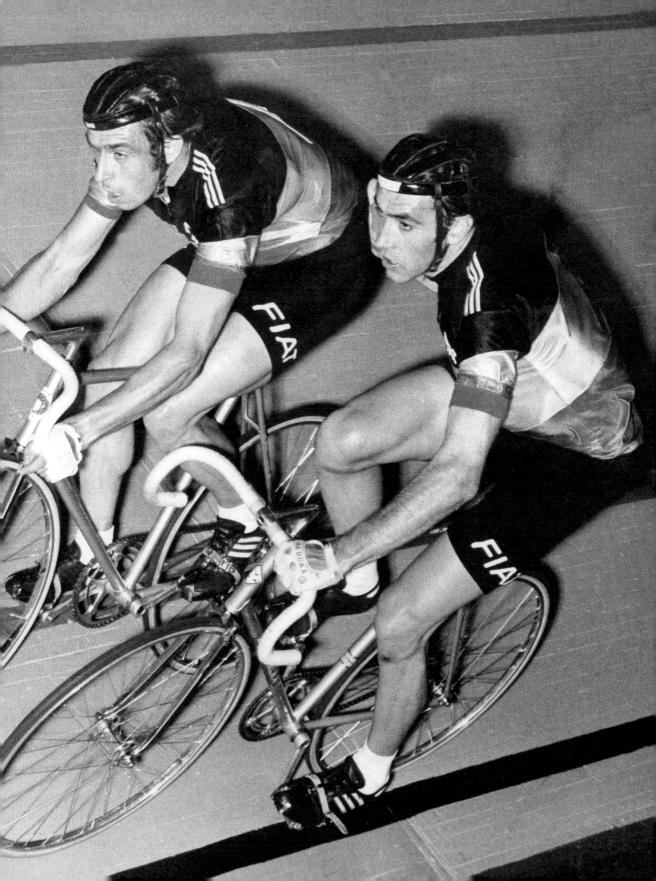

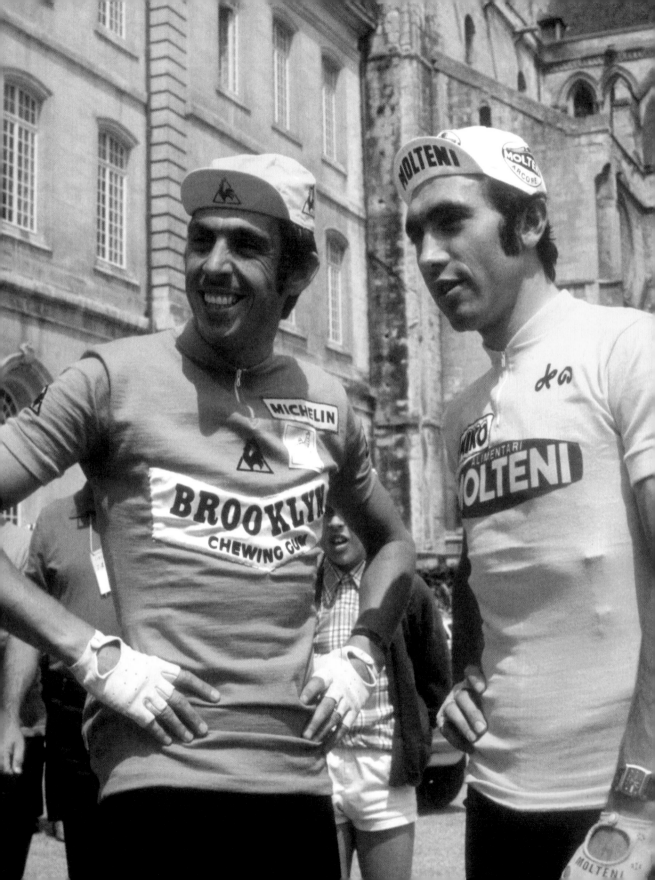

I think it's fair to say that school had never *really* been my thing. However, through Merckx, Ballerini and Induráin I'd begun to take an interest – albeit a highly specialised one – in geography. I wanted to know where these riders were from and where the races took place, and as a consequence I developed a better understanding of the continent.

As I discovered more about cycling's heartlands, I began to understand that there was a symbiotic relationship between the races, the climate and landscapes. The cycling calendar, the way the season evolves, is a masterpiece, not because it's particularly innovative, but because it isn't. Its rhythms have developed organically over a hundred years, the timing and positioning of the races informed by Mother Nature.

Belgium fascinated me above all else and, though it sounds ridiculous, the fact that I'd been born there did wonders for my cycling ego. We'd moved to London when I was two, but I liked to

In the points jersey with Merckx at the 1974 Tour de France.

pretend – to myself, admittedly – that I'd absorbed some of East Flanders's cycling culture. In that part of the world, cycling remains the most popular sport, more popular even than football. That may take some believing, but it really is more than just a sport over there. It's wrapped up in the Flemish identity, so traditionally – and actually – it's been one of the means by which they've expressed their character and heritage.

That appealed to me, and I was romantic enough to kid myself that my having been born there legitimised me as a cyclist. I was convincing myself that I was, in some way, dyed in the Flemish wool, because it suggested kudos.

I T TURNED OUT THERE WAS A GRAIN OF TRUTH in my hare-brained, dyed-in-the-wool theory. Sort of . . .

At the heart of East Flanders is Gent. I'm fairly sure there's a statistic that nowhere per capita is home to more cyclists, and for a brief while it was home to the Wiggins family. As a baby, I'd been taken to Het Kuipke, the town's famous velodrome, to see my dad riding.

The Kuipke was – and remains – one of the great citadels of European track cycling in general, and six-day racing, or *Zesdaagse*, in particular. While all over Europe the Sixes have been dying, the Gent Six remains as popular as ever. *Kuipke* means 'tub' in Flemish, and that's exactly what the velodrome is. During the Six, it's a tub of noise, cycling tradition, low-brow Flemish culture, alcohol and entertainment. At 166 metres in length it's one of the shortest tracks in cycling and that, allied to the proximity of the crowd, gives it a unique intimacy. People go there for much the same reason they go to concerts, films or the theatre. They want to be *entertained*, and the riders are remitted to do just that.

I often think that road cycling tends to be a bit too worthy, and that as a sport it takes itself terribly, terribly seriously. It's forever dripping on about how glorious all the suffering is, but we shouldn't lose sight of the fact that sport is also about having *fun*. If you can't have fun at a six-day race, you're probably not human, and Gent is the perfect example of the form.

Back in the day, most of the big road stars rode the track, and that partly explains why it was so popular. During the 'golden age' after the war they'd do the road from March until October, all the while participating in track meets and criteriums to supplement their income. Then during the winter, Flemish superstars like Rik Van Steenbergen and Stan Ockers would ride omniums and Sixes, and this in turn enabled the public to get really close to them.

There were packed velodromes all over France, Belgium, Italy, Germany and Switzerland. The track specialists became famous as well, so there was a symbiotic relationship. Sprinters like Antonio Maspes and pursuiters like Guido Messina didn't often ride the Sixes, because they didn't need to. They made a lot of money doing challenge matches, weekend meets and omniums, and rode for pro road teams in the spring to supplement it.

Unfortunately, track and road cycling started to go their separate ways in the mid-1950s, when the UCI started actively prioritising the road – the roadies were discouraged from taking part in track cycling, and in their absence the gate money dwindled. With less gate money there was no way they could entice the big road champions, so you had a classic vicious circle.

Partnered by Merckx at a Six – a formidable team.

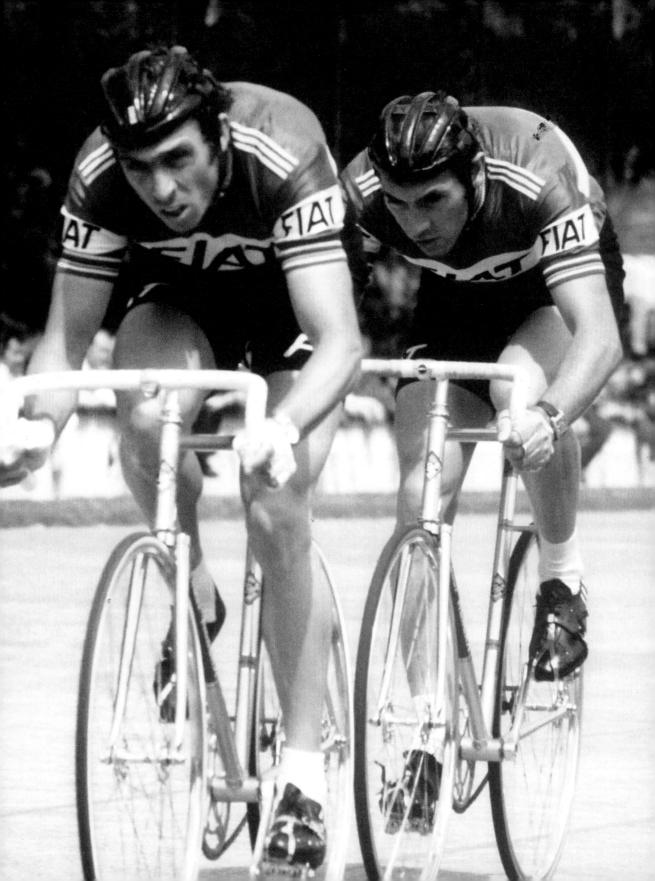

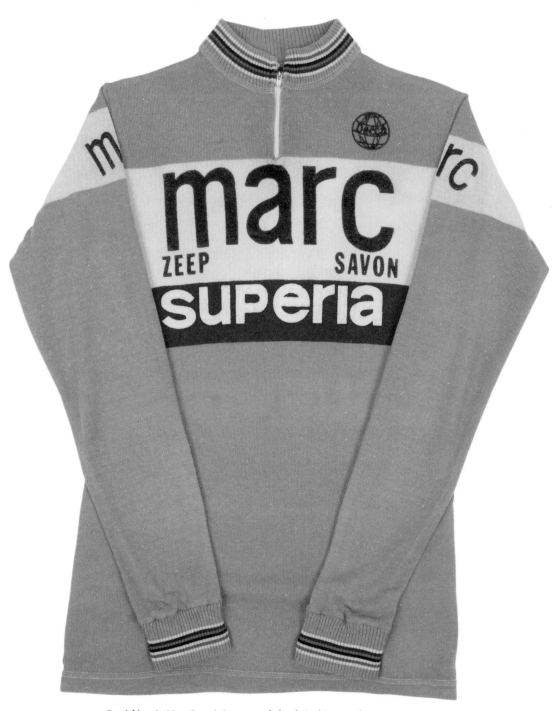

Patrick's 1980 Marc Superia jersey; my dad rode in this team the same year

Sad to say it, but nowadays track and road are poles apart. They're not quite rugby union and rugby league (at least not yet), but there's very little crossover between the two of them. Hardly any of the roadies I raced against rode the track, or even contemplated it. That's another reason why the Sixes are so few and far between now, and why the track is such a poor relation. To my mind, as a cycling 'historian' and somebody who's done both, it's a travesty. In fact, it almost beggars belief, because as anyone who's witnessed it first-hand will tell you, there's nothing like the electricity of track cycling.

By now you're probably asking yourself what on earth all this has to do with my visit to the Kuipke as a toddler. The answer is everything, because it was there that I 'met' (or was at least held by) a true great of six-day racing.

For those of you unfamiliar with Patrick Sercu, he won Olympic gold in 1964, and three rainbow jerseys. On the road he won the points jersey at the 1974 Tour, and 11 stages at the Giro. More importantly, though, he was probably the greatest six-day racer in the history of cycling. Between 1961 and 1983 he took part in 233 of them (that's about three and a half years of his life) and won 88. The first one he won was with Merckx, and over the years they won 15 together. Then he was partnered with great trackies like Peter Post, Didi Thurau, Albert Fritz, René Pijnen, you name them.

When Patrick started out, Post was the 'boss' of the six-day circuit. They won a lot of Sixes together, and when Post retired it was Patrick who assumed his role. They nicknamed him 'The Phenomenon', because that's what he was. So while admittedly my connection was a bit tenuous, it was good enough for me.

In 1998 I won the junior world championship for the individual pursuit and finished fourth in the seniors at the Commonwealth Games. The following October, I was selected to ride the team pursuit in the World Championships in Berlin. I was just 19, but we finished fifth and I rode well.

By then Patrick was organising the Gent Six. I'd been a couple of times and had made no secret of the fact that I wanted to ride it. I guess I was quite unusual in that sense, but I already felt a sort of desire and responsibility to try to honour the history of the sport.

The Sixes have their own arcane rules and strictures, and as such they were always something of a closed shop. There's no question that the scene was already in decline commercially, but the races were much more popular than they are today. You still had good fields, and a dozen or so high-class riders travelling around Europe making a living from riding them. People like Gilmore, Madsen, Villa, Risi, Baffi and Collinelli constituted an authentic 'Blue Train', because they were all specialists. They were hitters, and you had to be extremely good to break into their circle. Patrick liked me as

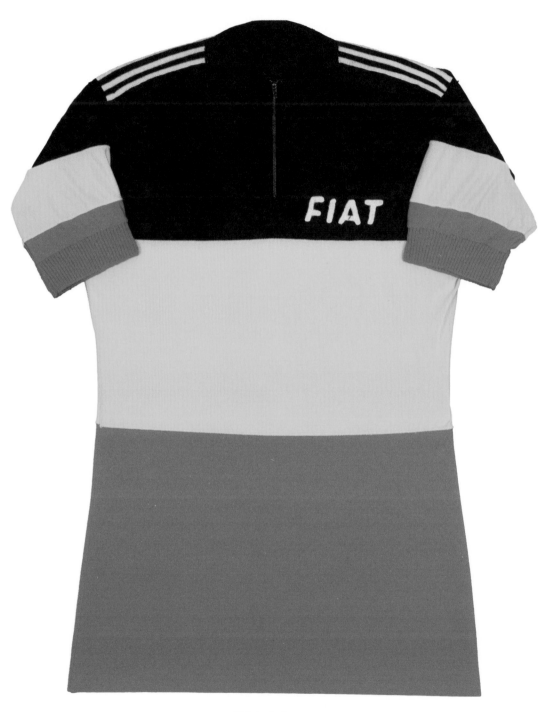

Fiat six-day jersey

a rider, though, and obviously there was a certain emotional attachment. After Berlin he said, 'OK, I'm going to give you a contract, because we won't know whether you're any good unless you try.'

The Gent Six. Brilliant.

To operate in that environment you needed to understand your place in the hierarchy. That meant following the choreography and having a degree of complicity in what unfolded. I was partnered with Rob Hayles and we finished last overall, but that wasn't important. I was strong, I won a couple of individual events and I proved that I was capable of holding my own. Part of that was not getting in the way of the people the public were there to see, being able to do a madison sling without wiping people out, and generally playing your part in the performance. I loved it, and Patrick subsequently offered me contracts for Zurich and Berlin, two of the most historic Sixes of all.

Zurich was fantastic. There was a 100-kilometre chase, a 100-minute chase, and then a 75-kilometre handicap chase. The handicapping was based on how many laps you'd lost, and Rob and I started 20 laps up on the leading team, and finished 13 down. So we lost 33 laps, because it was just ferocious. People were just attacking lap after lap after lap and the crowd was going berserk – the whole thing was just mad. It was one of the hardest things I'd ever done physically, but also one of the most exhilarating. I loved every minute of it, and I remember thinking, 'If I could make a living just doing this, I would.'

Silvio Martinello ran the Sixes, or at least orchestrated them. He didn't necessarily say much, but he didn't need to. Like Sercu before him, he was one of the best, most influential riders, and also a natural leader. For me he was a hero anyway, because he'd been Olympic and world champion in the points race. He taught me that if the star rider attacked with ten laps to go on the Saturday night, the last thing the public wanted to see was some nobody chasing him down.

So when I say there was an element of complicity it's perfectly true, because everybody had to make a living. Now some would argue that the Sixes weren't 'pure' sport, but I'd take issue with that. In road cycling most of the people are paid to help someone else win, ergo to lose. The Sixes were different, but without becoming too philosophical about it, there were similarities. In any sport the cream rises, and the Sixes were no different. Everyone had a mutual interest in ensuring the event worked commercially, and everyone knew they were part of the entertainment industry. Their livelihoods depended on it, and it was good for business that the best riders were going for the win. They were the reason people bought tickets, but that's not to say they weren't extremely competitive. They were, because as with any walk of life, the more successful they were the more they earned.

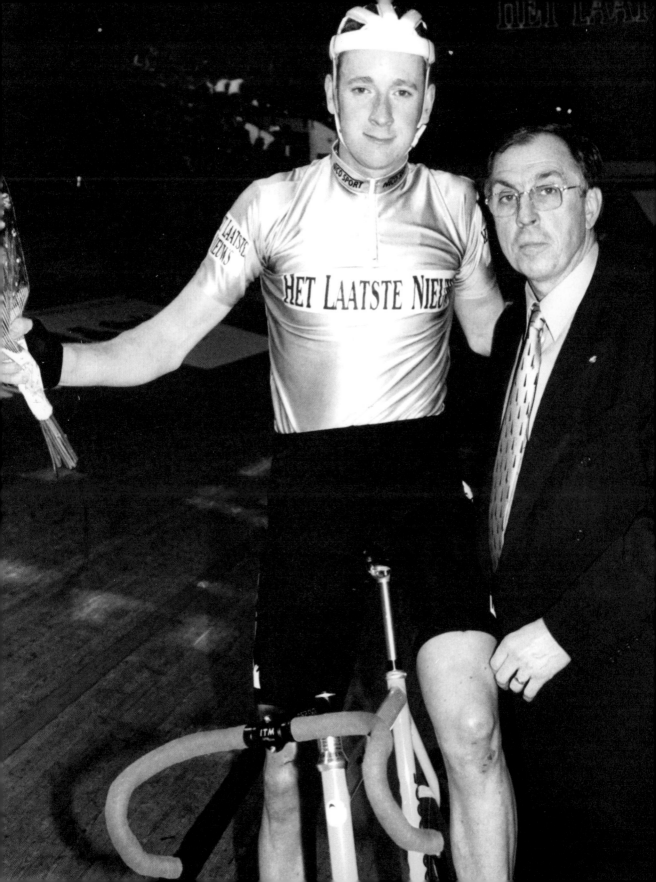

The people who really *knew* cycling understood that, and when the Sixes were at their most popular it was intrinsic to the narrative. There was a lot of suspense because you'd try to second guess what was happening, how the pecking order was evolving and how the show would play itself out. So while the *cognoscenti* understood that there was an element of stage management, only a fool would think that what they were witnessing was 'fixed'. Certain scenarios were constructed and certain results 'engineered', particularly on days one to five. For the track aficionados, though, that was always the point. Much of the fascination lay in what was happening behind the scenes, and in trying to unravel the mystery of it all. That was also one of the reasons the bookies did so well out of it.

And, of course, people could go along and get absolutely lathered.

So it's no coincidence – what with my heightened sense of theatre and all – that my last two races were the London Six and the Gent Six, with Mark Cavendish as my partner.

The fact that I finished my career at the Kuipke tells you everything you need to know about my feelings for Flanders, for the Gent Six, and for those, like Patrick, who made the legend. I'm always going to hope that the Sixes will return to their former glory. Unless someone is prepared to invest vast amounts of money, the roadies are unlikely to change course. That's a shame, because I know for a fact that guys like Elia Viviani love doing them, and if they are managed correctly they can be really good training. It would be great to see Sagan, for example, at the Kuipke. But Gent will survive regardless. Even if the others disappear, the *Zesdaagse* is so deeply embedded in the Flemish psyche that it's inconceivable it will go the same way.

Whether we'll ever see another Patrick Sercu, however, is another matter entirely. Phenomenal . . .

Me and Patrick 'The Phenomenon' Sercu. Truly the greatest six-day racer in the history of the sport.

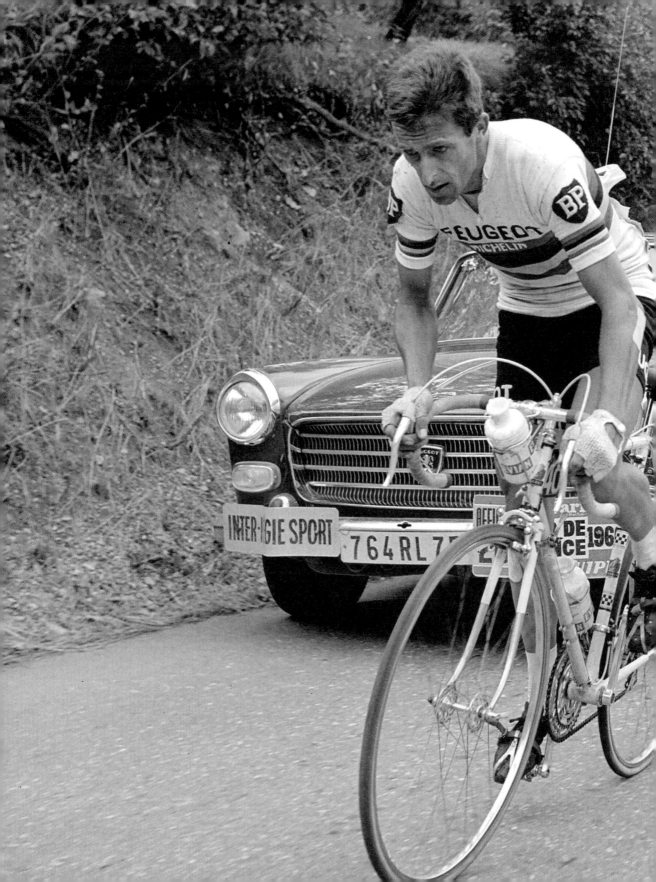

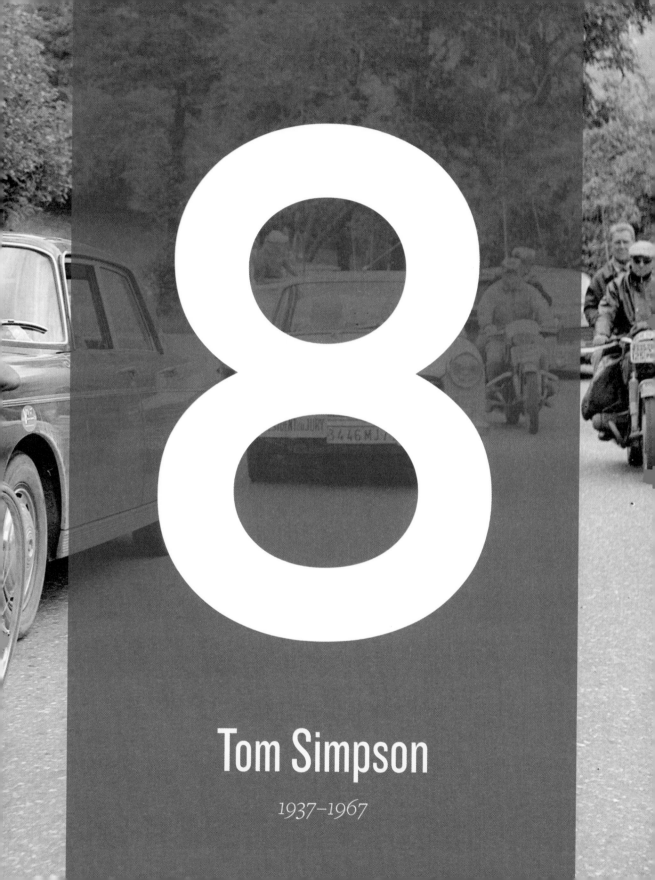

8

Tom Simpson

1937–1967

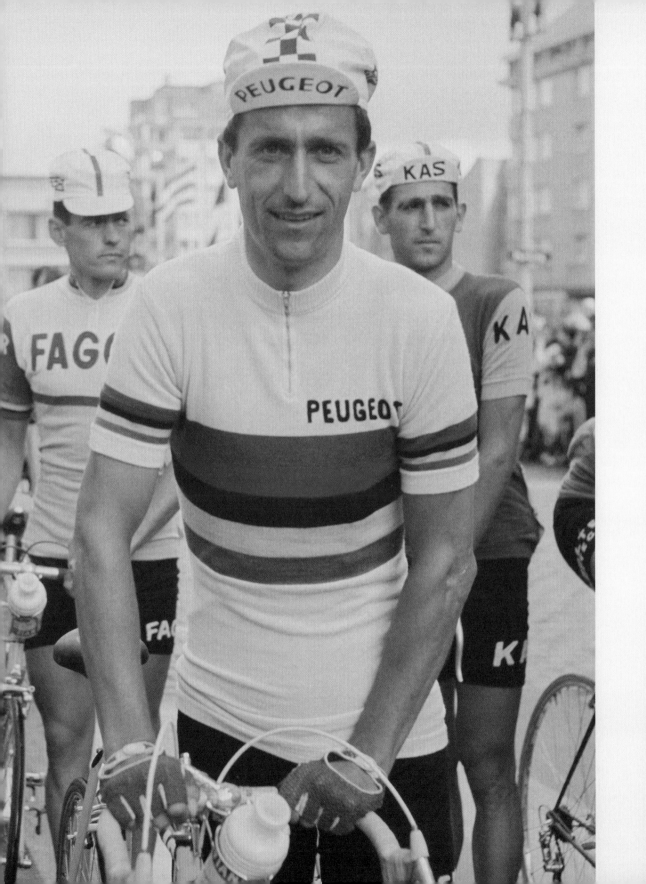

There's a bust of Tom Simpson at the Kuipke. My mum had told me about it, and explained how he, Vin Denson, Alan Ramsbottom and other English-speaking riders had made Gent their home in the 1960s. The town had become a sort of beacon for starry-eyed Brits, and a steady stream had gone over to try their luck. Most of them came up short, but a few clung on and made cycling their career. That was one of the reasons Mum and Dad had ended up living there, and why I'd been born there.

As I progressed I read bits and pieces about Simpson in the magazines. Like most cycling people I assimilated some of the rudimentary facts, a rough sketch of his life. I knew he'd been a very good, very popular rider, and that he'd won some of the biggest races on the continent. I learned that he'd been world champion in 1965, and most of all about how he'd died during the 1967 Tour de France. He'd ridden himself to death on Mont Ventoux. People said it was because

of amphetamines, but I didn't know anything about that and I wasn't much interested. I was a teenager, and I was focused on the here and now. For me that meant Induráin, Pantani and Ballerini. For me, the 1960s were pre-history.

When I went to the 1999 Gent Six, the place was full of former cyclists, and they seemed to be magnetically drawn to this one particular café. It had such character and its owner had been hugely important in Tom's story and, though I hadn't yet realised it, in my own. His name was Albert Beurick, and the week I spent with him fundamentally changed my perception of – and relationship with – the sport of cycling.

Tom as world champion at the 1966 Tour de France.

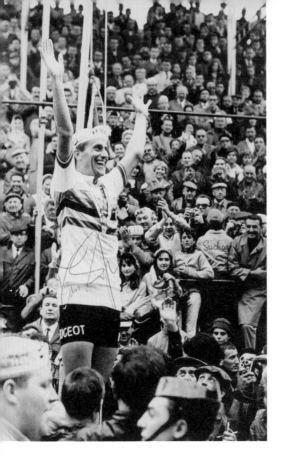

There's a famous photograph of Tom on the podium at San Sebastián. He's just been given his rainbow jersey and winner's medal, and as usual he's grinning from ear to ear. Just off to the right is this guy Albert, and the two of them are looking at one another in apparent disbelief. Tom has become world champion and Albert has been, by turns, his protector, friend, number one fan and confidant. He probably knows him as intimately as anyone at that point, and I think it's fair to say that he also idolises him.

He'd met Tom at the 1958 Worlds in Paris. Later that winter, Tom had visited Gent to race at the Kuipke, and had stayed with Albert while he was there. Albert ran the Café Den Engel, a bar and boarding house in Mariakerke, so when Simpson subsequently moved to Gent it was his first port of call. Denson and Ramsbottom, struggling to make ends meet across the border in Troyes, decamped there in 1963, and others would follow. Needless to say, they were all popular – as high-class pro cyclists they'd honoured Gent by choosing to live there – and none more so than Tom. He was a great champion, and an honorary Gentenaar.

It may seem banal to people brought up on Chris Hoy, myself, Cavendish and Froome, but he prospered at a time when British cycling was light years behind. With his bowler hat, his tea-drinking and his 'city gent' antics, the press loved his Englishness. He was *extremely* patriotic, but he also understood that cycling was partly show business. So both his nationality and his outgoing personality informed his legend.

I think it's important to contextualise what he did as a rider, because without that you can never truly understand the magnitude of it. The guys he was riding against – and beating – grew up in places like Lombardy, Brittany and Flanders. They were born into

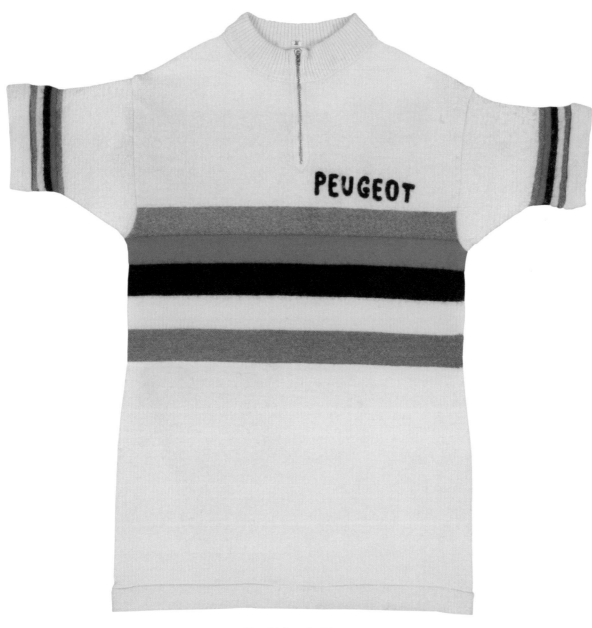

1966 world champion's jersey

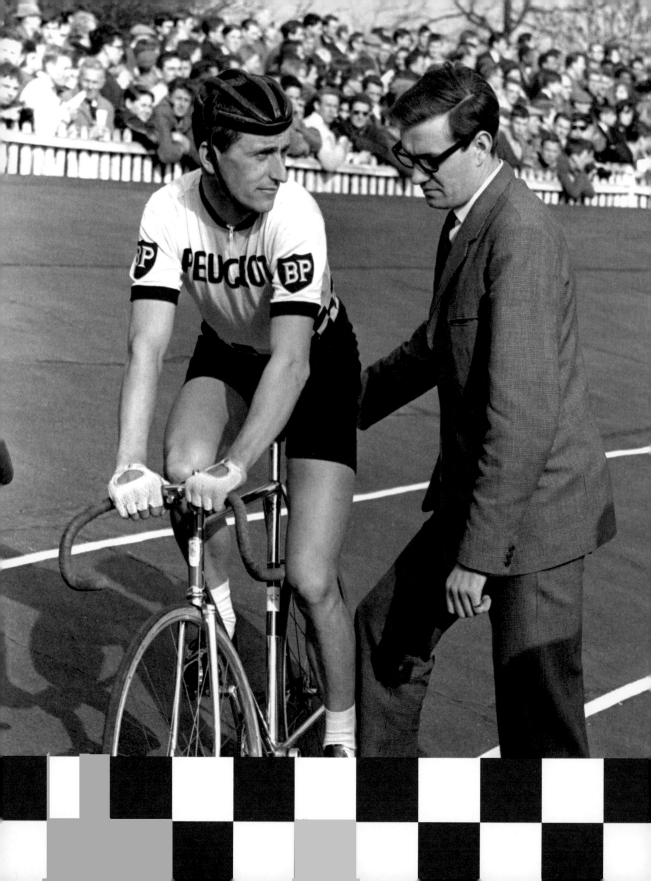

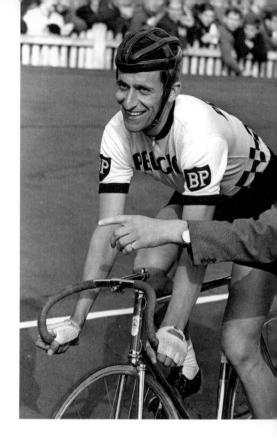

an old road-racing tradition and emerged as the best of a large talent pool. Tom Simpson wasn't, and didn't. He was the 'Four-stone Coppi', a slight, small, skinny guy who came from a northern, English mining village. And yet in 1960 he almost won Paris–Roubaix as a first-year pro.

The following year, at the age of 23, he won the Tour of Flanders. It's indescribably hard to do that in the 21st century, and it's something I could never have dreamed of back then – for someone like him to have done it in that era almost defies belief. You had guys like Rik Van Looy and Rik Van Steenbergen, massive engines backed by extremely powerful teams. The system was feudal, Tom was just starting out, and on the bike he looked more like a little Spanish climber than a Flemish classics rider. So, all things considered, the odds against him being able to win *that* race, *then*, were colossal. Add in Milan–San Remo, his masterpiece at the Tour of Lombardy, Paris–Nice and the rest, and you have arguably the most complete British road cyclist of all time. Cavendish was – and still is – a better sprinter, I was a much better time triallist, and Tom couldn't climb like Robert Millar. However, none of us could have won so many big, important and widely diverse races, and it's very unlikely anybody else from these shores ever will.

That explains why, over time, a visit to Albert's became an intrinsic part of the Gent Six experience. The week represented an annual gathering of the clans, and each November old friends from across the Channel would drop by. Former riders and fans would catch up, ruminate on the sport in general and, overwhelmingly, what with British cycling's affinity with the place, reminisce about the swinging 60s. Given that Tom was synonymous with that time, talk inevitably centred around what he'd represented and the extraordinary life he'd led.

Opposite and right: Tom at Herne Hill, where I started my career 35-odd years later.

That said, there used to be very little information about Tom in the public domain. There was no biography, he didn't feature in any of the films I'd bought, and stuff like YouTube didn't yet exist. There had always been an awareness of his story among cycling people of a certain age, but it hadn't really percolated down to my generation. Maybe it was because his death had been so shocking, and because the British cycling 'movement' tended to be quite insular. Cycling wasn't a mainstream sport in Britain, and the people who did it tended to be a bit 'other'. They were generally fairly uncommunicative, and by definition a bit non-conformist. A lot of people thought they were just plain weird, and as often as not they weren't too far wrong.

In retrospect there were maybe other factors, too. Prior to the Festina Affair at the 1998 Tour, cycling's doping issues had been its dirty little secret. Doping was bad news and, rightly or wrongly, Tom was linked to it. As such the sport saw no particular value in celebrating him, I assume because to have done so would have appeared hypocritical. I use the word 'appeared' deliberately, because in reality the exact opposite was true. Tom Simpson made the ultimate sacrifice for the Tour de France, and it wasn't his fault the sport had developed a drug problem. The real hypocrisy, as everyone now knows, lay in *not* celebrating him and not examining the causes of his death.

By 1999, three generations of British cyclists had come and gone since his death on the Ventoux. The British presence at the Kuipke was virtually non-existent, with only Rob Hayles earning occasional invites to the Sixes. The well had run dry. So when I showed up, Albert took me under his wing instinctively and gleefully. Not only did he make me feel like I belonged, but also like I was part of something – a tradition – that really mattered. That week, however, Gent became a genuine part of me, and I of it. I fell in love with the place, with its history and its cycling culture. For all that 32 years had passed since his death, Tom Simpson was absolutely central to that.

On the surface there was nothing revelatory about Albert, nor his café. It was a simple, down-to-earth sort of a place with decent, unpretentious food. The same could be said for the proprietor, because Albert was just a good-hearted man who lived for cycling – and for cyclists. He felt blessed to have spent the best years of his life supporting, as best he could and as selflessly as any man could, a true giant of the road. He loved the Brits, although I'm not sure he'd have described himself as an anglophile as such. My guess is that it would have sounded a bit contrived to him, and a bit pompous. As anyone who's spent time among the Flemish will know, that's not a good look over there.

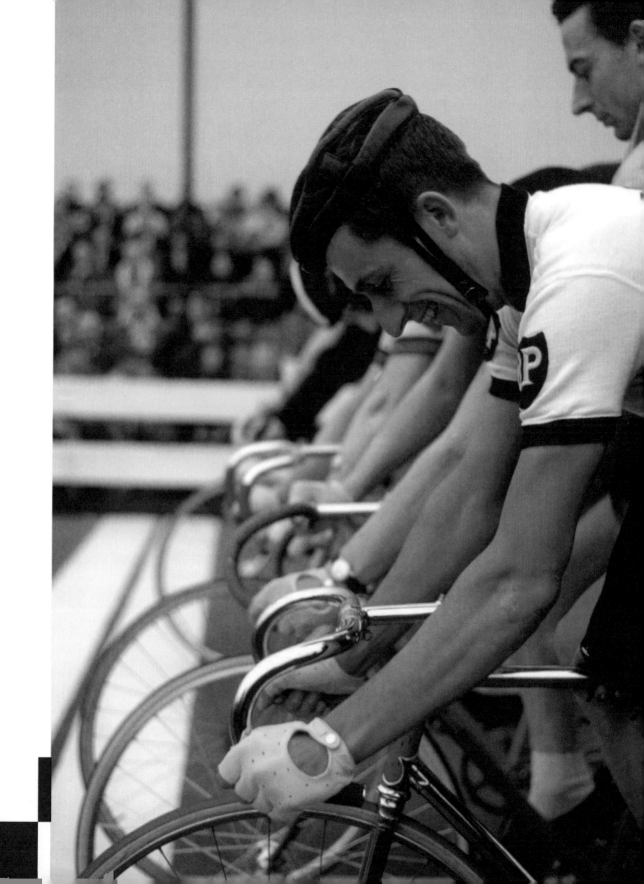

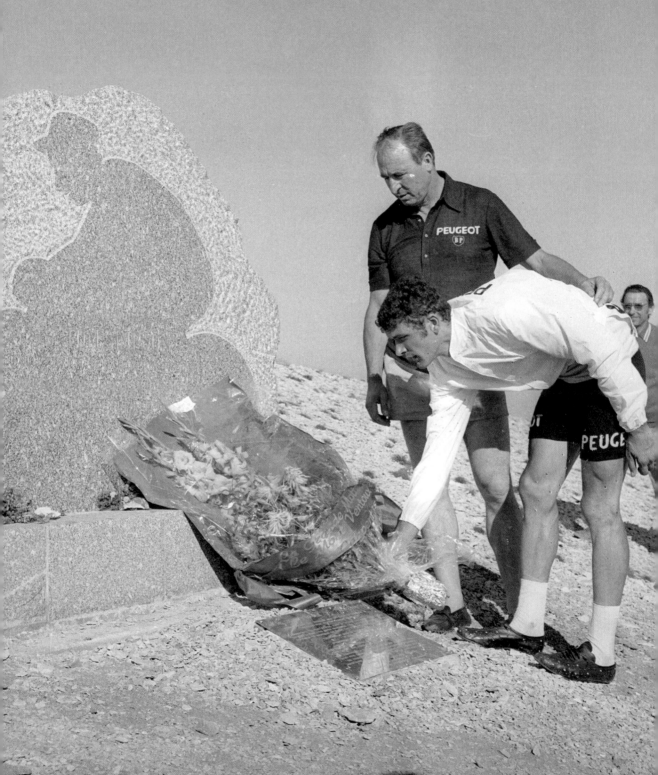

What happened was that Albert started to tell me about Tom and, having done so, he never really stopped. The memories were precious to him, but he shared them eagerly and generously. He was never boorish, and he wasn't a man who tried to place himself at the heart of everything. Gradually he painted a picture of Tom's world, and it was fascinating. It had previously all seemed a bit abstract, but now the magnitude of his achievements began to dawn on me. I'd been familiar with elements of his life, but Albert's joining up of the dots, and my being immersed in the culture and traditions of Gent, brought it to life. Suddenly it became apparent just how important a figure he'd been, and just how deeply everyone in cycling had been wounded by what had happened to him.

When I got home from Gent I found an old copy of *Cycling Is My Life*, a short autobiography Tom had written in 1966, having won the Worlds and the BBC Sports Personality of the Year award. Then I tracked down *Something to Aim At*, a documentary film about Tom made by Ray Pascoe. As chance would have it, Chris Sidwells, Tom's nephew, wrote a book about his life that was published the following year. By then Chris and Dave Marsh had started a Tom Simpson Memorial Fund, and I developed a profound respect for their efforts to keep his memory alive. These were essentially a small group of volunteers, well-wishers and the Simpson family.

News about Tom amounted to periodic notices that the monument on the Ventoux was in need of restoration, and that the Memorial Fund was scratching about for the money to fund it. Beyond that there was a small display of memorabilia in Harworth, Tom's village, and an annual Tom Simpson memorial race.

In 2002 another Simpson biography was published, this time by William Fotheringham. It did very well, and the Simpson 'legend' began to filter into the newspapers. They say that with distance comes understanding, and now the British cycling fraternity, for all that it was small and parochial, started to pay heed to the context in which Tom had lived and died. It was as if a light had come on. It was also abundantly clear that the people I was riding with, my fellow professionals from around the world, were largely ignorant of it all. I wouldn't say I found that shameful, but it did irk me. Here was a great champion who'd given his life for their sport, and yet they seemed to know little or nothing about him. The Tour de France would pay lip service when it went up the Ventoux, but there was no real conviction.

The last stage of the 2007 Dauphiné finished at the summit of the mountain. It was a nothing stage for me, and I was out the back with David Millar. As we passed the Simpson memorial he and I both took off our caps in deference to what Tom had been and what had happened. It was just an instinctive thing – because how, as a British cyclist, could you not do it? – but somebody took a photograph and there was a story

Bernard Thévenet and Gaston Plaud place a wreath beside the monument to Tom Simpson during the 1972 Tour de France.

written about it. From then on I started receiving messages from the family, people who'd known Tom and people who'd been part of his story.

Two years later the Tour was back on the Ventoux for a summit finish on the penultimate day. It was the last 'real' stage and, a podium contender at last, I was fourth going into it. Tom had been seventh on GC the day he died, and I felt his presence more keenly and more urgently than ever. I felt I was going to need him because I was heading into unchartered territory – it was a stage I'd been fearful of, and I was on the limits both physically and mentally. I'd never even raced the Tour for GC before, so I asked one of the team staff to print off a photo of him and stick it to my top tube.

I'd been hoping to overhaul Lance Armstrong for third, and on the approach to the Ventoux I felt like Tom was guiding me in some way. That sounds hopelessly romantic, but the Ventoux is the Ventoux. It doesn't actually do romance, yet it's almost spiritual, and by the time we reached the memorial I was almost hallucinating with fatigue. Lance was really strong, and I had Klöden, Schleck and Nibali breathing down my neck for fourth. I was yo-yoing off the back and yet somehow, miraculously it still seems, I found some energy from somewhere and rejoined them just as we reached the Simpson memorial.

I'm not really one for 'out-of-body experiences', but I turned myself inside out to get back on. For me it was due, without question, to Tom's presence, and there was something profoundly spiritual that day. I felt it – it will remain with me forever – and it's a fact that without it I'd have cracked. I finished the Tour de France fourth, but without that belief in Tom I'd have been sixth at best.

The following year my objective was to better that fourth place. In advance of the race, Chris Sidwells cut the sleeve off the undervest Tom had worn at San Sebastián and gave it to me. Now a sleeve may seem strange, but he wanted me to have something small that I could stow in my jersey pocket as I rode. In the event it didn't come together for me, but that's cycling. As I said before, it's the great sporting metaphor, and Tom's own tribulations at the Tour would be testimony to that. Having worn the yellow jersey and finished sixth in 1962, he'd been convinced he could challenge for the overall. After that, though, it was generally a Calvary for him. There's a hell of a lot that can go wrong, and for Tom something always did. So, while 2010 was a disappointment, I consoled myself with the fact that I was in good company.

The events of the 2012 Tour are well known, and I'm not going to recount them all again here. All I will say is that Tom Simpson and I won that Tour de France together, and that nothing and nobody will ever break that bond.

Obviously I never knew him, so to a degree the Tom I know is the one I've imagined into being. I know that it's an idealised version, and of course his having died young is an

Trying to achieve what Tom set out to do.

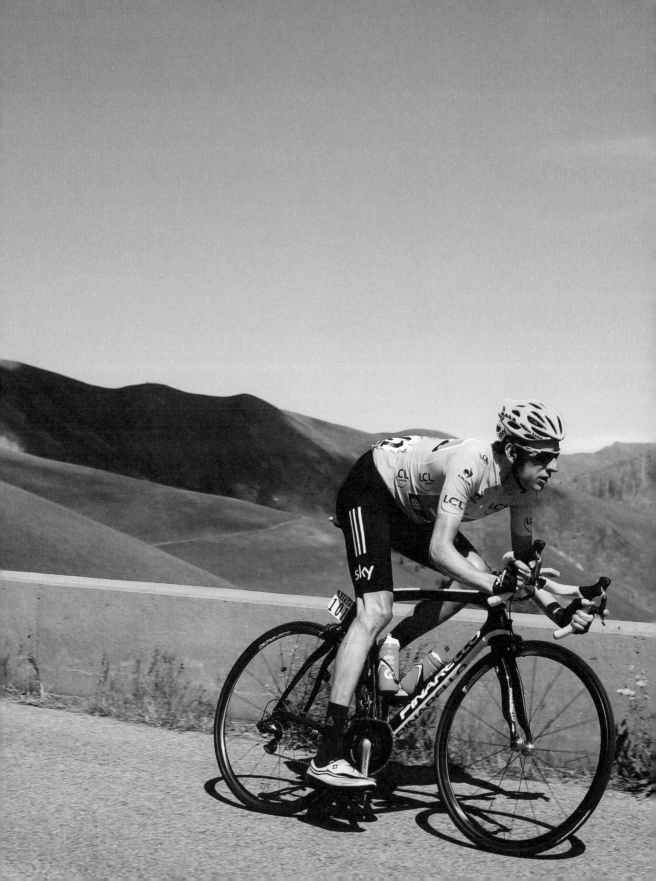

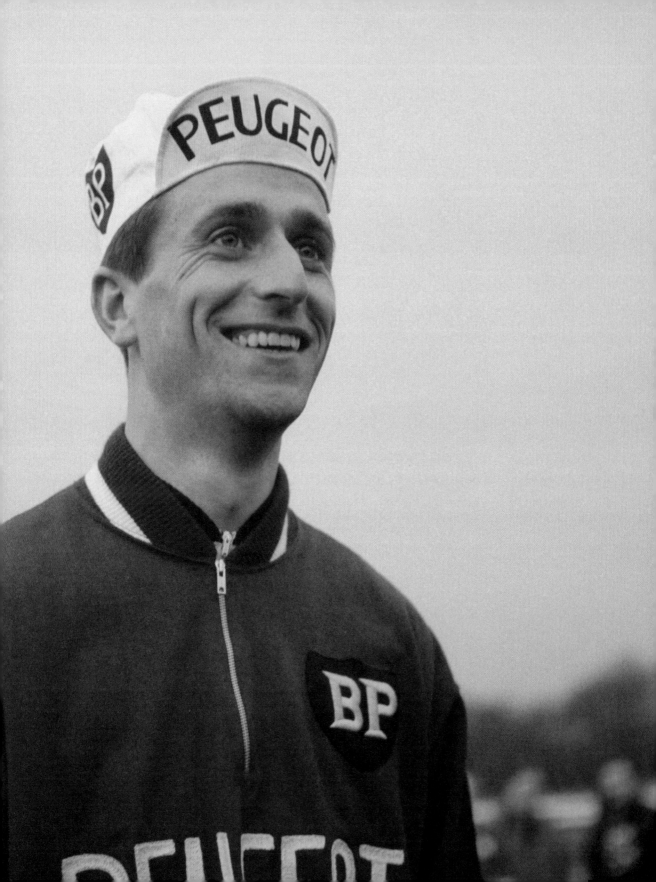

essential part of the mystique. In this sense he's cycling's Elvis Presley, its Jim Morrison or Marilyn Monroe. That said, for me he's much more than the tragic figure who suffocated on Mont Ventoux. From the age of 19 I was inspired by his journey, and that shaped the kind of cyclist I aspired to be. As I matured I became a husband and a father, and I had to try to balance that with the career of a professional racing cyclist. One way or another I was spinning quite a lot of plates, and in simple terms it's very difficult to do all of it. Being a good pro cyclist just isn't conducive to being a good, present father, and vice versa. It's an itinerant life that can leave you feeling a bit lonely, and also a bit inadequate. As a professional athlete you're quite insecure anyway, and as often as not it's the small things that make the biggest difference. Tom's smile was one of those small things, and it helped me no end.

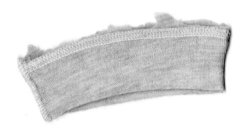

Part of the undershirt Tom wore when he won the World title

Winning the Tour de France is the dream of every cyclist, but I'd be lying if I pretended there weren't strings attached. There's no question that the good far outweighs the bad, however, and becoming a sort of ambassador for Tom Simpson is seriously, seriously good.

Through all the peaks and troughs, and through all my own misadventures, if I can be a conduit through which his story is told then I'm one very proud former racing cyclist.

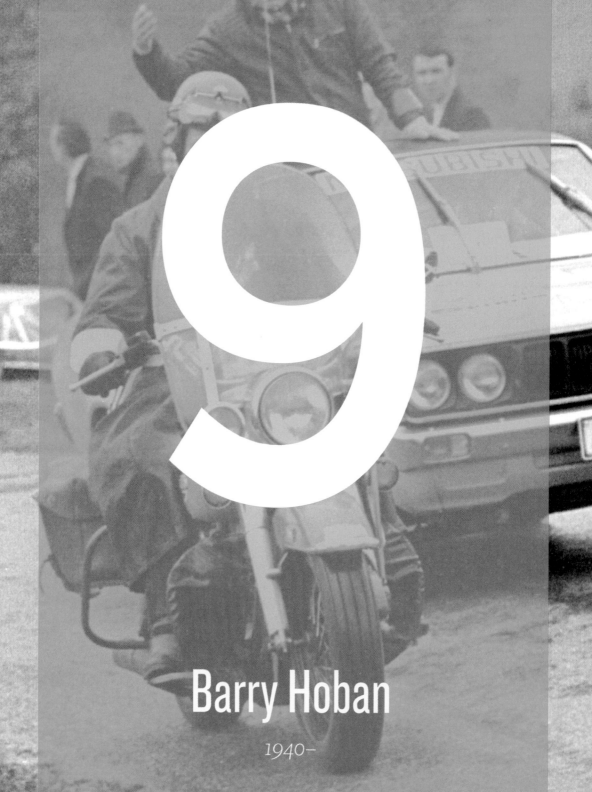

9

Barry Hoban

1940–

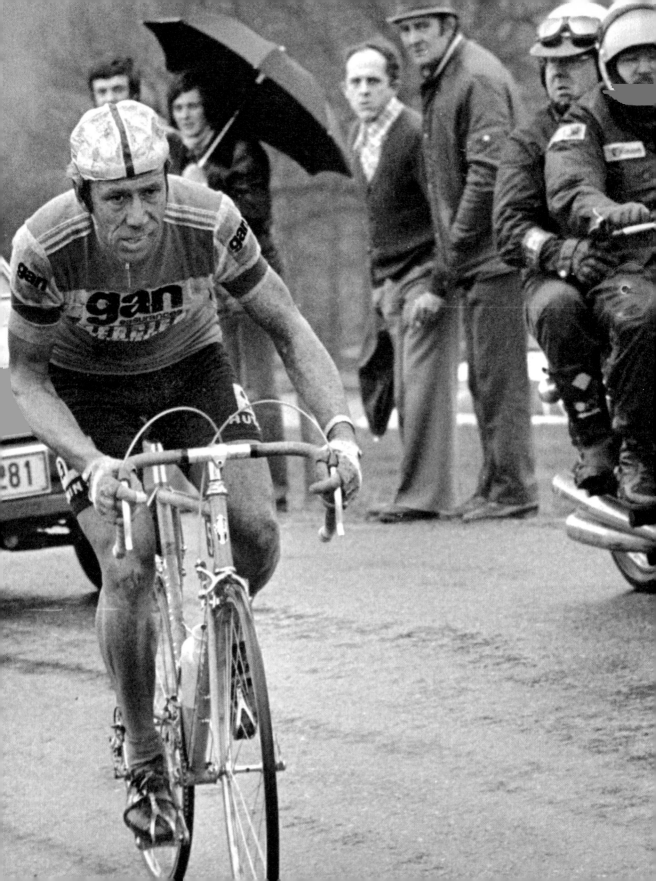

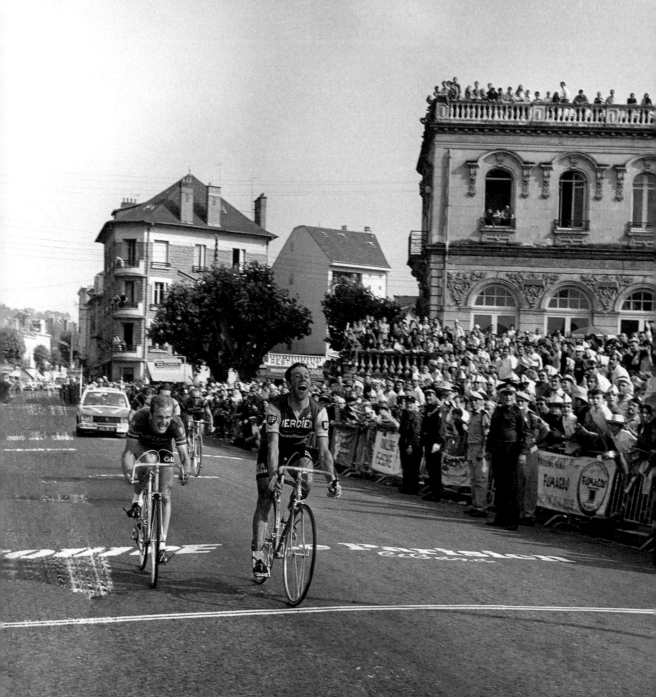

One of the first things you learn as a professional cyclist is that you need to be good at something. That may seem ridiculous, because you only *become* a pro if you're good. Riding in France, however, you quickly learn that there are hundreds of would-be professionals waiting to take your place, and thousands if you include Italy, Belgium, Spain and the rest. In that sense elite cycling is no different from any other elite sport, but it explains why so many guys only manage two or three years as professionals.

When you set out you're under constant physical and psychological stress, and you've got a short time-frame – maximum three years – in which to establish yourself. You've got to prove that you have something special to offer, because if you don't you're going to be useless to your team. You're going to be anonymous, and then you'll be added to the long list of ex-pros who are out of the sport before their 25th birthday.

Cycling is hard. It hurts a lot of the time, and often you're doing things that 'normal' human beings wouldn't and couldn't even contemplate. When I started in France I was constantly tired, because my body wasn't accustomed to the workload. Then I was always on the move, and I wasn't getting the psychological benefit of results. I knew, however – because they kept telling me – that the only way to improve was to keep hurting myself day after day. That probably doesn't seem like much of a career choice, but in point of fact I was one of the lucky ones!

Mother Nature had given me a good engine. It was a diesel and it needed a lot of work, but I had the potential to become a good time triallist and prologue rider. Only thing was, I had to prove that to the people that actually mattered, the people signing the cheques at the end of the month . . .

Crossing the line ahead of Evert Dolman in Brive to win Stage 19 of the 1969 Tour de France.

W HEN TOM SIMPSON DIED ON THE VENTOUX he was riding for the British national team. With cycling in mourning the following day, one of his team mates was able to ride unopposed to the stage 'win'. That rider was Barry Hoban, and he's a perfect example of a smart, talented and resourceful bike rider making himself indispensable to his team.

Tom cast a long shadow in death, just as he had in his life. He was a big champion with a big personality, and he was universally loved within the peloton. His loss left a huge void, and no Brit was ever going to fill it. Vin Denson and Alan Ramsbottom were good riders but not prolific winners, and they were at the end of their careers anyway. Derek Harrison was a talented guy, but his career was short because he had bad luck with injuries. The Glaswegian Billy Bilsland was another. He was outstanding in Britain, but after three years 'over there' he came home without having made a name for himself. That left Hoban as the one Brit truly established on the continental circuit – and that, more or less, would be the context for the rest of his career.

Barry was a cracking sprinter and an exceptional *rouleur*, but he wasn't Simpson. There were any number of riders with similar characteristics, and by then Merckx was beginning to dominate the sport. That meant fewer chances for everyone else, all of whom had to review their ambitions. Or, to put it another way, they had to find a way to survive. Some gave up altogether, but not Hoban. If there's one word that defines Barry, it's 'survivor'.

The first post-Simpson Tour was contested, once again, by national teams. The British had nobody riding for the overall classification, and so Barry didn't have to work for anyone else. The conditions were right for him to go for a stage win, but the same could be said for dozens of other guys as well. They all understood that the importance of a stage win is immeasurable, but it was Barry who broke away in the Alps to take one. Even the French had to admit that his ride was a masterpiece. They probably hadn't realised he could climb quite so well, but they understood what it meant. It was very nice and very prestigious, but it didn't exist in isolation. The *consequences* of it were what really mattered: to win a stage was to find a platform and establish oneself as a name in the sport – for sponsors and teams, sure – but for fans and observers, too. For the people watching and seeking that emotional escapism that comes with watching cycling; those who are inspired by seeing the cyclists 'do their thing'.

The 'thing' is something that makes an individual cyclist stand out, and it doesn't always entail victory. For example, in guys like Adam Hansen, the Australian who's broken the record for consecutive grand tours, you see a similar sense of determination and tenacity to that of Barry Hoban. Adam's not a champion, but he's

Victorious on Stage 19 of the 1968 Tour de France. Most of Hoban's wins were sprints and it was unusual for him to win in the mountains.

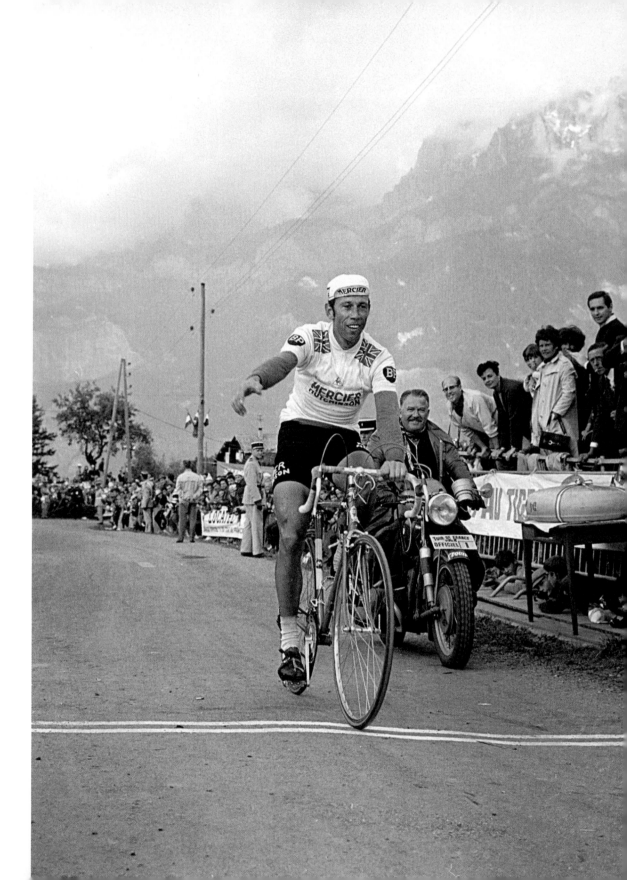

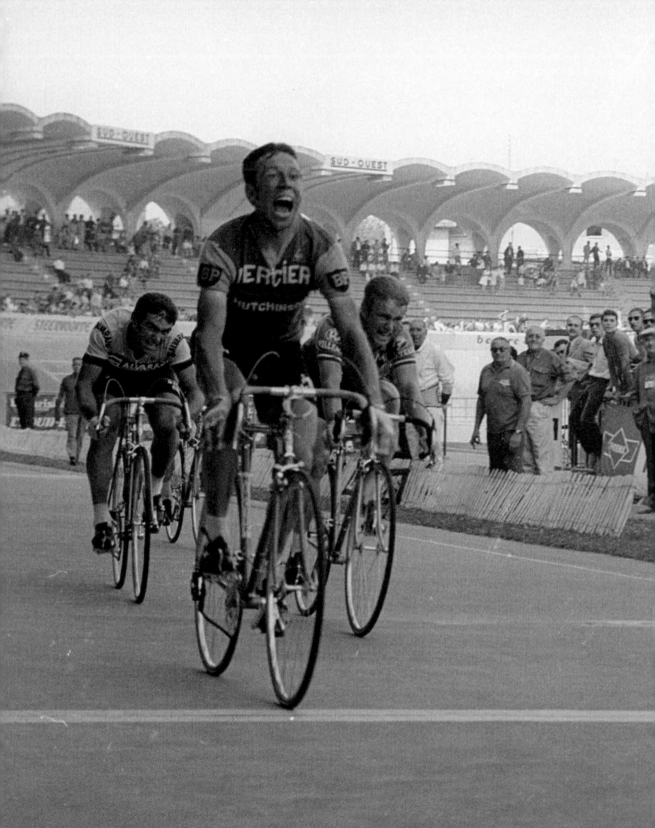

made a career out of staying upright and embracing his major talent – determination. He attracts attention and therefore guarantees his team column inches, so they keep supporting him. Steve Cummings is always at the back – or front – because he knows he's invisible in the middle of the bunch. Thomas De Gendt is a great breakaway specialist, Thomas Voeckler's gurning was pure theatre, and so it goes on.

In a cycling context, I grew up with Charly Wegelius. Like all professionals he was talented, but not quite enough to win any races. Instead he turned himself into an outstanding *gregario* for some of the top Italian teams, making a virtue of not winning. Another Brit, Roger Hammond, made himself the best northern classics rider he could be. He never rode the Tour or the Giro, but he was always visible at Paris–Roubaix and Flanders.

Back in the day, making a name for yourself was crucial. Cycling was much bigger in relative terms, but there was much less media. You needed to get yourself into the newspapers, because if you didn't, you'd be back to the farm or factory in no time. That explains why the riders always seemed to be clowning around for the cameras, why so many of them tried to invent catchy, clever nicknames for themselves and why they tended to keep their newspaper clippings. They needed to prove to the fans and to prospective team managers that they would deliver visibility, and their scrapbooks were their portfolios. A few filled them by winning the biggest races, but the majority were constantly searching, like me when I started out, for something to distinguish them from the rest of the pack.

In that respect, Barry Hoban was one of the best. He lived on his cycling wits, never once took a step backwards, and like all the best riders he was as stubborn as a mule. He also understood – and here's the key – that the Tour de France was the centrepiece of the season. A stage win there meant a big pay day, rich pickings at the post-Tour criteriums, and a virtual guarantee of continued employment. The others knew that as well, but knowing it and being able to deliver it were different things entirely.

You needed to get selected for the Tour first, and for that you needed to prove that your legs were good. You didn't want to hit peak form until you got there, however, and getting that balance right can be extremely precarious. Get it wrong and it can turn into a nightmare that goes on and on, for three miserable weeks. Having finished fourth in 2009, my job in 2010 was to get on the podium. I arrived thinking I was in good order, and in fact I was in good order. That was the issue, though, because I'd been so desperate to do well I'd overdone it. By the second week I felt flat, and by the third my form had deserted me completely. I'd peaked far too early, and with the best will in the world there's nothing you can do about that.

To have any chance whatsoever you've got to get the balance right, and that requires dedication, rigour and attention to detail. Barry won this stage because he

Winning Stage 18 of the 1969 Tour de France in Bordeaux.

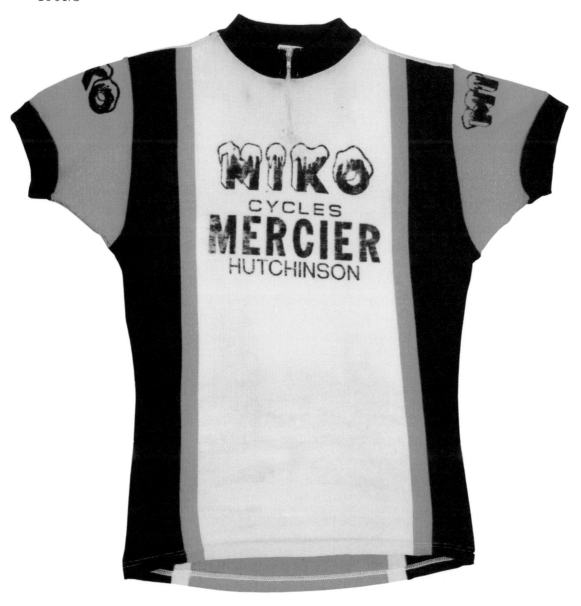

Tour de France jersey, frame number and team classification winner's pennant
from Hoban's last Tour in 1978

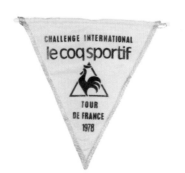

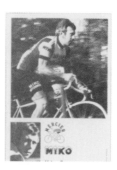

possessed all three, and he went even better the following year. He won successive stages at Bordeaux and Brive by getting his form spot on and being smart enough to get in the right breaks. It all sounds very matter-of-fact, reeling off two Tour stages in succession, but it's impossible for all but a tiny minority. Barry was a smart, talented and resourceful bike rider and what he had done was exceptional.

By the time he retired he'd perfected it so well that he'd won no fewer than eight stages of the Tour. To put this into some sort of perspective, it's one more than the great Raymond Poulidor, three more than all riders from Poland combined and six more than me. Barry Hoban won more stages than Sweden, Canada, Austria and Slovenia put together, and it's worth reiterating that he wasn't a 'pure' sprinter like Mark Cavendish. He was pretty quick, but he won across all types of terrain, utilising different tactics across a full range of racing circumstances. He also beat Merckx and co. to win the 1974 Gent–Wevelgem, finished third at Paris–Roubaix and came second in the British national championship aged 39(!). Whichever way you look at it, his was a brilliant career.

When Barry agreed to let me have a jersey, I arranged to meet him in Chester. We sat down for a cup of tea and then, typical him, he never stopped talking. I barely got a word in edgeways, but I didn't mind a bit. I like Barry, and I think his is a story well worth the telling. It's classic British, but also unique. It's also so far removed from the 21st-century Team Sky/British Cycling model that it almost beggars belief. The opening act was conditioned absolutely by Simpson, while Act Two ran parallel to and was indivisible from Tom's. The final act, post-Ventoux, was – and remains – unprecedented in the history of British cycling.

Barry was two years younger than Tom, and he grew up near Wakefield, about an hour's drive away from Harworth. By the time he started racing in the mid-1950s, Tom already looked set for the stars. In 1956 the two of them took part in a 25-mile time trial near Doncaster, and Tom put four minutes into 16-year-old Barry. By then Simpson was a shoo-in for the Melbourne Olympics, where he'd win bronze in the team pursuit. In the process he'd become an inspiration not only for Barry, but for young riders the length and breadth of Britain.

Simpson had strength, stamina and incredible willpower. He was everything Hoban aspired to be, but Barry was more mature than I'd been in my juvenile admiration for Sean Yates. He was no starry-eyed daydreamer, but rather a tough, resolute, ambitious Yorkshireman. In one important respect he shared a bike-racing heritage with hundreds of Frenchmen and Belgians. Tour de France cyclists had been emerging from the pits for decades, and Barry had started his working life at the colliery. No wonder he viewed Tom, himself brought up in a pit village, as a trailblazer.

Put simply, where Tom went, Barry made it his business to follow. By the time Tom won the 1961 Tour of Flanders, Barry's mind was firmly made up. In the spring of 1962 he caught a ferry to Calais with a fellow young Yorkshireman, Bernard Burns. They settled in another mining community, this one an hour's drive south-west of the Belgian border, and began the long march.

Hoban and Burns arrived in France on the coat tails of Simpson and another stubborn Yorkshireman. Brian Robinson had come from Mirfield armed with not much more than a cast-iron will, and had won the Dauphiné Libéré and two stages of the Tour. Tom's win at Flanders had shown that a Briton could win one of the classics, but the odds remained unfavourable. Britain was still a fledgling cycling country in the early 1960s, because time trials had been the only form of competition before the Second World War. In terms of road-racing development, we were literally 50 years behind the continent.

The upshot was that, like all the Englishmen abroad, Barry needed a helping hand to get him started. His came from Ron Kitching, a former time triallist from Harrogate who'd become an importer of continental racing equipment. He started selling frames and components with fancy French and Italian names, and for the cool kids they were *de rigueur*. Kitching was a bit of a visionary, and one of his suppliers was Bertin, a frame builder based half an hour inland from Calais. Like all cycling companies, they agreed to sponsor young riders like Barry for one reason and one reason only – they believed it would help them to sell more bikes.

This 'sponsorship' generally amounted to a racing licence and a club, a bike (obviously), a few jerseys and a very small allowance. It's a familiar story, and you often hear it from that generation. The money wasn't enough to live on, but that was the point. Even today they reckon a hungry bike rider is a committed bike rider, although back then the hunger was probably actual as well as metaphorical!

Barry would have struggled with the speed, the language, the culture, the food and the missing. The world was a much, much bigger place back then, and northern France would have seemed a world away from West Yorkshire. I found the move hard almost 40 years later, and by then both communication and living conditions were a lot more advanced. There were days when I wanted nothing more than to pack it in, go home to London and just ride the track, because hardship – and *hardness* – were implicit in French racing.

Barry had to hit the ground running to survive, because he needed to start earning some money. That meant racing hard, often against French guys determined that no rosbif was going to pocket the prizes. It took two years, but by 1964 he had a contract with Raymond Poulidor's team, Mercier. That April he won two stages at the Vuelta, and the following month he added another at Midi Libre, a very important stage race.

First in a bunch sprint in the Bordeaux velodrome, Stage 8 of the 1975 Tour de France.

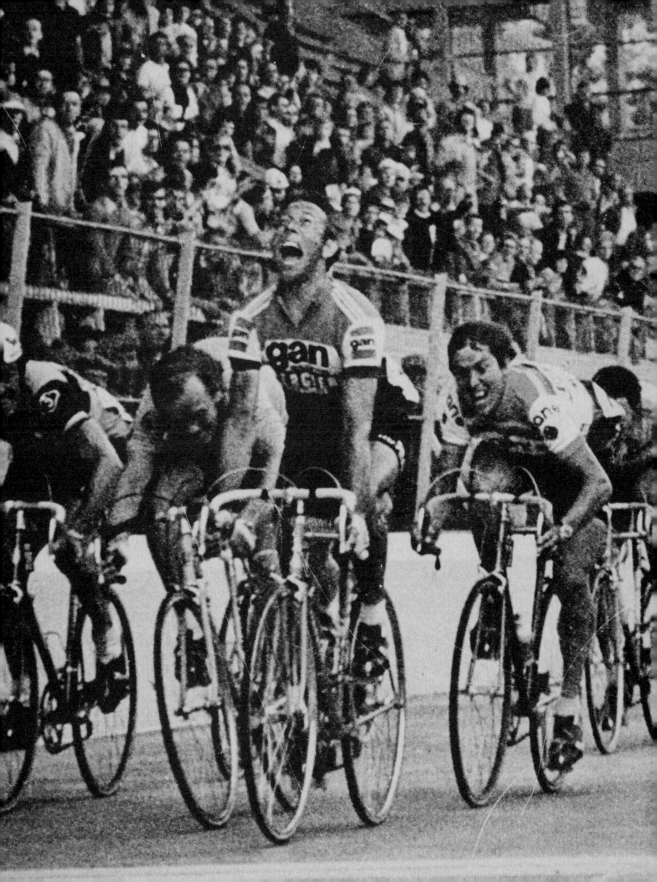

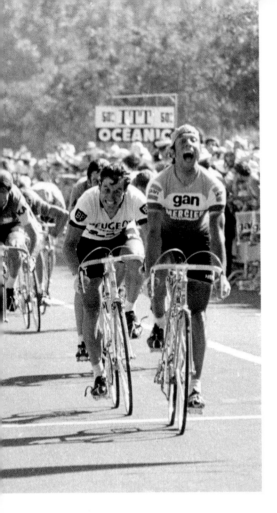

He also won the King of the Mountains prize there, so there was no way they could leave him out of the Tour.

He almost won the sprint in Bordeaux, and so he got to ride some of the crits. The problem was he hadn't had any sort of a break, so he was exhausted. He fell out with his team manager, Antonin Magne, over his workload, and Magne made him pay by leaving him out of the 1965 Tour. That forced him to re-evaluate his career, and he spent July and August riding kermesse races in Belgium. This was the only way he could earn a bit of money, but travelling back and forth was both tiring and expensive. The cost of living in Belgium was much lower, so, with Simpson again acting as both pathfinder and professional benchmark, he upped sticks and moved across the border. He found a place in Zomergem, just north of Gent, helped Tom to win the Worlds in Spain, and the following spring achieved his biggest victory yet, at the Henninger Turm in Frankfurt.

The rest is the history of one of Britain's greatest ever roadmen, and certainly her most underrated. It goes without saying that Barry Hoban isn't as famous as Tom Simpson. He never won a classic as big as Flanders, Lombardy or Milan–San Remo, or a stage race as important as Paris–Nice. He never wore yellow at the Tour, and never crossed over into the wider public consciousness as Tom did after the World Championships in 1965. Cycling never made a martyr of him, but instead, between 1970 and 1977, he was the one and only British rider to honour Simpson's memory at the Tour.

It's no coincidence that Barry was the only British constant during the era of Merckxism, or that he outlasted even Eddy. All told, he survived a staggering 18 years at the top of the sport, in an era when even the very best seldom managed ten.

Eighteen years, and eight Tour de France stages. As hard as nails.

Left:
Taking the win for Gan-Mercier ahead of Jacques Esclassan and Patrick Sercu in Montpellier on Stage 13 of the 1974 Tour de France. Hoban claimed 11 victories for the team between 1972 and 1976.

Opposite:
At Stage 2 of the 1974 Tour de France in Plymouth, the first time a stage of the Tour had been held in Britain.

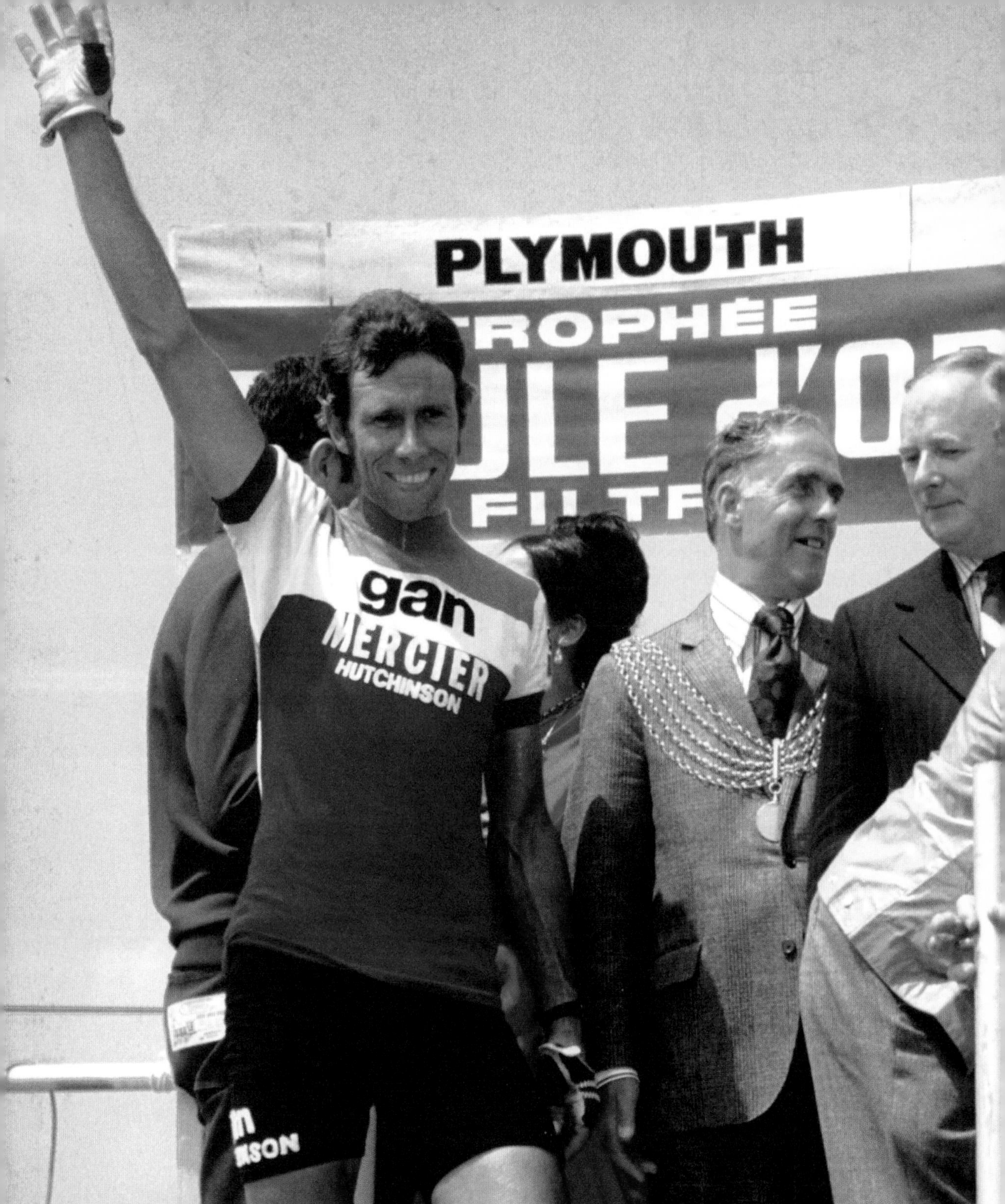
PLYMOUTH
gan
MERCIER
HUTCHINSON

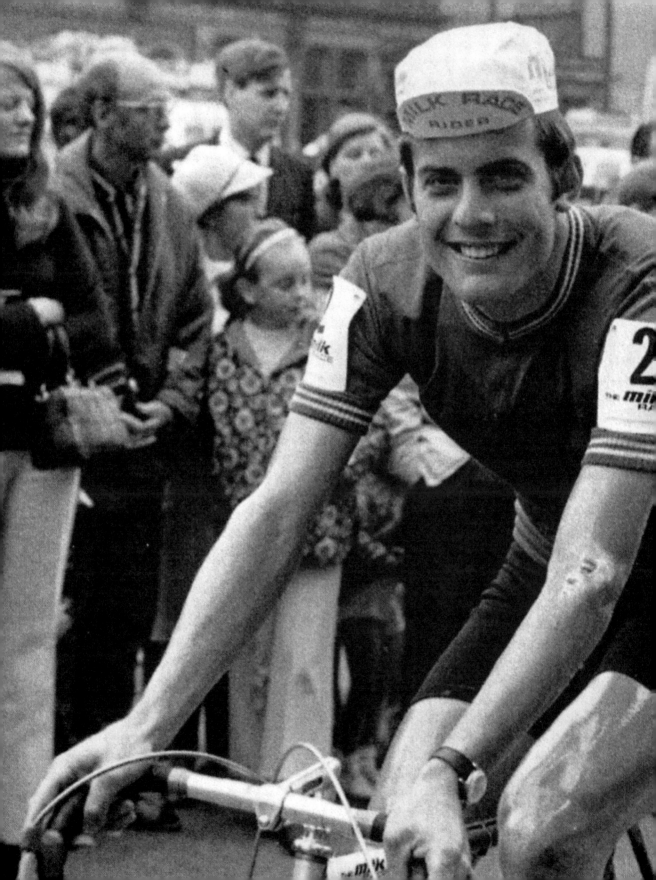

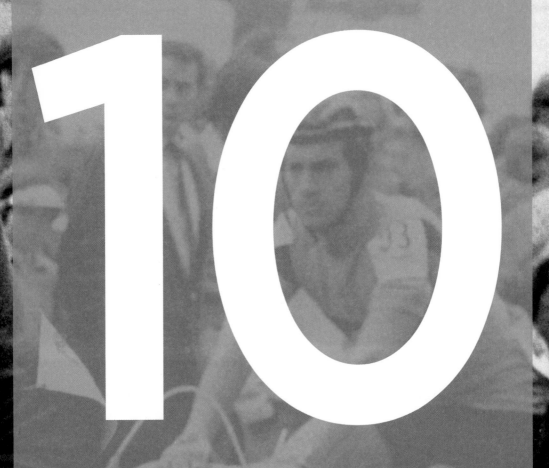

10

Phil Edwards

1949–2017

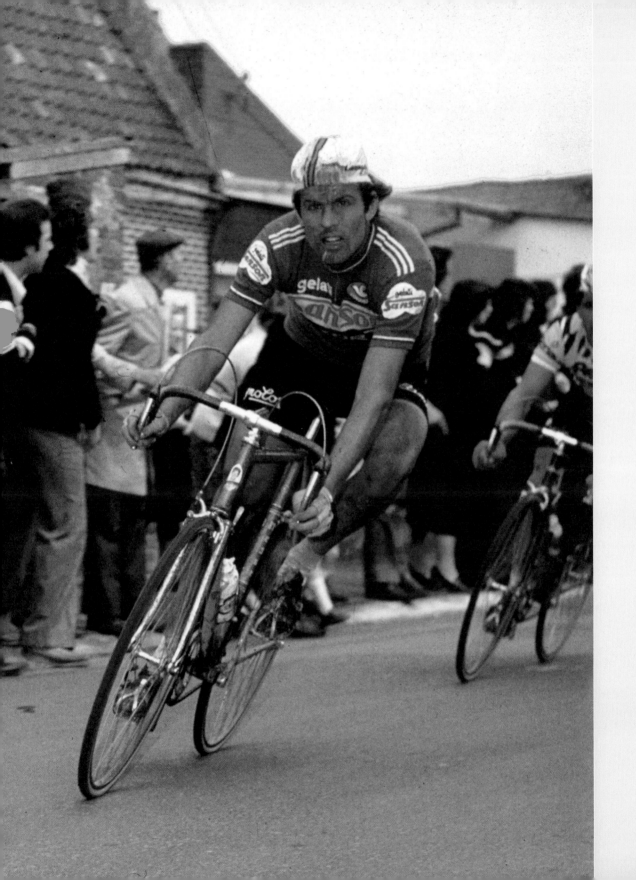

I never met the late Phil Edwards. I never saw him race, and I knew nothing about him as I was growing up. By the time I started riding he'd been retired over ten years, and he wasn't someone they wrote retrospective articles about. In that sense he was no different to thousands of other ex-bike riders. He was gone and almost forgotten by all but his friends, his family and a small group of well-wishers.

Just as Barry Hoban was no Tom Simpson, Phil was no Barry Hoban. As a matter of fact, he was just about as far removed from someone like Barry as any bike rider could ever be. Where Barry was relentless in his ambition, Phil had to renounce all his aspirations for personal glory. That was just as well, because he wasn't paid to win bike races. It could even legitimately be argued that he was paid *not* to try to win them, and if you think about that it's a different concept entirely. I mention it because as far as I know it's a concept unique to cycling; I can't think of another sport where the participants are explicitly instructed not to attempt to win.

Phil was paid to *shape* bike races but, unlike almost everyone else in this book, it wasn't his place to go interfering when the final reckoning was made. That explains why you can count his professional wins on the fingers of one hand and still have enough fingers to pin a number on your jersey. It also explains why he's the least famous rider in this book, but I make no apologies for that. Cycling's not just about its champions, and without guys like Phil there would be *no* champions.

And besides, you don't have to be a champion cyclist to be an iconic one.

Phil during
Paris–Roubaix.

T O UNDERSTAND PHIL EDWARDS, it pays to understand a little about cycling in general, and Italian cycling in particular. Put simply, Francesco Moser was its greatest champion between 1975 and 1985. He dominated the scene over there, and that's why he's on our list. We're going to cover him in the next chapter, but I mention him here because Phil, the last of our Brits, spent five years working for him.

I'm going to assume that quite a lot of you have never heard of Phil. He hardly ever won, but in 99 per cent of the races he was working as a *domestique* for someone else. His job was to plough Moser's furrows, and to put that into some sort of perspective, I'm going to tell you the story of a race I did at Crystal Palace when I was 16 years old. Bear with me on this one . . .

By May 1996 I was quite a good junior bike rider, so they used to let me race with the seniors. This one particular night I broke away with another guy, and like everyone else he was much older than me. He was in his mid-30s, and he'd ridden professionally in Italy back in the day. Now he was making some sort of a comeback, and he was really strong. I wanted to ride bit-and-bit with him, but it was hard. I was only a kid, and he really didn't like the idea that a spotty teenager would be able to come through and do a turn.

So all I could do was cling on as best I could and then try to win the sprint. I *did* win the sprint, and he wasn't at all happy about it. He gave me a bollocking afterwards, saying that I had nicked it because I hadn't done a turn. I remember thinking that wasn't really fair because he hadn't actually *let* me do a turn, and I'd only just turned 16. And anyway, what else was I supposed to do?

He had ridden for Francesco Moser, and with that in mind – and with this book in mind – I asked Moser about the two of them, Edwards and the other fella. This is what he said:

'Over the course of my career I had two Englishmen working for me, and they were as different as night and day. Edwards – "Filippo" as we called him – couldn't really sprint, and he wasn't much of a climber. He was strong, though, so he was very useful for

28-5-96

Crystal Palace Lge

PROMISING junior Bradley Wiggins (Archer RC) got the better of ex-professional David Akam (Wembley RC) in a sprint to win the fourth round of the Crystal Palace Tuesday League.

Starting in the third category group, Akam jumped across to the juniors in the early stages of the 50km race and formed a partnership with Wiggins — the reigning national juvenile points race champion on the track — which nobody could match.

Bradley Wiggins (Archer RC); 2, D. Akam (Wembley RC); 3, M. Lee (London Fire Brigade CC); 4, P. Mill (Olympia Sport); 5, B. Elcombe (Festival RC); 6, B. Taylor (Bournemouth Arrow).
Overall.- Mick Lee 35; 2, S. Joseph (Catford CC) 32; 3, G. Hughes (Addiscombe CC) 32; 4, Elcombe 29; 5, Mill 22; 6, Wiggins 20.
Juveniles.- Peter Keil (Woolwich CC); 2, T. Morley (Surrey RCC); 3, K. Storey (Chelmsford CC); 4, C. Sellen (Woolwich CC); 5, S. Mazreku (Old Portlians CC); 6, N. Harman (Woolwich CC)
Overall.- Peter Keil 20; 2, Morley 16; eq 3, M. Tunnell (Addiscombe CC) & Mazreku 5; eq 5, G.

Left:
A couple of newspaper clippings from that momentous day at Crystal Palace.

Opposite:
Clinging on at Crystal Palace in 1996!

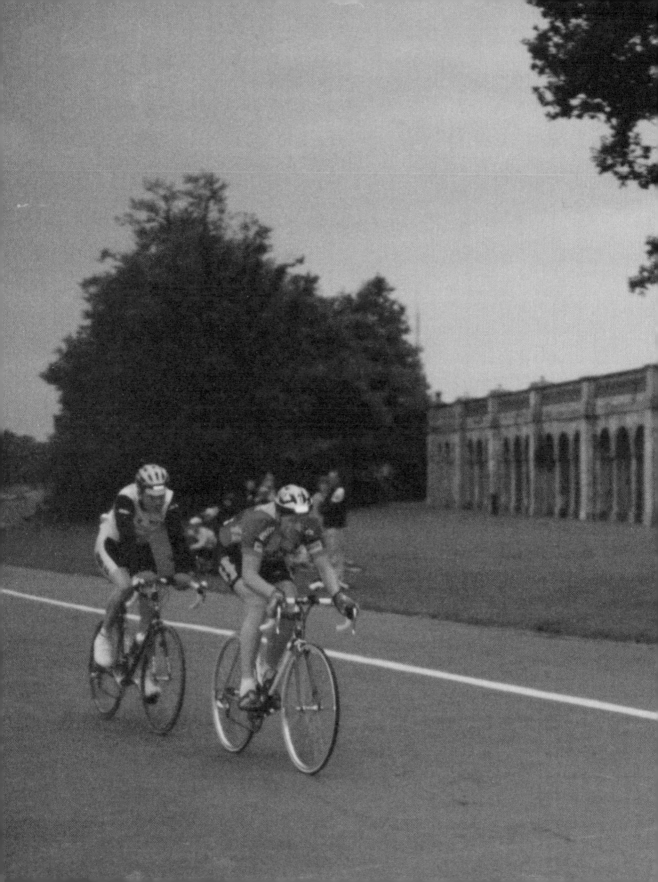

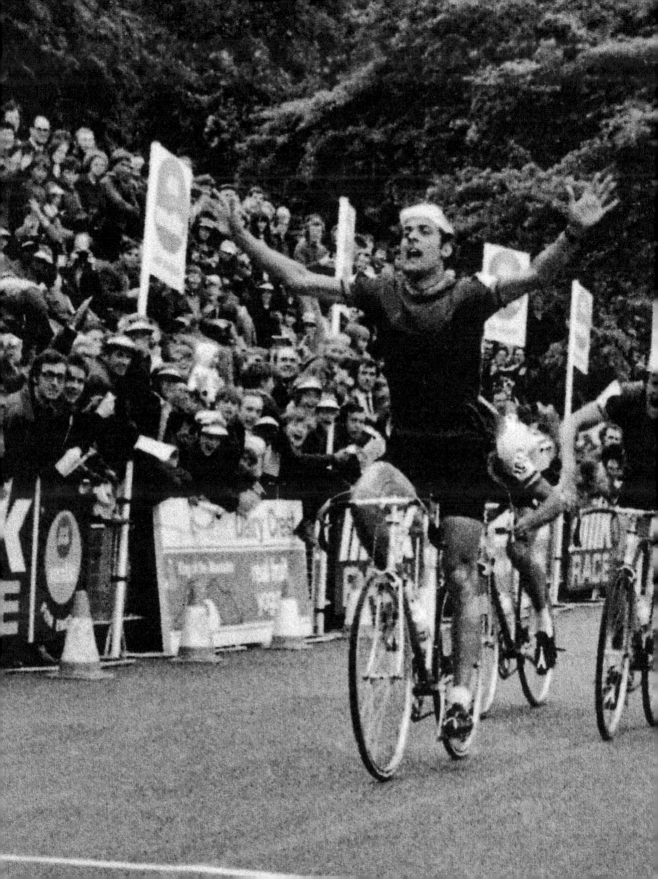

a certain type of racing. You tended not to see him at the finish, because he did most of his work in the early part of the races. He was a very good *gregario*, because that was his nature. He was a person who was predisposed to help others, and he took pleasure in it. He was also very likeable, he learned to speak Italian and he was smart enough to realise that he wasn't talented enough to be a champion himself.'

And the guy I beat at Crystal Palace?

'He was strong, but I had no idea what to make of him. He'd been used to riding in France, and he seemed to think he could just do as he pleased. It was impossible to get through to him, and in the end I gave up trying. He had the physical ability to be a rider, but he wouldn't listen. He only did two years with us, then he went to PDM, and then he disappeared.'

And that was it. Moser hadn't said that much, but he hadn't needed to.

Phil Edwards came from Bristol, but his story is rooted in wartime Treviso. They make Campagnolo and Pinarello there, but in April 1944 there was a massive Allied bombing raid. In five minutes the Americans dropped 2,000 bombs, killing 1,000 people and gutting 80 per cent of the town. Brinley Edwards was a sergeant in the Royal Air Force. After the war he was deployed to Treviso to assist in the clean-up exercise. While he was there he met a girl named Maria Caratti. He fell in love with her, and by the spring of 1948 she'd made an honest man of him. By September 1949 they were back in Bristol and had a baby boy, Philip.

During the school holidays they'd go to Italy, and over time Phil developed an appreciation of the place. His uncle lived behind Pinarello's shop, and like most Italian males back then he was mad about cycling. Having grown up with Gino Bartali and Fausto Coppi, it couldn't really have been otherwise.

By and by Phil was given a bike of his own, and one day while he was out riding he met a group from the Western Road Club. They asked him if he was interested in joining, and he said he was. He started racing – ironically enough on a disused airfield – and the rest is a fairly standard cycling adolescence. Although it happened in the 1960s, it's not so dissimilar to my own story – at 14 he was regional schoolboy champion, and from there on in he'd one thing and one thing only on his mind. And no, it wasn't girls.

By 1967 he was an apprentice at British Aerospace, but he hated being cooped up indoors all day. He was fixated on racing, and he was winning a lot. Like me, he became national junior road race champion, and they even put him on the shortlist for the Mexico Olympics the following year, although in the event they didn't feel he was quite ready. He resolved to ride the Games come what may, however, and for him that meant pinning everything on Munich in 1972.

Back then the British Cycling Federation was a world away from the wealthy,

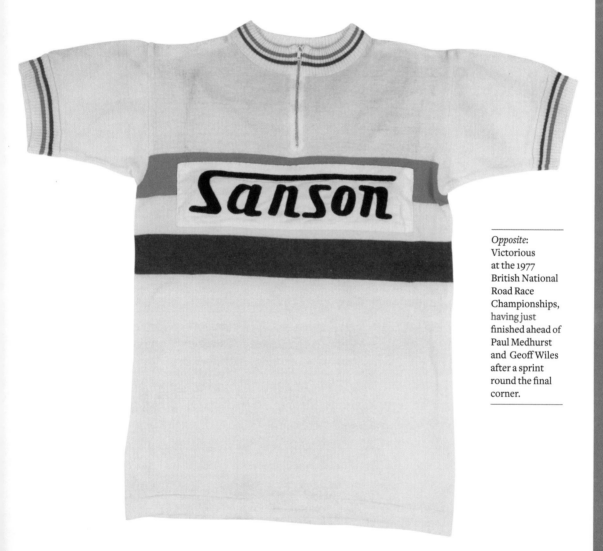

Opposite: Victorious at the 1977 British National Road Race Championships, having just finished ahead of Paul Medhurst and Geoff Wiles after a sprint round the final corner.

1977 national champion's jersey

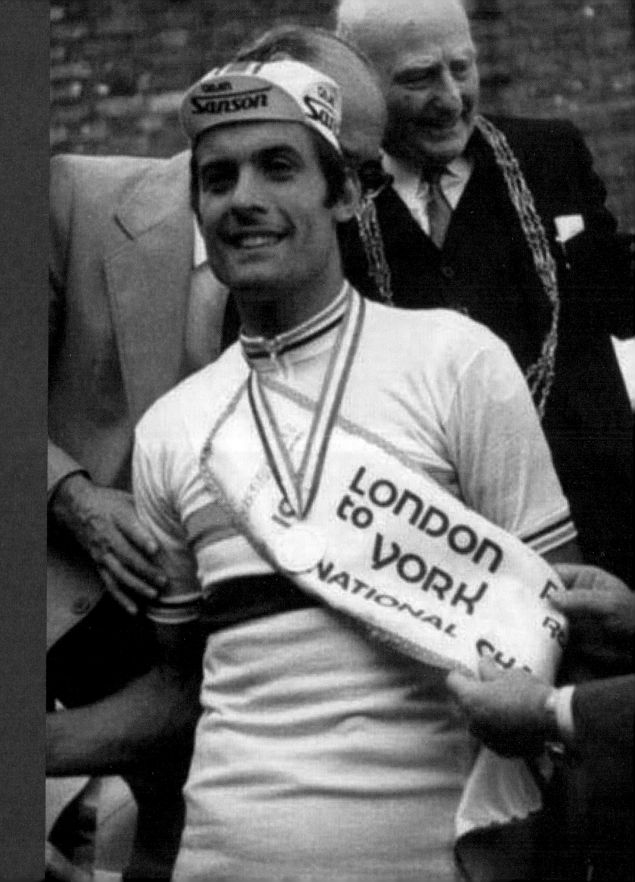

highly calibrated organisation of today. It was staffed by enthusiastic amateurs, but somehow they cobbled enough money together to get Phil a cycling 'scholarship'. In 1969 he went to Holland for four months and rode criteriums. These taught him how to stay out of the crosswinds, and how to look after himself in a fast and furious bunch of riders. He went back the following year, and by 1972 he was a proper racer. He won the Lincoln Grand Prix and the Essex Grand Prix, and also a stage at the Milk Race. He finished fourth on GC there, the best of the Brits. He was one of the best British amateurs, but more importantly he was holding his own with the best Europeans.

The start list for the 1972 Olympic road race is a who's who of 1970s cycling: Hennie Kuiper, Moser and Freddy Maertens would all go on to become world champions, Giovanni Battaglin would win the Giro, and the Pole Ryszard Szurkowski was probably the greatest amateur rider in the history of the sport. In the event Kuiper won, but Edwards and Englishman Phil Bayton finished fifth and sixth. It was a good result, and later that month Phil went up against the best in Europe again, at the Tour de l'Avenir. He wasn't a climber, and the Tour de l'Avenir takes place in the Alps, but he came second in a couple of stages and finished ninth on GC. To put that into context, Battaglin was eighth and Kuiper tenth.

Managing the post-Olympic period is one of the hardest things to do as an athlete. Lots of people really struggle with it, and I know from personal experience that you're left with a big hole in your life. It's easy to fall into a state of depression, because if you pin everything on that one event you feel bereft afterwards. It happened to me, and I was one of the lucky ones. I'd won gold, and by comparison with someone like Phil I had plenty of support and plenty of options.

Moving abroad was difficult, uncertain and uncomfortable. It meant quitting your job, your friends and your family, and statistically there was a high probability you wouldn't make it. Edwards and the other Olympic Brits had a decision to make. John Clewarth remained amateur, but Phil Bayton turned professional with the new TI-Raleigh team. The problem was that Raleigh had little or no distribution in Europe, and the team mainly rode at home. Edwards had different ideas.

At that point no Brit had ever ridden for an Italian professional team, but Phil had a smattering of the language. The story goes that he had his mum write a letter to Ernesto Colnago, the famous Italian frame builder, and he helped to place him in an amateur team.

The first problem was that England is basically flat and Italy basically isn't. It's all hills and mountains, and he wasn't accustomed to that. It took him two years to come to terms with it, but by 1975 he was winning a lot of races. He was also more or less fluent in the language, people liked and trusted him, and he'd developed a nice little sideline

Busting a gut for the Sanson team in 1976.

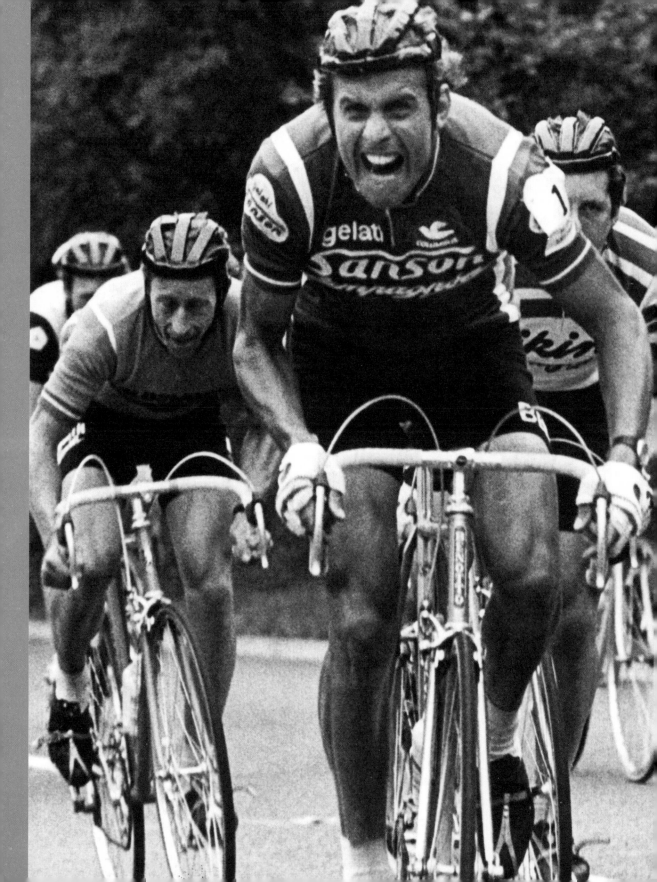

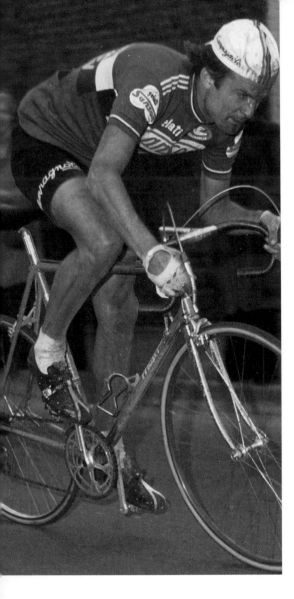

with his brother. Phil would ship fancy Italian kit home, and Mark would sell it on.

By then Moser was a star, and the ice-cream company Sanson wanted to build a new team around him. They needed a strong, willing *passista*, and there was nobody more willing than Phil Edwards. His persistence, character and work ethic got him the job, but it was insanely hard. In Britain the standard had generally been pretty poor. Italian amateur racing had been harder and faster, the terrain completely different and the riders more tactically astute. He'd learned to cope with all of that, but now he had to come to terms with a new kind of cycling. It meant much longer distances, better riders, incredible top speeds and brutal changes of rhythm. He once said that his first two years as a professional were 'like being punched repeatedly in the guts', and I can well imagine. Been there, done that . . .

Over time he learned to chase down breaks and to keep Moser out of the wind. He towed him up the climbs, hurt the climbers on the flat, generally did the fetching and carrying that you never saw on TV but which were crucial to the team.

These days we're used to watching races like Tirreno–Adriatico, Milan–San Remo, Lombardy and Strade Bianche. Cycling has become a global sport, and there's a huge amount of media coverage. Back then it wasn't, and there was little or no continental cycling on British TV. For the die-hards there was a very good monthly magazine, *International Cycle Sport*, but that was your lot. Even the Giro, for all that it was generally a more interesting race than the Tour, may as well have taken place in a black hole for all the British public knew. For an Englishman to be riding professionally in Italy was about as likely as an Italian off-spinner turning out in the county championship.

Do it he did, though, and he became so good at it that Moser insisted that the Italian Cycling Federation pay his air fare for the World Championships in Venezuela. Moser was also best man when Phil got married, and that probably tells you everything you need to know about Phil both as a bike racer and as a human being.

Moser demanded total loyalty from his *gregari*, but it takes a certain kind of human being to deliver that. You only turn professional because you're ambitious, and because you're used to winning. It's not easy to renounce that personal glory, and in Phil's case it meant a change of mentality on top of everything else he'd been subject to as a foreigner in Italy. There was no value in him getting ideas above his station, though, because those who did tended not to last very long in Moser's world.

By 1982 Sanson was folding, and 'Filippo' was struggling with a persistent wrist injury. But the bike business he'd established was thriving and he was well connected. The American mountain-bike market was about to boom, and the manufacturers had designs on Europe. Phil began distributing Specialized, and five years later Trek. He played a major role in the growing popularity of carbon frames and did extremely well off the back of Lance Armstrong's Tour de France wins. He moved to Monte Carlo and opened a restaurant, but died in 2017 aged just 67.

The jersey I have of his tells the story of his professional cycling journey. In 1977 he rode the Giro for Moser, and then flew home to Britain. He then made a beeline for the glamour and glitz of the South Mimms service station, starting point of the National Road Race Championship. It was his annual British outing, and the one time each year that he got to ride exclusively for himself. Eight and a half hours and 193 miles later one extremely proud, half-Italian Englishman pulled on the mythical red, white and blue, with sponsorship provided by an Italian ice-cream company.

Fantastic.

RIP Phil Edwards.

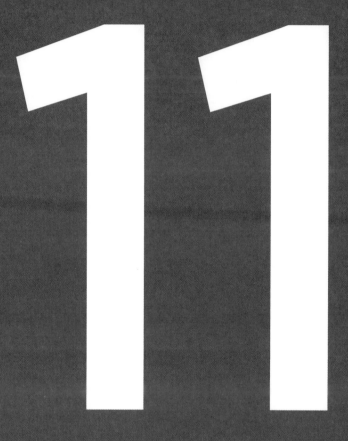

11

Francesco Moser

1951–

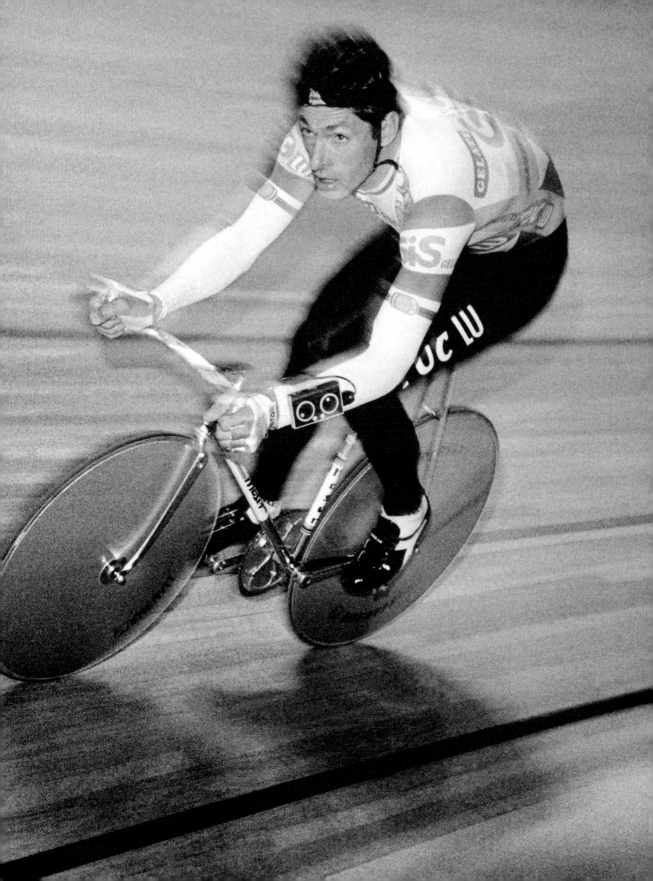

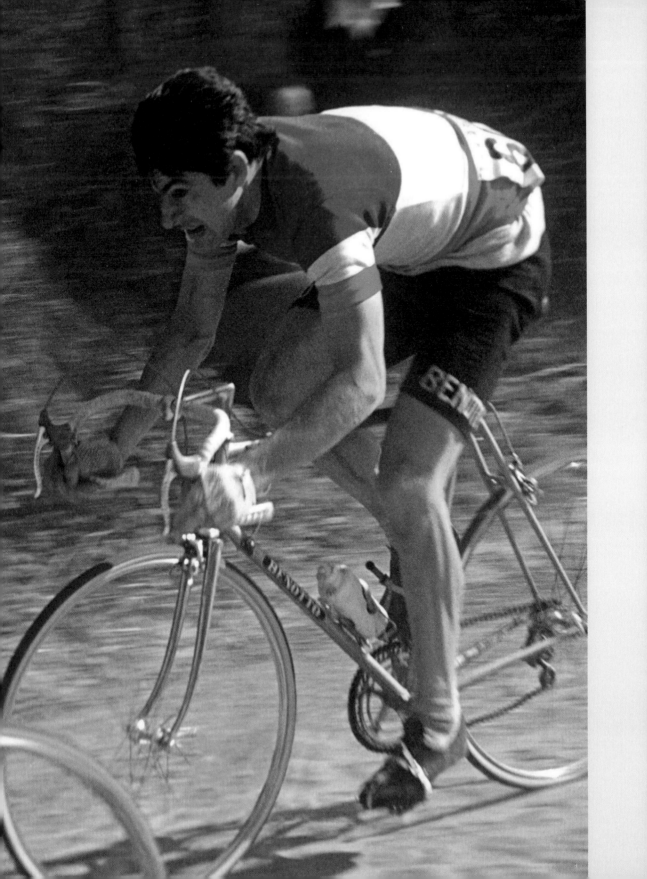

In the Ballerini chapter, I mentioned feeling like an extra in *A Sunday in Hell* when I packed it in at Roubaix. The film was Leth's third cycling documentary, and as a kid I'd spent many evenings watching it repeatedly and probably unhealthily. Back then it was a cult thing, but it's become very popular recently. To my mind there are three main reasons for that. The first is that it's brilliant, the second is that cycling has become fashionable, the third that Paris–Roubaix is probably the only race that hasn't fundamentally changed. It hasn't needed to, because it's perfect.

There's an amazing sequence at the start, where the mechanic is building Francesco Moser's bike. It goes on, without commentary, for four or five minutes, and it's hypnotic. Later you see Moser at the team meeting, and then they load the bikes and head off to the race. Moser was one of the strongest riders in the world, and Sanson one of the strongest teams. And yet they have this tiny little van with three blokes squeezed into the front. It's all really simple, particularly when you think about all the infrastructure and personnel that modern cycling teams cart about. We've come a hell of a long way in terms of preparation, performance and 'professionalism' over the last 40 years, but the further we seem to have come, the less it feels like bike racing. Cycling always was a business, but it now sometimes feels like the business just *happens* to be cycling.

Later in the film you see Moser racing in his *maglia tricolore*, his Italian national champion's jersey. He always looked utterly beautiful on a bike and it's a timeless image, but for me it represents a lot more besides. That's because, quite simply, there's a lot more to cycling than cycling.

Wearing the national champion's jersey.

ROAD CYCLING WAS INVENTED TO SELL THINGS, and as a rider you learn pretty soon that you're a moving billboard. That being the case, you've to try to choose your races carefully, although in reality not too many riders have that opportunity. When I started out they'd send me here, there and everywhere, as often as not to races the team had no chance in and no particular interest in. I was making up the numbers, because a number was pretty much all I was. I would get a kicking most days, and a lot of the time I was in a sort of mindless bubble. Sometimes I literally had no idea where I was. I knew it was a hotel somewhere in France, but that was about it. It's a glamorous life, cycling.

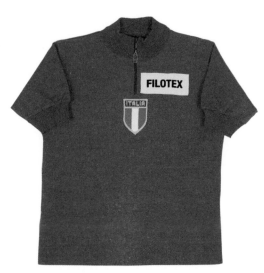

Filotex Italian national team jersey worn at the 1974 World Championships in Montreal

As you develop you start to specialise, and then the races start to choose you. What I mean by that is the management figures out where you're likely to be most effective, and they plan your racing accordingly. There'd have been no point in them sending me to the Tour of the Basque Country, because it was just never going to happen. I went once, in 2010, but it was miserable. I was as much use as Contador on the cobbles at Paris–Roubaix or Cavendish at Lombardy. Even the best cyclists only ever win a tiny fraction of the races they compete in – unless they're called Merckx – so wasting time and energy on the ones where you can't perform isn't a smart move.

At a certain point, if you're both extremely good and politically astute, you might become part of that decision-making process – here we're only talking about the absolute best, essentially the team leaders. The majority have no choice but to do as they're told, because if they don't they'll be out of a job.

So cyclists don't generally have much influence over cycling. To quote a famous current politician, they're generally rule-takers, not rule-makers. The calendar is fixed by sports administrators around a few cardinal points, and the races don't generally alter much. In order to get funding they have to do what they say on the tin, so Milan–San Remo has to go from Milan to San Remo, Paris–Nice from Paris to Nice. The Tour of Flanders is a cultural and political event as much as a sporting one. It's a

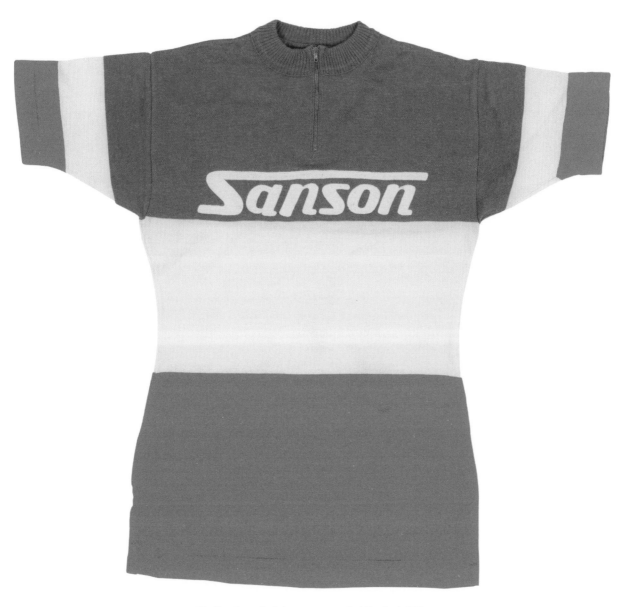

1976 Italian champion's jersey – as seen in *A Sunday in Hell*

promotional vehicle for, well, *Flanders*, and its job is to show the place at its best. The Tour de France is a tour of France and . . . OK, you get the picture.

Cycling and politics always were – and always will be – indivisible. The cyclists themselves are important, but not *that* important. They get sent from race to race, and the vast majority don't have a hope in hell of winning any of them. The public wants to see the big stars, but even they come and go. When all's said and done they're pawns in a much bigger game, and in the big picture they're mainly decorative. Aren't they?

Francesco Moser was the youngest of four cycling brothers, an authentic bike-racing dynasty. The oldest of them, Aldo, rode the Giro 16 times and carried on until he was 40. Enzo, the second brother, wore the *maglia rosa* at the Giro, and later became a very successful sporting director. Diego was next, but Francesco was something else entirely. He was easily the most charismatic, easily the most popular and easily the best.

He turned pro in 1973 and the following year he won 18 races. He was handsome, uncomplicated and likeable, and you didn't need to be a rocket scientist to understand then he was going to be a major star. He was a man's man, and the Italians quickly deduced that he was the great national hope for the post-Merckx era. That was all well and good because he was immensely strong, but he was too big and too heavy to compete with the natural climbers. He knew it, and he also knew that because of it the Giro d'Italia was going to be a big, big problem. Given that the Giro was *the* bike race in Italy, he needed to find a solution. He needed to find a way to bend it to his strengths and to his will, because otherwise it would cost him.

Vincenzo Torriani was the boss of the Giro. He'd been running it since the war, and he was both an institution and a cultural icon. Torriani was one of the most famous people in Italy, and in a sporting context one of the most powerful. He wasn't actually much bothered about the racers themselves, because as he saw it most of them were interchangeable. They were merely the orchestra; he was the conductor.

Now I can confirm – because I've hauled myself through the Giro – that Italy is a very mountainous country. In the south you have the great plateau of the Sila, with the Apennines forming the 'spine' that runs up the country. These two were a big part of the performance, but the grand finale always came in the much higher Alps and/or Dolomites, the great theatres of the race, which Torriani understood were intrinsic to the show.

By 1975 Merckx had won the Giro five times, but he was coming towards the end of his career and his monopoly had started to become tedious. Torriani realised that he had to be replaced by a new star, ideally an Italian. Merckx had been untouchable, but in general terms foreign winners were really, really bad for business. Given Moser's limitations in the mountains, the climbers Gianbattista Baronchelli and Giovanni Battaglin seemed the men most likely. If they could mount a decent challenge, then

Francesco's brother Aldo in the snow on the Stelvio Pass. The unremitting steepness of the Dolomites meant that Francesco Moser always played second fiddle to the climbers on mountain stages.

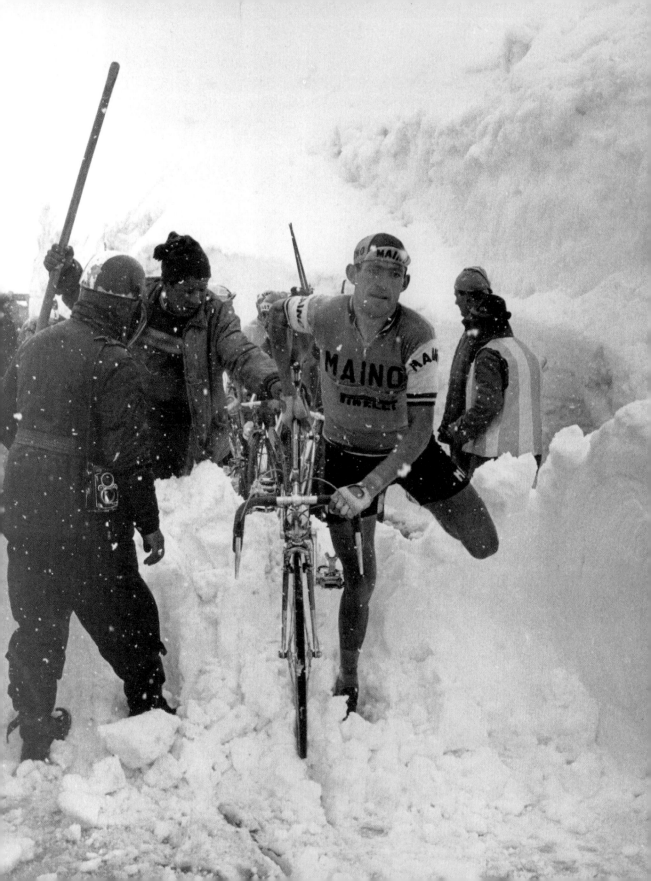

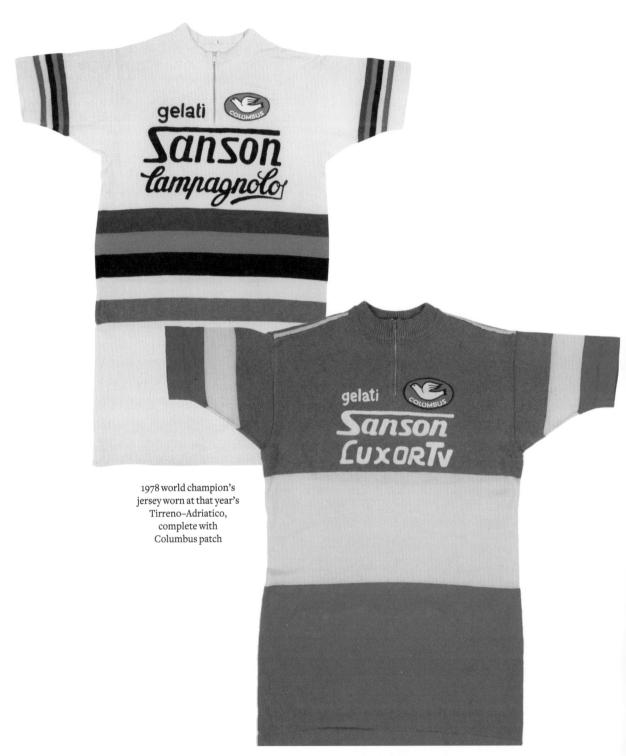

1978 world champion's
jersey worn at that year's
Tirreno–Adriatico,
complete with
Columbus patch

1980 Italian champion's jersey

the *Gazzetta dello Sport*, the race organiser, would sell more newspapers, and state broadcaster RAI would increase its viewing figures and ultimately its coverage. With that in mind, Torriani created a mountainous Giro and announced that it would finish 2,700 metres above sea level at the top of the Stelvio Pass. He was gambling on the Dolomite weather holding up, and on either Baronchelli or Battaglin exploiting it to dethrone – or at the very least unsettle – the great man.

Now Torriani was a brilliant race director, but the *percorso* amounted to a kick in the teeth for Francesco Moser. Baronchelli and Battaglin were his immediate rivals, and as he saw it Torriani had sided with them and not him. He therefore did something incredible and truly, truly outrageous. He announced, at the age of 23, that he would be boycotting the greatest sporting institution in the country. He said he'd be riding the Tour de France instead, because Torriani's route amounted to a betrayal of Italian cycling. Bloody hell.

It was a huge strategic gamble, but part one worked brilliantly. Merckx fell ill and didn't ride the Giro, and both Baronchelli and Battaglin failed badly. An unknown *gregario* named Fausto Bertoglio came through to win the thing, and that was unsatisfactory for everyone.

Everyone, that is, except for Francesco Moser.

Part two, the Tour, was much harder. Italians had been failing there for years, but if Moser could deliver he'd have the public on his side. That would force Torriani into a rethink, and into engineering the Giro around his strengths. In the prologue he went up against Merckx, and beat him by two seconds. He took the yellow jersey, kept it for a week, won another stage, and finished up in the white jersey. More importantly, his popularity grew with each passing day, because he was the opposite of Baronchelli and Battaglin. They were both shy and withdrawn – proper old-school climbers – but he was open and engaging. By the time he got home it was mission accomplished, and by the end of the season he had the *maglia tricolore* of the Italian champion and the Tour of Lombardy. His popularity was limitless, and so Torriani was left with no choice but to build the Giro with him in mind. A Giro without Moser was no Giro at all, and everyone – journalists, fans, advertisers, sponsors – understood the value of his being centre stage. The race became flatter with each passing year, because Torriani daren't risk his defecting to the Tour again.

Moser didn't win the *A Sunday in Hell* Paris–Roubaix, but between 1978 and 1980 he would become the only rider in history to win a hat-trick of them. He also won the 1977 World Championships and, having deposed Baronchelli and Battaglin, developed a ferocious rivalry with Giuseppe 'Beppe' Saronni. It was even more spiteful than Coppi and Bartali, and the *tifosi* couldn't get enough of it. Cycling had been losing popularity

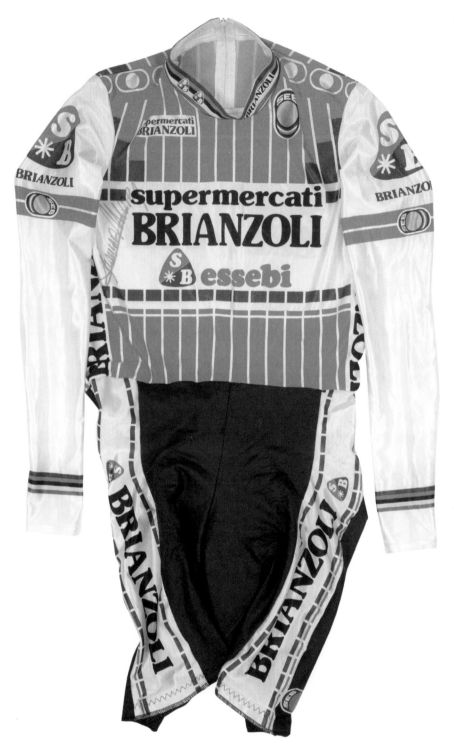

Moser's Hour Record skinsuit from his failed record
attempt in 1986 at the Vigorelli Velodromo (*opposite*)

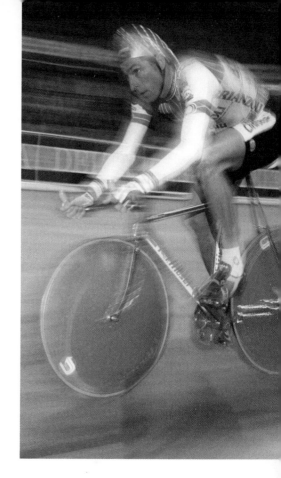

for over 20 years, but these two had the fans and the sponsors flooding back. They were great riders, but more importantly they were skilled politicians and great showmen. Saronni was faster and cleverer, but Moser was stronger and more popular. Over his career he would win a mind-boggling 273 professional races, but his genius lay in the fact that he determined the trajectory of an entire cycling movement. Moser was known as 'The Sheriff', because in Italian cycling nothing and nobody moved without his say so.

Not content with dominating at home, Moser would later turn the whole sport on its head. Bernard Hinault was a much better stage racer than him, and so was Saronni. By 1983 both Hinault and Saronni had each won the Giro twice, and Moser still hadn't accomplished it. Torriani had reconfigured it around him, but Italy is Italy. It's mountainous, and so Moser had to make do with stage wins and the points jersey. No other cyclist has ever been more inventive, however, and Moser had an idea up his sleeve.

Saronni had dominated the 1983 season. He was six years younger than Moser, and the rivalry seemed to have run its course. Most considered Moser to be past his best, but he'd started to figure out the correlation between science and performance. In preparing for an attempt at the Hour Record he engaged an elite group of doctors, scientists, technicians and aerodynamicists led by Francesco Conconi. They developed tests for threshold power output and assembled the most efficient aerodynamic bike ever built. It was a genuine revolution in the way cyclists thought, trained and prepared, and in January 1984 Moser travelled to Mexico and smashed Merckx's record out of sight. This was Moser's second coming. Or, to put it another way, the coming of a new and completely different Moser, and a completely different way of thinking about cycling.

That June Moser finally won the Giro, and Italy went nuts.

Ten years on from Mexico, Moser would come out of retirement for another attempt at the Hour Record. He'd ride a kilometre further aged 42 than he had at 32, which demonstrates the sheer speed of the changes he brought about. He had the best technology and the best preparation, and by now science and sport were operating in tandem as never before. It was an incredible ride, but then Francesco Moser was one incredible human being.

It could be argued that others have been better, and certainly they've been more complete. That's as maybe, but none – Coppi and Merckx included – have ever been as influential.

Francesco Moser was a cycling colossus.

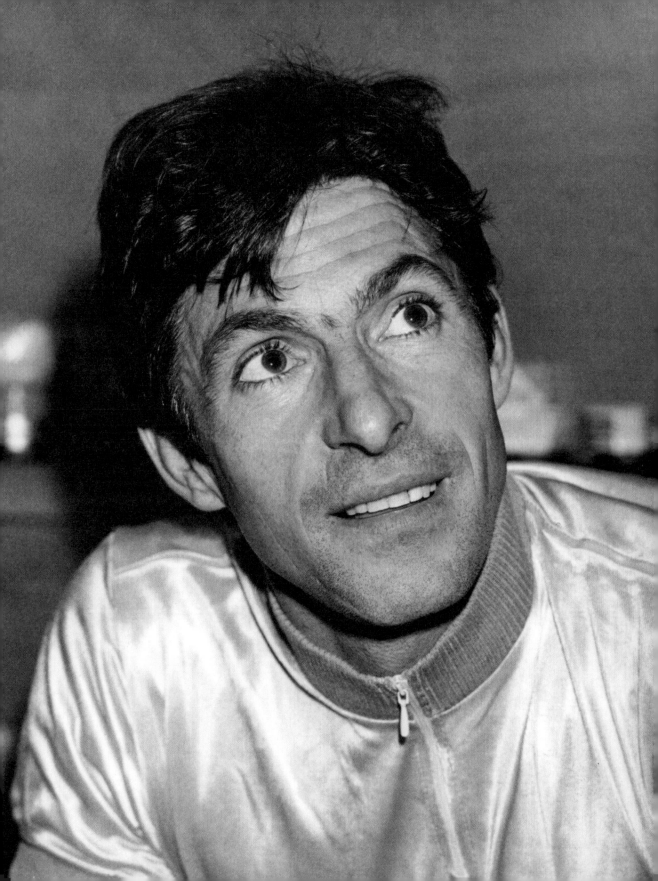

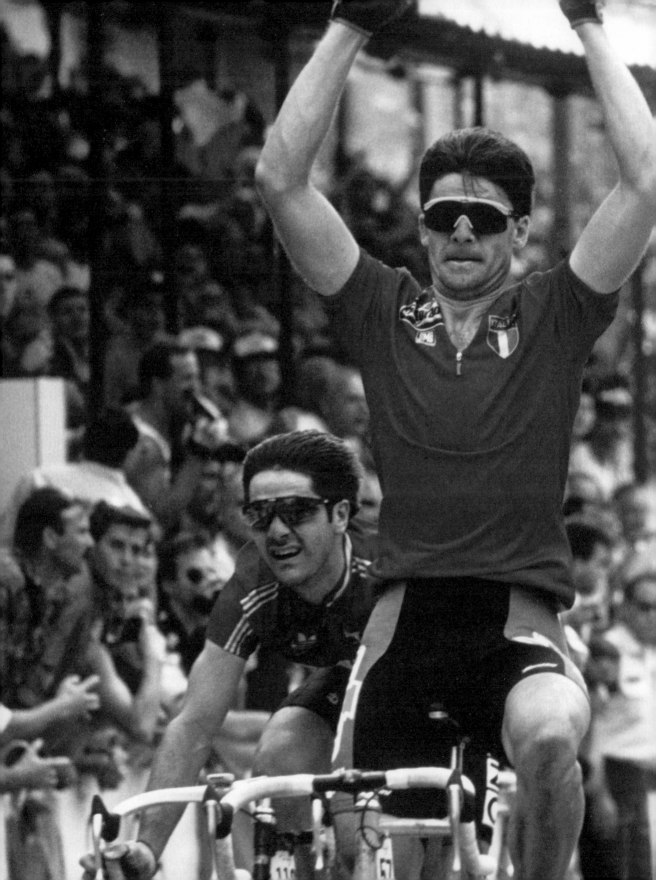

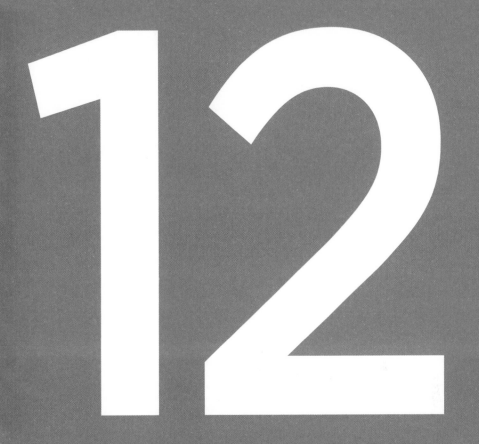

12

Gianni Bugno

1964–

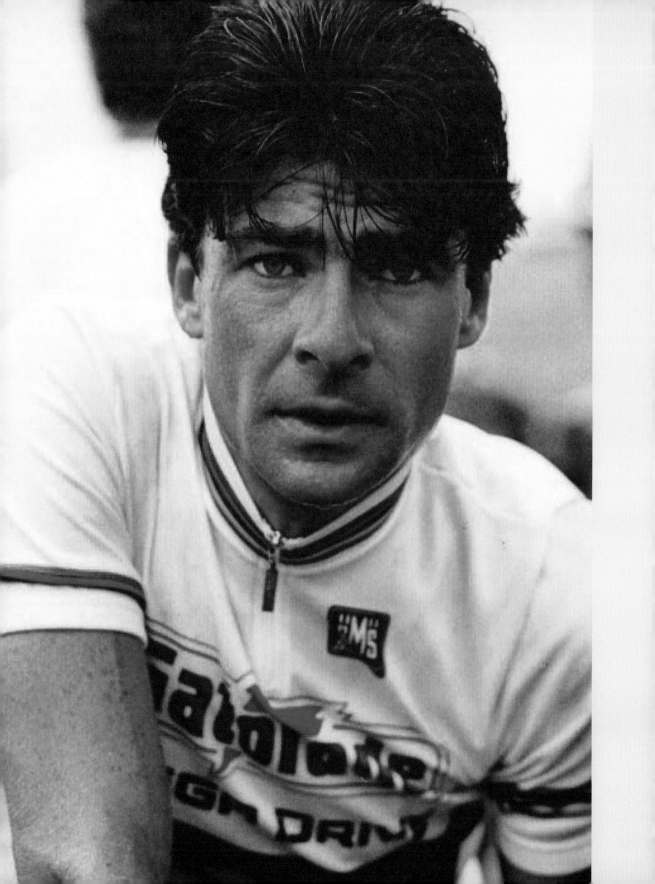

Open YouTube and watch the 1992 World Championships Road Race. It's in Benidorm, and there's a group of about 15 guys coming to the finish together. In it you have people like Induráin, Rominger, Luc Leblanc and Steven Rooks. It's the cream of world cycling, because the merely very good have long since been dropped. The reason is that at 260 kilometres the course is long and hard, they've been up and down for six and a half hours, and it's as hot as hell. At times like that it can feel like you're riding in a kiln.

Among them you have three overwhelming favourites. The first is Laurent Jalabert, the Tour de France green jersey. He's one of the classiest bike riders on earth, and he's lightning fast. The others are a very talented Russian named Dmitri Konyshev, and Gianni Bugno, the reigning world champion. It's a slight drag up to the finish, but objectively one of these three is probably going to win because on paper they're the best sprinters.

Given that it's hot, it's uphill and they're exhausted, the finale seems to take place almost in slow motion. As a bike rider you know how it feels to be scraped out, so it's quite a tough watch. They get out of the saddle and, as best they can, attempt to summon something resembling a sprint. Some of them sit up straight away, because they know they can't get a medal and their tanks are completely empty. Others keep flailing away at it, but in reality they're just grovelling – they look like they're riding through quicksand. A couple actually produce a passable impression of a sprint, but one seems not to be sprinting at all. While the rest seem to be breaking their necks simply to get over the line, he looks like a tourist. His cadence doesn't seem to alter, he doesn't seem to be extending himself, and yet somehow he just seems to float away from them.

Ladies and gentlemen, I give you . . . Gianni Bugno.

A slightly haunted, Italian-handsome rider with jet-black hair, a rainbow jersey and the thousand-yard stare of a troubled genius.

WHEN I STARTED GOING OUT ON CLUB RUNS, talking about the pros was one of the things that helped me feel like I belonged. I probably didn't have that much else in common with some of the others, but with cycling I felt I could speak to them on equal terms. As an adolescent finding your way, these things can be important because you're looking for your place. I see it in my own kids, this search for identity, and that's one of the reasons I couldn't not have Gianni Bugno in this book. There was nobody even remotely like him, and I was in awe of him as a bike rider. He was astonishing, but he was also the first sportsman that really fascinated me as a human being. I spent a lot of time pretending to be him on the bike, but also imagining what it must have been like to be him off it.

Bugno was just this beautiful, beautiful bike rider. Everything he did was immaculate, graceful and, to my teenage mind, quintessentially Italian. If the others wore helmets or caps, he didn't – he had perfect jet-black hair instead. When the others looked knackered, he looked totally fresh in his cool, black Bollé sunglasses. While they grimaced with the pain, he just looked smooth. When they got out of the saddle because the gradient steepened, he stayed sitting down. If the others were crouched down to ride on the drops, he'd be leaning nonchalantly on the tops. While they huffed and puffed and hauled themselves over the steepest climbs, he seemed just to glide up them. Where they had lurid, multi-coloured and multi-sponsored jerseys, he had the most sophisticated jersey of all, the rainbow stripes of the world champion.

Had there been a world championships for cool, he'd have won that as well. By a country mile.

There are two other famous Gianni Bugno sprints, and they're essentially the same. The previous year the Worlds had been in Stuttgart. The race had finished with a four-man sprint, but I always liken it to a bullfight. You had Bugno, the matador, and then Induráin, Rooks and Álvaro Mejía. I've seen it any number of times, and I still find it astounding. Induráin starts to sprint, but Gianni just glides by him. Now Miguel and Rooks are hell for leather. They're absolutely flat out to try to come round him, but he's just soft-tapping to keep them at arm's length. He has time to check over his left shoulder first, and then over his right. Then, as they approach the line, he checks over his left *again* and then, about 15 metres from the finish, he sits up. He claps his hands because he knows he's won, and then just rolls over the finish line.

It's an incredible thing to watch, and still more so because he hasn't ridden away from them. It's not as if he's a pure sprinter and they're a bunch of lightweight climbers, and at no point does he have more than a bike length. By the time he crosses the line he probably has less than a wheel, and he's broken every single rule in the sprinting book. Then again, cyclists as talented as him – if there *are* other cyclists as

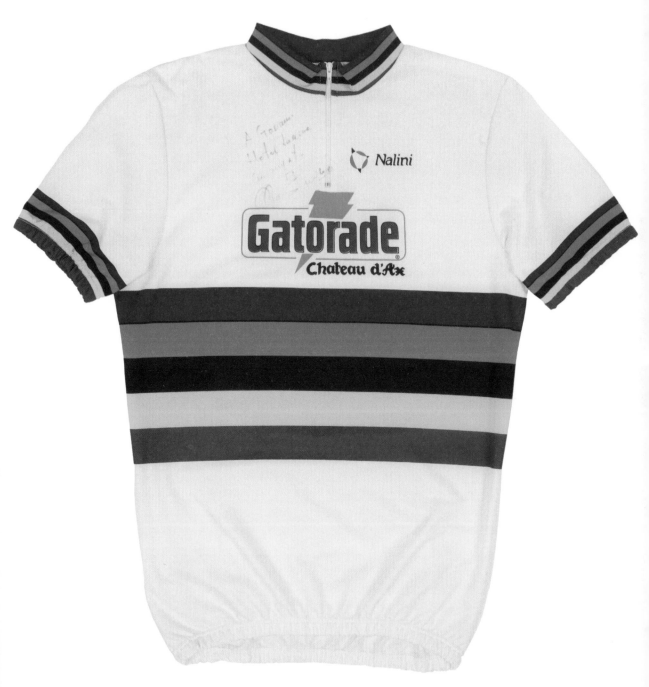

1991 world champion's jersey

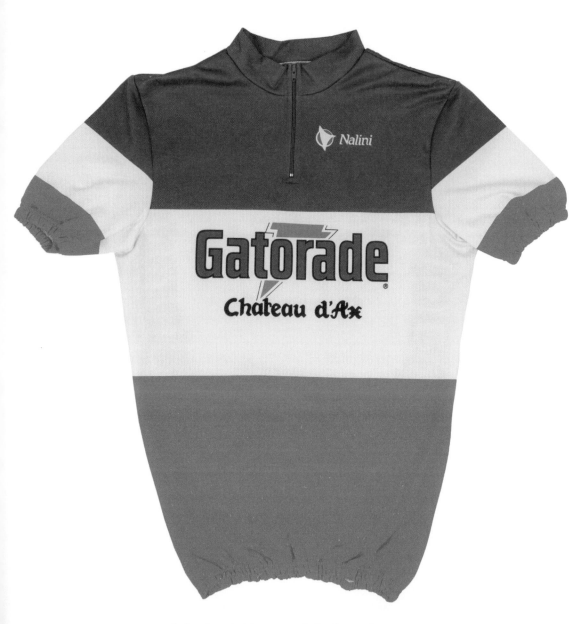

1991 Italian champion's jersey worn during the Tour de France

talented as him – can probably get away with it. Who needs boring old orthodoxy when you have sporting divinity?

The other one is the 1994 Tour of Flanders. Another four-up sprint, the difference being that he's up against Ballerini, Museeuw and Andrei Tchmil. They're northern classics specialists, and between them they account for four editions of Flanders and six of Paris–Roubaix. Bugno, on the other hand, has never really bothered with Flanders. Museeuw is rapier-fast, and yet once more Bugno is able to sit up well before the line. Once more it *seems* a close-run thing, but only because Bugno is doing the bare minimum. In the final analysis you have to conclude that he's in a class of his own.

We've established that Bugno won Flanders, just as he'd won Milan–San Remo, the national championship and consecutive rainbow jerseys. But so what? Tom Boonen won all of the above, Cancellara came close, and sooner or later Peter Sagan will complete the set by winning San Remo. What's more, Sagan has won three Worlds on the spin (and counting) to Bugno's two. Cancellara and Boonen each won Flanders three times, and Gianni only managed it once.

I think we can all agree that Boonen, Cancellara and Sagan are superstars. They're genuine cycling greats, but at this point it's worth asking ourselves a few questions. Is it plausible that Peter Sagan could win a grand tour? Did Boonen or Cancellara ever even contemplate the idea of riding one for GC? Would their physiologies have permitted it?

While we're doing rhetorical questions, here are a few more. What are the chances of Nairo Quintana winning the Tour of Flanders? How many single-day classics (let alone northern classics) did Alberto Contador and Ivan Basso accumulate between them?

By now you're probably asking yourself where this is going, because all of the above are so far-fetched as to appear ridiculous. It's inconceivable that any of the above could happen, so what, precisely, is the point?

The point is that in 1990 Gianni Bugno won the opening stage of the Giro d'Italia. He pulled on the *maglia rosa*, and then kept it for 22 days, all the way back to Milan. To put that into its rightful context, the *maglia rosa* was invented in 1931, and precisely one other person accomplished that feat before or since. His name? Édouard Louis Joseph Merckx.

In 1991 Bugno focused on winning three jerseys: the *tricolore* of the Italian champion, the yellow of the Tour and the rainbow of the Worlds. He won two of them, and came as close as anyone ever would to unseating the mighty Induráin at the Tour. He finished a brilliant second, and would podium again the following year.

We're often told that cycling has changed, that we're in the age of specialisation, that it's pointless to compare riders from different generations. It's a reasonable argument, and it's true that the cycling Bugno practised was completely different to that of Sagan, Froome and Quintana. The methodology has evolved, so has the calendar, and so too the physiology of the riders. That being the case, in order to fully understand Gianni Bugno we need to pose two further questions, and they're perhaps the most pertinent ones of all. Could Induráin, probably the greatest Tour de France rider in history, have ridden the Tour of Flanders with Tchmil and Ballerini? Could Johan Museeuw, the Lion of Flanders, have won the Giro d'Italia? Probably not.

Between 1990 and 1992 Gianni Bugno made winning the biggest bike races look ridiculously easy. Before that, however, he'd frustrated his fans, sporting directors and team-mates for years. They all understood that he was a once-in-a-lifetime talent, but psychologically he could appear fragile at times.

It wasn't until 1990, his sixth season as a professional, that he rode away to win San Remo. Maybe that was when the penny dropped as regards the magnitude of his talent, but I don't think he ever really embraced the pressure and responsibility that came with it. It didn't sit comfortably with him, and that's key to understanding his place in Italian cycling history. His reticence put Italians in mind of their great *campionissimo* Fausto Coppi, the first true superstar of European sport.

Coppi's bike had been his refuge. In 1954 he'd scandalised Catholic Italy by leaving his wife for a married woman, and after that his private life became a public pantomime. He was only truly at peace when he was riding, and many believe that Bugno was the same. Like Coppi he found the winning quite easy, but the consequences of it much, much harder. Nobody was pretending that Bugno was Coppi's equal – Fausto was cycling divinity – but it was impossible not to draw parallels. Like Coppi he was honest, decent and self-effacing, so it's no wonder the Italians worshipped the ground he rode on.

Moser, that other great Italian champion, was a significant part of Bugno's problem. When a character like Moser leaves the scene it always creates a huge void, and for five years no Italian had been able to fill it. It fell upon Bugno, but the two of them were as different as night and day. Where Moser had loved the spotlight, Bugno tolerated it as best he could, but he was never comfortable with it.

He also tolerated Claudio Chiappucci. Two months after Bugno's masterpiece at the Giro, Chiappucci almost won the Tour. That was a godsend for Italian cycling, and thereafter he was promoted as Bugno's great rival. Of course, rivalry is the heart and soul of professional sport, and the Italian media understood its commercial value. So did Chiappucci, and he stoked it for all it was worth. Being Gianni's 'rival' did wonders for his career. Bugno didn't much like it, but he understood it. He was smart enough to recognise that the champion and the journalist are interdependent, and that the rest of the sport relies on that relationship in order to function. The journalists need copy, because that is what, figuratively speaking, puts bums on seats for the sponsors.

At the 1991 Tour de France, where he finished second to Miguel Induráin, his best placing in the race.

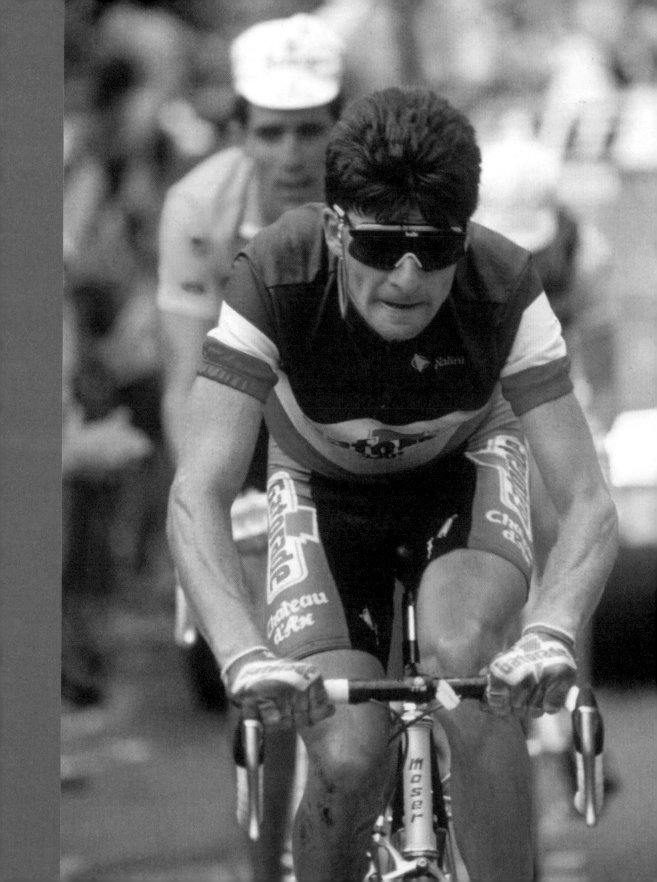

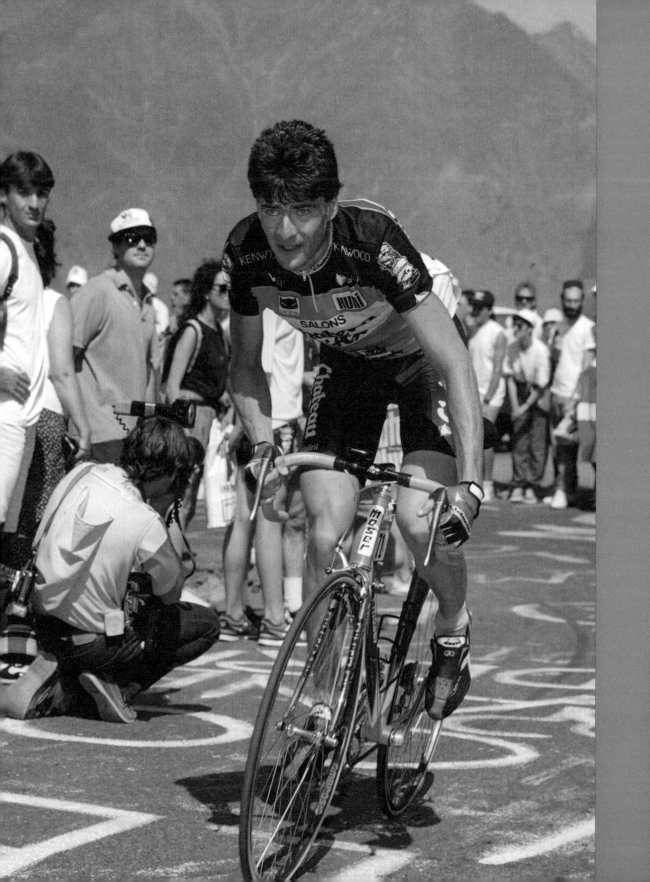

I know all about that, and I also know what it feels like when you no longer have control over it. By and large many people just believe what they read, and when they come after you you're essentially powerless. If you're good at sport you get fame and fortune, but it's swings and roundabouts. The fame is ephemeral, and there's a price to pay for it. The more famous you are, the higher that price is, and so it rolls on.

Bugno won Flanders in 1994 and afterwards he won sporadically, but he was past his prime and Italy had a new star in Marco Pantani. I remember one of the wins very clearly, a stage at the 1996 Vuelta, which I think illustrates his character perfectly. He broke away to win, but as he crossed the line he didn't even lift his hands from the bars. At the time I thought he just looked impossibly cool, like it wasn't worth celebrating because he was a great champion and it was 'just' a stage at the Vuelta. In reality, though, he wouldn't have wanted to appear ostentatious or arrogant. It was as if he'd been condemned to win, but he was trying to avoid drawing more attention to himself than was absolutely necessary.

By then I was riding with guys like Yanto Barker and Charly Wegelius, the best of the British juniors, and I remember discovering that he was their favourite rider as well. In fact, one of my abiding memories of Bugno is from that time, a stage of the 1997 Tour de Langkawi in Malaysia. Obviously he'd been a great champion, but he was at the end of his career and it was a nothing sort of a race for a guy like him. However, on this particular stage he got in a break with the Englishman John Tanner and a young Malaysian rider.

Now John Tanner was a seriously good bike rider, and Bugno was still just about Bugno. They rode bit-and-bit, but as they got towards the finish the Malaysian kid, for whom it was a *really* big race, started to struggle. He started to yo-yo, but Bugno waited for him and kept trying to push him back on. In the end the kid just couldn't do it anymore, and they had no choice but to leave him as they would have been caught otherwise. Bugno beat Tanner in the sprint, but I bet the Malaysian kid will never forget the day he was in a break with Gianni Bugno. It was beautiful.

All of which leaves two final questions. How do we assess Bugno historically, and will we ever see his like again?

When British people think about cycling in the early 1990s we tend to think of Induráin. The only cycling on terrestrial TV was the Tour, we all tuned into it and he dominated it. Although Gianni ran him fairly close in 1991, it's undeniable that Miguel was much the better stage racer. However, there's much more to cycling than the Tour de France, and while Miguel was universally admired, outside of Spain he never *really* enthused the fans. He never had Bugno's star quality, nor, truth be told, his finesse. Where Miguel was reliable and serene, Gianni was ethereal and fragile. Of

Racing in the mountains for Chateau d'Ax. Bugno pipped Greg LeMond to the line on Stage 11 of the 1990 Tour de France at the Alpe d'Huez for the team.

course, that only added to the mystique around him, but between 1990 and 1992 he was truly sublime.

I'm struggling to think of a natural successor, and someone like Laurent Jalabert would probably be the closest. Like Bugno he looked fantastic on the bike, and in 1995 he won a grand tour himself, the Vuelta. Jalabert never won Flanders, San Remo or the Worlds though. The late Frank Vandenbroucke probably had the God-given talent, but tragically he never made it.

Of the current riders, someone like Geraint Thomas springs to mind. G has a huge engine, and there's nothing he's not really good at. Michał Kwiatkowski would be another one, but that sort of tells its own story. Kwiatko is an insanely talented cyclist, but I'm not sure he's Bugno-talented. And we know about G now!

At the risk of stating the blindingly obvious, this book and this collection are a love letter to cycling. More specifically they're a love letter to *cyclists*, those who helped to form my own career. At the risk of appearing conceited, everything I ever tried to do as a cyclist was rooted in the history of the sport, because I've been totally immersed in it since I was 12 years old. That immersion also explains why I commissioned a great artist named Karl Kopinski to paint me three oils. The first is of Eddy being Eddy Merckx, smashing it to bits in his Molteni jersey. The second is of Tom, for obvious reasons.

The third is of a slightly haunted, Italian-handsome rider with jet-black hair, a rainbow jersey and the thousand-yard stare of a troubled genius.

I think it's a masterpiece.

A typically introspective shot of Bugno, taken in 1994.

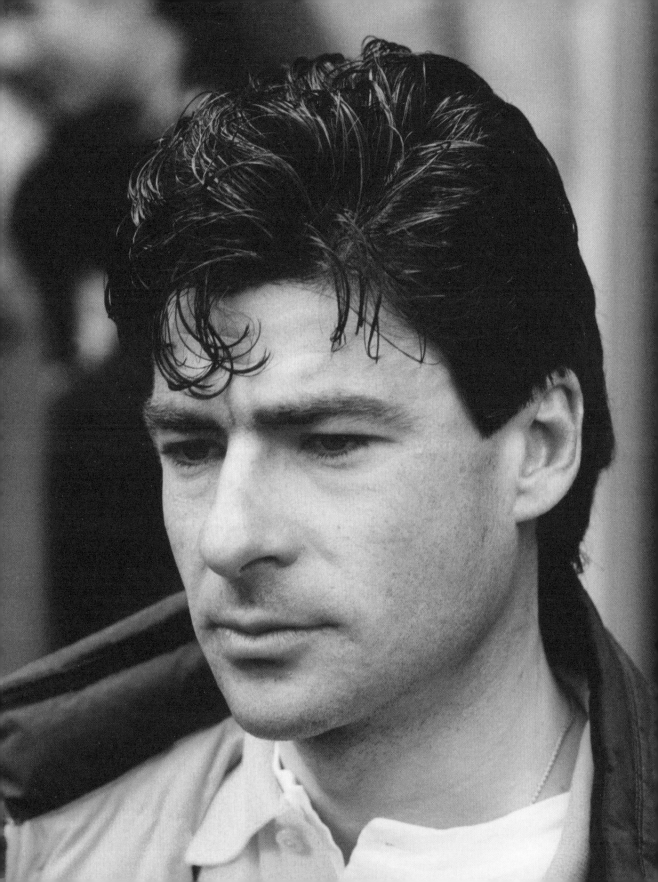

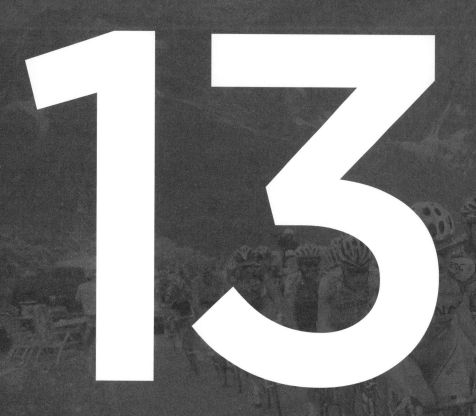

13

Lance Armstrong

1971–

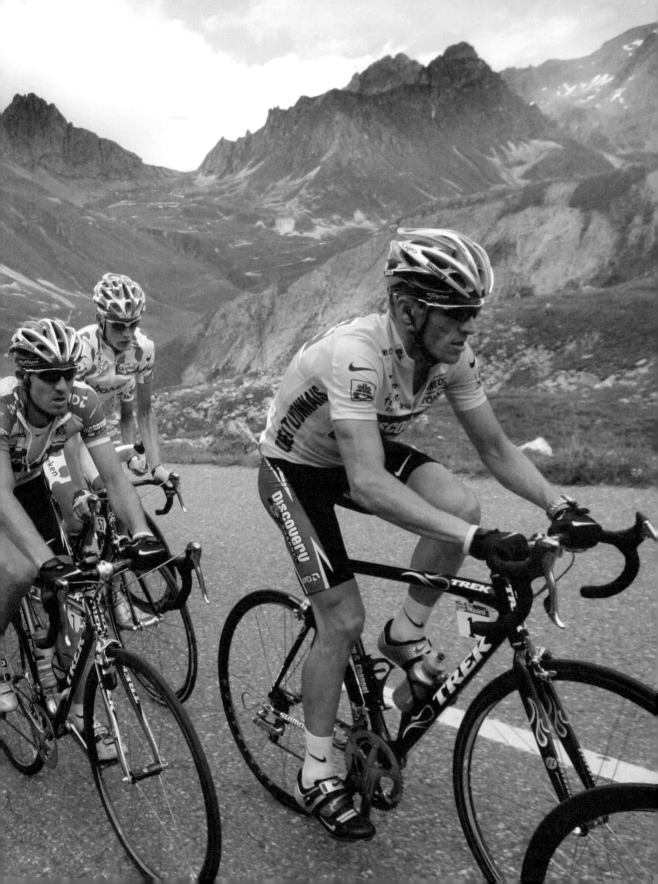

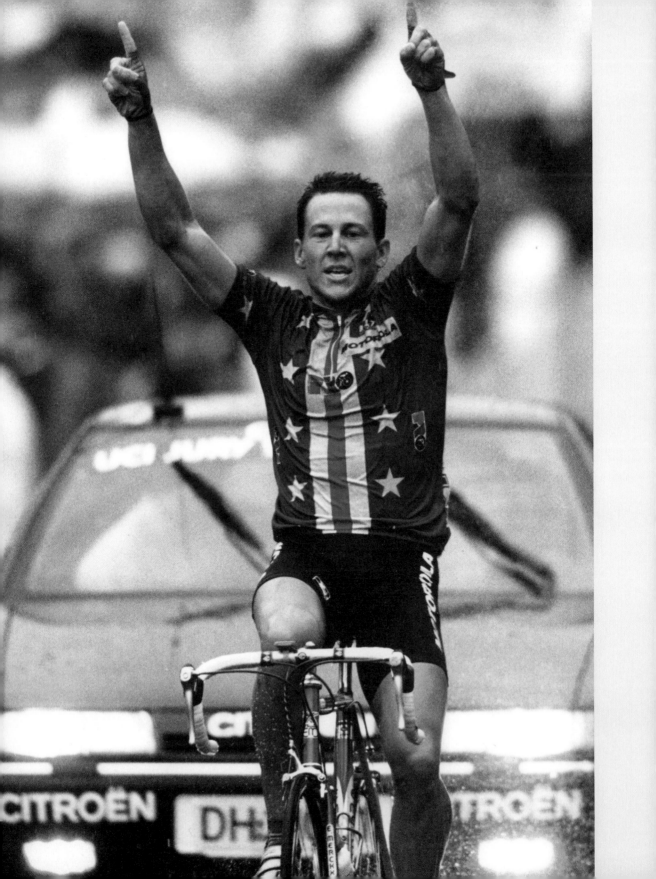

I experienced those Bugno Worlds after the fact. It was in August 1993 that I discovered cycling had World Championships, and that year they took place in Oslo. Eurosport showed the whole race, and Oslo being Oslo it was belting it down with rain. The favourites were the usual suspects, but with two laps to go a Norwegian guy named Dag Otto Lauritzen attacked off the front. The fans went berserk and old Duffers, the commentator, could barely contain himself at this point. Neither could I. In cycling there's nothing more thrilling than those moments when you think it might just stay away, and this was one of them.

They caught Dag Otto, and then this meaty-looking American attacked. I didn't know who he was, but he looked an absolute beast on the bike. In weather like that you're supposed to get yourself warm. You're supposed to get wrapped up in gloves, rain cape, thermal hat, all the gear. You're supposed to try to stay dry, but he didn't bother with

Victorious in the rain at the 1993 World Road Race Championships in Oslo.

all that European cycling stuff. He just had this mad stars and stripes jersey on. And no matter how hard they tried – and they tried bloody hard – they couldn't reel him in.

I remember racing at Eastway the following week under a deluge, so I guess you know what's coming next. In club cycling, everyone's pretending to be someone else at least some of the time. They might not necessarily let on, but that's the way it is. I had a bit of split-personality issue, because when I was climbing I'd be Bugno or Induráin, and when I was 'sprinting' I fancied myself as Wilfried Nelissen. I can assure you that it was quite a lot to cope with, being the most complete cyclist in the world, but now I had to add a new cycling persona to my repertoire.

His name?

I think you know his name . . .

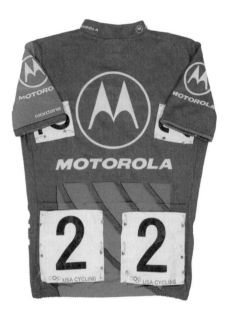

1992 Olympic Trials jersey

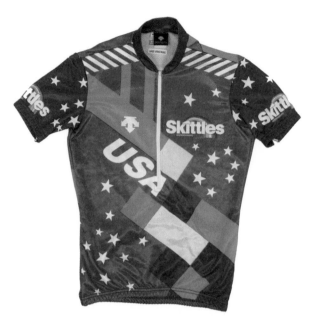

1992 Fitchburg Longsjo Classic US national
team jersey, also worn in the Tour DuPont

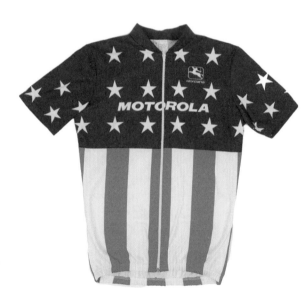

USA amateur national
champion-issued jersey –
extremely rare, only one or
possibly two were made

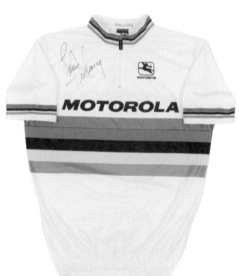

1994 Tour of Flanders,
world champion's jersey

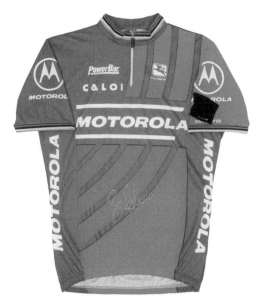

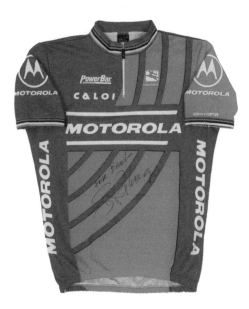

1995 Tour de France jersey, worn in
third week, complete with black patch
pinned on in memory of Fabio Casartelli;
sleeves cut to accommodate his arms

1996 Tour de France Stage 4 jersey

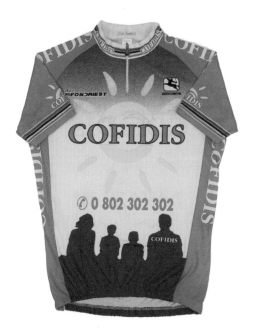

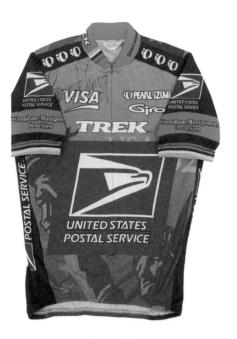

1997 press photoshoot jersey

1998 Vuelta jersey

L OOK AWAY NOW IF YOU'RE EASILY OFFENDED.
I'll never forget the first time I 'met' Lance Armstrong. It was during a bike race (oddly enough), and he came up and rode alongside me. He said, 'How you doin' there, Wiggo?' or words to that effect, and smiled at me. I felt ten feet tall because ... well, because he was Lance Armstrong. Am I allowed to say that, or does it make me some sort of cycling heretic?

During the 2009 Tour, when I was effectively starting my road career in earnest, he was very encouraging. He was losing the physical and psychological war with Contador, and the consequence was that he was scratching about for a podium place with the likes of me. It was a bike race like any other, however, and I didn't have the impression he was trying to shaft me or psyche me out. If anything he probably had me believing I was better than I actually was, but I don't think it was part of some Machiavellian plot to ruin my career and my self-esteem. Maybe I'm deluded, though, and maybe it *was* a Machiavellian plot after all. Maybe I was just too dumb to notice ...

Lance's story has been told *ad infinitum,* but for me one of the most interesting aspects is his transformation from classics rider to post-cancer grand tour rider. It's interesting because, as a young cyclist, you tend to fall into certain ways of riding and of thinking. Sometimes they're suited to your physical attributes, and sometimes they just aren't. Transforming yourself into something else altogether can be difficult but not, by definition, impossible. People who don't understand cycling would like to *pretend* that it's impossible, but it's just a question of power to weight. Prior to winning the 1968 Giro, Merckx was considered a classics rider. He reinvented himself, and so did Beppe Saronni. He was a track rider who went on to win the Giro twice, while Ercole Baldini, Evgeni Berzin and Hugo Koblet were time triallists/pursuiters. They all evolved into grand tour winners, and so did I. Obviously, Lance was stripped of his Tours, and everyone has an opinion on that. What's fascinating to me is that seven Tours de France equals about 160 days of it not going wrong, in addition to all the weeks and months preceding the race. During the race you can get caught behind a crash, have a really bad day, have a mechanical failure when it's on, get blown out the back when a gap opens, make a tactical error, anything. Then you've your opponents to deal with, in Lance's case Ullrich, Pantani, Zülle, Heras, Basso and Beloki.

Whether you like cycling or not, Lance is fascinating as a 21st-century cultural and social phenomenon. There are any number of books analysing his career, the corporate interests behind it and the context in which it took place. It's unbelievable in the most literal sense, but it's also interesting as regards the way cycling defines itself as a sport. Legend has it that Henri Desgrange, the 'Father of the Tour', envisaged a 'perfect winner'. He was of the idea that the ideal Tour de France would have one

Sergio Paulinho leading Armstrong and race leader Alberto Contador in the *maillot jaune* up the Col du Petit-Saint-Bernard, Stage 16 of the 2009 Tour de France. I'm riding for Garmin-Slipstream, just behind Contador.

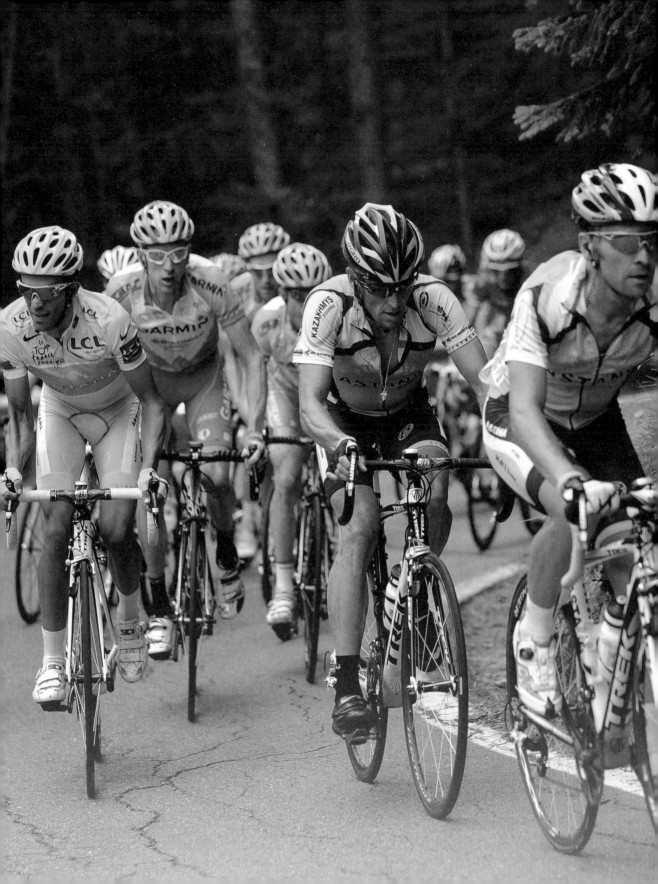

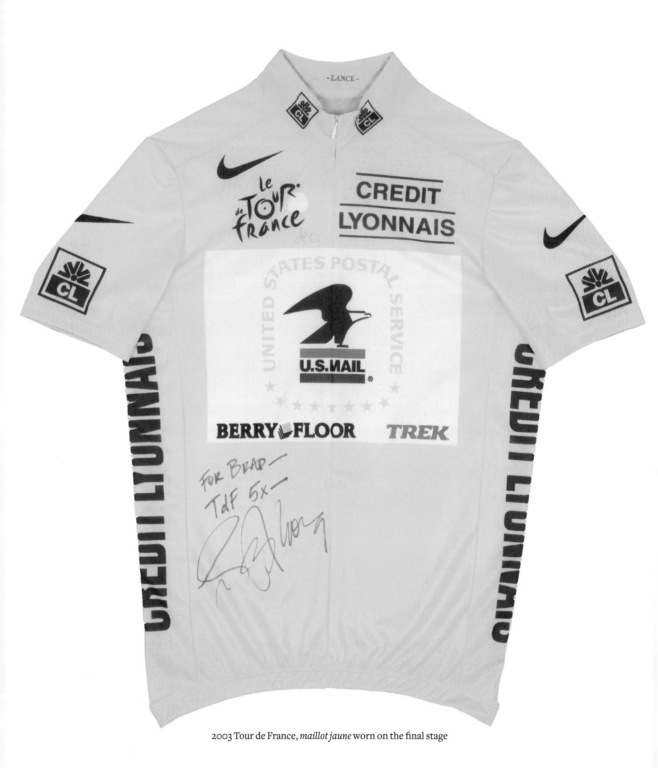

2003 Tour de France, *maillot jaune* worn on the final stage

finisher, a type of super-athlete who would not only defeat his opponents, but also whatever nature might throw at him. It was an extreme version of cycling, and a very French one. It also explains why Tour de France winners tended to be masochistic, obsessive and, on occasion, borderline sociopathic.

The Italians – and by extension the Giro – always preferred shorter, faster races. For them cycling was about stealth as well as strength, intelligence as well as speed. Tactics and cunning were important, because they viewed sport as an extension of 'normal' life. Cycling was hard, but then so was life in a poor country like theirs. To prosper you needed to be clever, so the riders often took shortcuts, both literally and metaphorically. That was to be expected because they were ordinary, working-class, home-spun blokes. They were human beings who had undertaken to do extraordinary things, and they needed all the help they could get.

When they rode the Giro they became ambassadors for their village or province. They set off with their bikes, rode around the peninsula and came home with amazing stories about the things they'd experienced – the great cities, the different people and dialects, the strange food they'd eaten, the scenery they'd witnessed and so on. The organisers liked the stages to finish in bunch sprints, because that way they sold tickets for the stadiums and velodromes. They saw the riders as 'personalities' and promoted them as performers in a great travelling circus.

The French weren't much interested in cycling as *spettacolo*, and their perception of it was fundamentally different. They felt no particular need to cultivate the riders as personalities, because the mere fact that they were riding the Tour did that. The stages were biblical, so it went without saying that they were super-human. With little or no public transport, your average Frenchman wouldn't and couldn't *conceive* of travelling 400 kilometres, let alone riding that distance on a pushbike. In 1928 the Tour was 5,400 kilometres, the Giro 3,000 kilometres. Only one in four of the Tour starters made it round, but more than half completed the Giro.

The point is that the Tour de France was always an extreme sporting event, and it was always contested by extreme human beings. They were extraordinary *by definition*, and people like Gustave Garrigou and Henri Pélissier, the winners in 1911 and 1923 respectively, were cases in point. The peloton was full of madmen, and they were probably the maddest of all.

Over the decades the racing has evolved more or less in line with society. The stages are much shorter and more human, but as a consequence the racing is much, much faster. Things like nutrition, training and machinery are virtually unrecognisable from how they used to be, and in truth the modern Giro is probably harder than the Tour. I think the basic premise is unaltered, though, because the Tour remains the

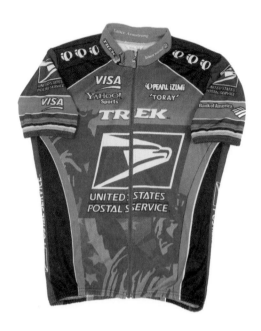

1999 Amstel Gold Race jersey

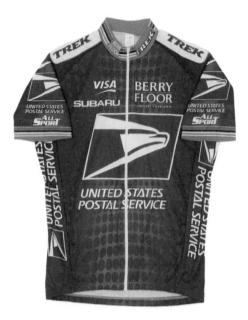

2003 Tour de France Stage 7 jersey

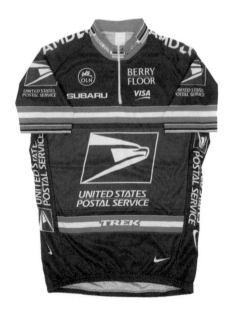

2004 press ride jersey

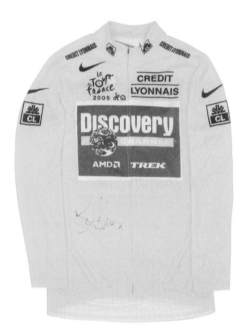

2005 Tour de France Stage 5 podium jersey

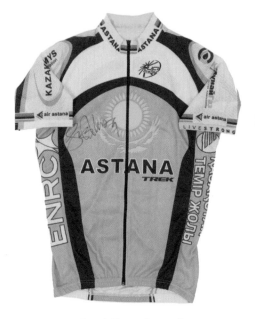

2009 Tour de France Stage 17 jersey

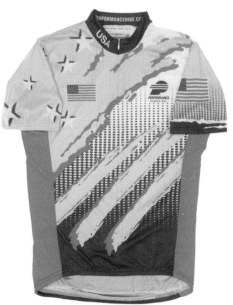

2000 Sydney Olympics road race jersey

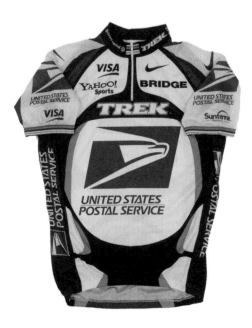

2000 Tour de France Stage 10 jersey

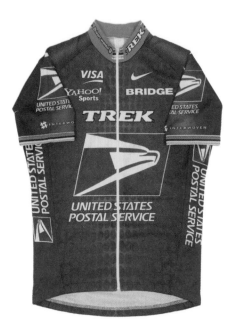

2001 Tour de Suisse jersey

pinnacle of cycling achievement. As regards prestige and global reach it's still way, way ahead of the Giro and the Vuelta, and always will be. Its public is bigger because it takes place during the summer holidays, France is much richer than Italy or Spain, commercially it's a juggernaut and it has cultivated its legends extremely well. It's won, almost without exception, by the best stage racer in the world, and he is always a very special, very driven human being.

Therein, I think, lies the paradox of Lance's having been stripped. His opponents didn't necessarily like him, but guys like Ullrich, Pantani and Michael Rasmussen sure as hell *respected* him. He was the archetypal Tour de France cyclist, and he was *precisely* the sort of winner Desgrange had in mind 120 years ago.

I can't say that I really know Jan Ullrich, Lance's great rival. I do know, however, that he was one incredibly gifted athlete and that he won the 1997 Tour at the age of 23. Everyone in cycling was convinced he'd go on to win a load more of them, because there was nothing he couldn't do on a bike. He was immense, and he inspired awe among fellow riders and fans alike.

Lance would tell anybody prepared to listen that Jan was much more talented, and he was probably right. He respected Ullrich and feared Ullrich, and that fear was a big part of his make-up. Winning the Tour (or not losing it) was existential for him, and most seem to agree that the need to win mutated into a sort of siege mentality. I think Bill Shankly said something like, 'Football isn't a matter of life and death – it's more important than that,' and for Lance cycling was probably the same.

I don't think Lance is a football fan, and my guess would be that he's not familiar with Shankly's 'life and death' quote. Regardless, in his case it seems entirely appropriate.

What was it Sir Alex Ferguson said?

Cycling. Bloody hell.

Lance on the
podium in 2005.

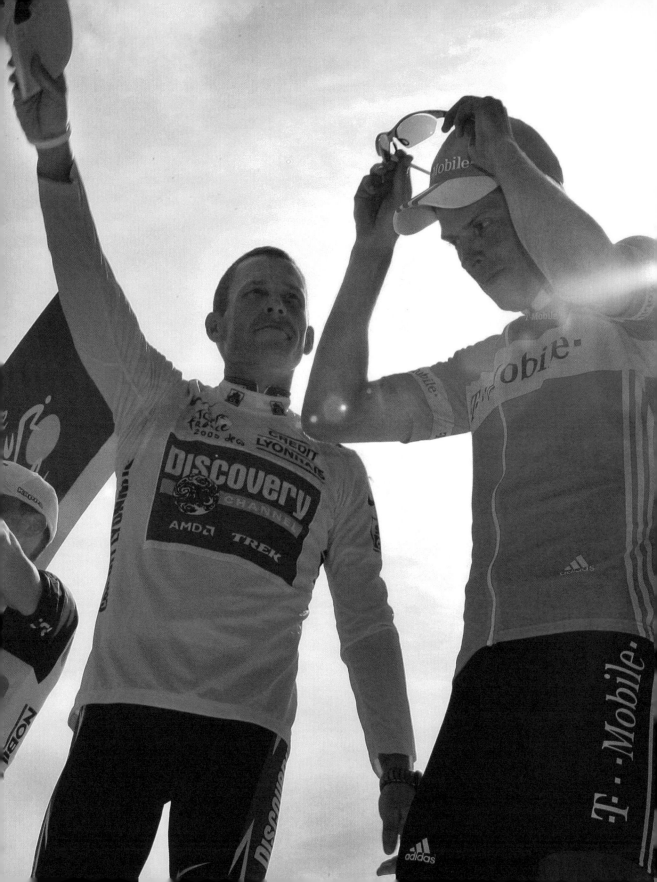

14

Jacques Anquetil

1934–1987

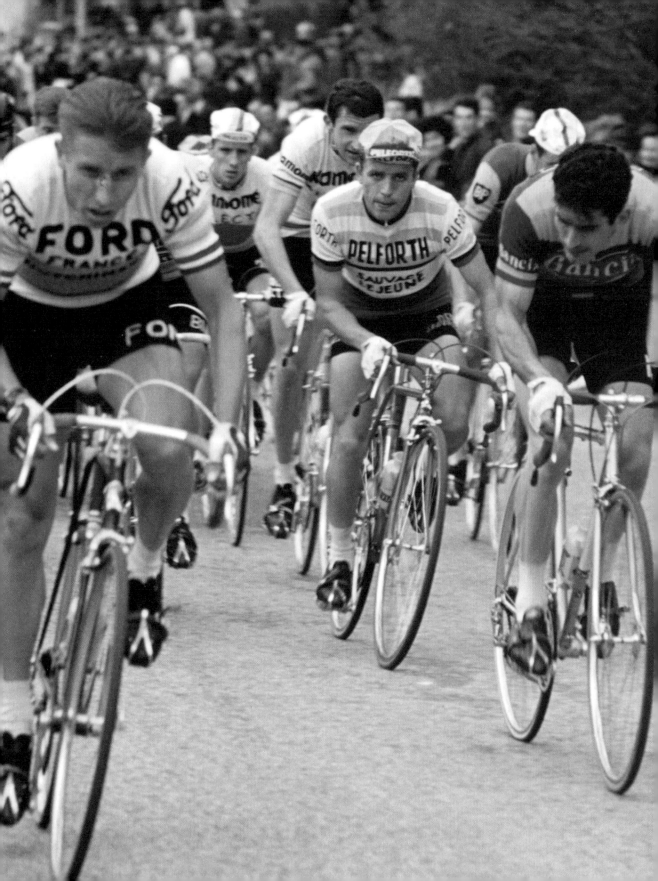

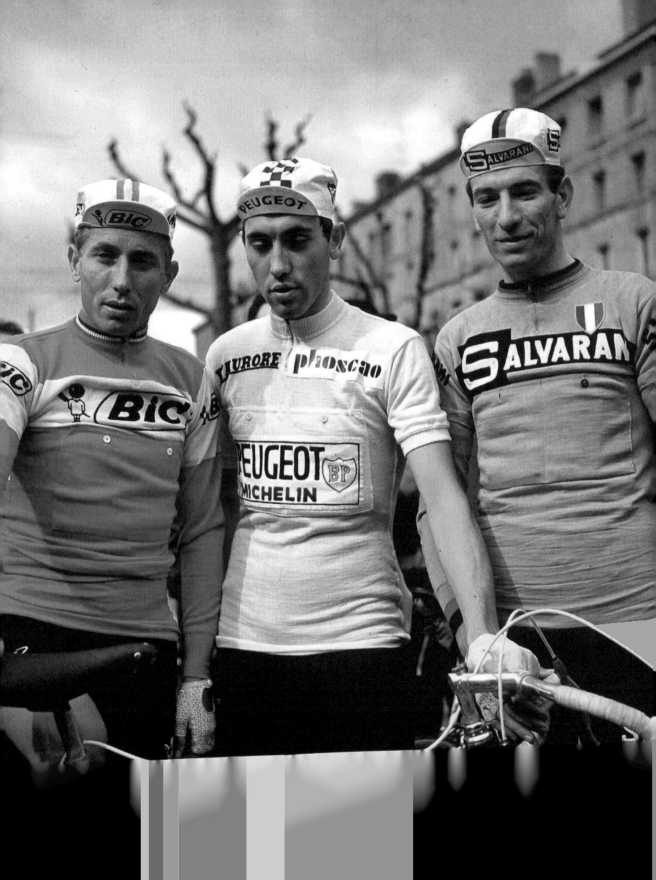

I've always lived cycling 360 degrees, and that's been both a blessing and a burden. A blessing because I developed a reasonable understanding of the sport, its journey and its story, and a burden because that understanding started to condition everything I tried to do.

To the best of my knowledge there's no one in the current peloton who's as dialled in to the history of cycling as I was. Of my generation, Cancellara, Cavendish and Pozzato were to varying degrees, but for the most part riders don't take the time or trouble to familiarise themselves with it. That's something I never really understood, because everything they are as riders is a consequence of the history and evolution of cycling. I'm not suggesting my way is necessarily better, but nobody ever needed to *tell* me about what the races meant. Like the true obsessive I am, I'd spent years trying to contextualise them all.

Three Tour de France winners: Anquetil, Merckx and Gimondi, pictured together in 1970.

A prime example would be 2012. Having won Paris–Nice I went and won the Dauphiné, and afterwards someone said, 'You do realise that you've won Paris–Nice and the Dauphiné in the same year?' I said, 'Yes, of course I do, and I also know what it *means* to win Paris–Nice and the Dauphiné in the same year.' Now to certain sectors of the cycling press I'd have come across as a bit of a bighead for saying that, and some of them portrayed me as being full of myself. That's perfectly understandable – and back then I probably *was* a bit full of myself – but I knew that Jacques Anquetil had done it, and that was one of the things that motivated me.

What I wasn't suggesting was that I was as *good* as Anquetil, because I very well understood that I wasn't and could never be. But cycling is all I was and all I lived for, and for a person like me to have something in common with a person like him was just . . . well, crazy.

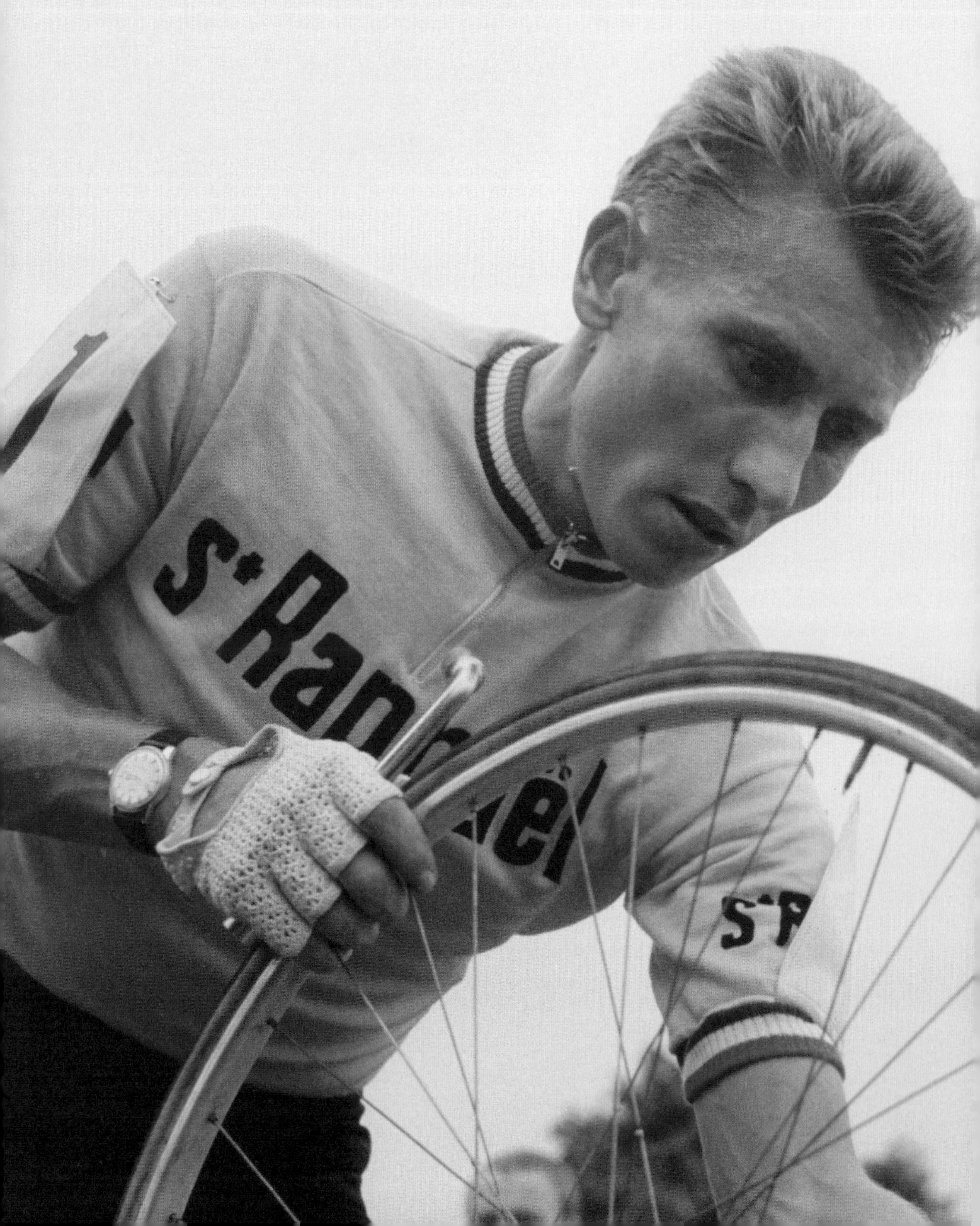
St Rap

WHERE ON EARTH DO YOU START WITH ANQUETIL? If you wrote his story up as a screenplay and took it to a Hollywood producer they'd probably dismiss it as too far-fetched. In that respect he has a lot in common with Fausto Coppi. They were both immensely talented stage racers, they were both capable of superhuman feats and they both had very complex relationships with the media. That was partly because they had very complex relationships with women and with social convention. But there's much more to them than that.

Anquetil's five Tour wins – and his rivalry with Raymond Poulidor – are one of the abiding images not only of 1960s cycling, but of 1960s France *itself*. The Tour is a celebration of French identity and French customs, and Anquetil and Poulidor embodied all of that. Anquetil was perceived as northern and Norman, detached and rational, Poulidor of the people and of the *France profonde*. In reality, Jacques was much more popular in the peloton, where it actually mattered.

The Anquetil–Poulidor saga finished, symbolically as well as practically, the day Tom Simpson died on Mont Ventoux. It was a line in the sand, the end of cycling's 'age of innocence', and a full-stop to French cycling's greatest era. By then Jacques was in his mid-thirties, Merckx was starting to dominate and the Pandora's box of doping had been flung wide open. In May '68 Paris burned, and a completely different kind of society began to emerge.

Preparing his bike for a meet at Herne Hill, 13 June 1964.

We measure the great champions in all sorts of ways. The first is obviously statistical – what they win. Then you've got to factor in who they beat, how they did it and how long they did it *for*. That lot, along with their personalities and the moment in time, informs the impact they have both on the public and on the sport as a whole. There are loads of Tour de France winners who, for one reason or another, never really captured the imagination of the wider public. They may have won on the road, but they never crossed over into the mainstream of public consciousness.

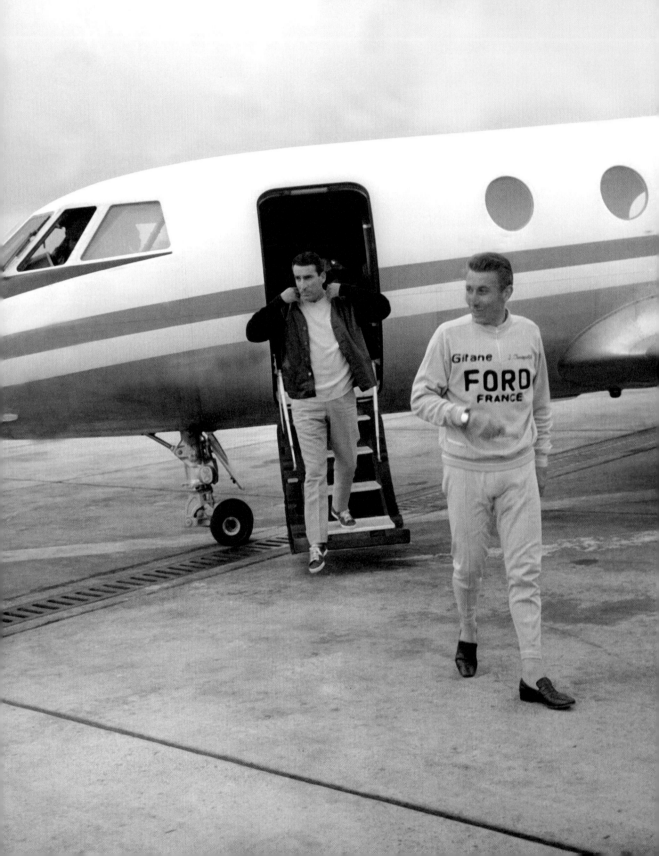

Roger Pingeon is a case in point. He won the 1967 Tour brilliantly, but events conspired against him. The French were used to winning, Pingeon wasn't particularly high profile, and Simpson's death overshadowed everything. He never won again, and as a consequence very few people remember just what a classy rider he was. On the other hand, 'one-hit wonders' like Jan Janssen, Jan Ullrich and me became household names. That was mainly because we were the first from our respective countries to win, and cycling back home enjoyed a huge boom as a result of our wins. The three of us also became tabloid commodities, but that's another matter entirely . . .

Jacques Anquetil ticks all the boxes we know about, and a load we probably don't. Was he charismatic? Check. Were both his public and private lives controversial? Check. Did he have a caustic rivalry? Check. Were his achievements ground-breaking? Check. Did he revolutionise the sport? Check. Did all of the above enrapture and infuriate the fans in equal measure? Check. Did his retirement create a void? Check. Has his legacy endured? Check.

When I started out in France, Marc Madiot told us about his time riding under Jacques for the French national team. One of the things I most remember was him trying to explain the sheer presence of the man. Madiot said everywhere they went people would just stop and gawp. He said that regardless of whether they knew much about cycling, they knew who he was and what he represented. He said they'd just stand, open-mouthed and awestruck, and I can well believe that.

The imagery you see of him on the bike is incredible. If you want to distil cycling's appeal right down, it's essentially a combination of grace and power. Everyone in this book possessed both, but the ratios differ from rider to rider. Bugno, for example, had the grace in spades, while nobody ever matched Merckx for brute force. I think that in Anquetil you see those two elements in total harmony. His position is perfect, his pedal-stroke is to die for and he's immensely strong. Add the aesthetic of his time and the whole thing just works. I've watched the colourised versions of his Tours de France, and they're beautiful. Then when you see Jacques off the bike he reminds you of a movie star, not some half-bred bike rider. You have the château, the blonde wife, the cars, the champagne. Then the way he looks in his clothes, the way he listens before he speaks, the way he moves and the way he stands still. The way he's never less than immaculate, never less than Jacques Anquetil.

Hollywood good looks. Anquetil on the runway at Bordeaux Airport in 1965, with his *directeur sportif* and former racer Raphaël Géminiani stepping off the plane.

Obviously, he's most famous for the Tour. He was the first to win five of them, and the first to win four in a row. In reality, Poulidor only came close to beating him once, the famous 1964 race when they went shoulder to shoulder on the Puy de Dôme. Other than that, he never *really* troubled Jacques, but he was the housewives' choice and everyone benefited from the idea that he might beat him. He wasn't in Anquetil's class, but there was no shame in that because neither was anybody else.

At the 1961 Tour, the second that Anquetil won, there was a split stage on the first day. In the morning a 15-man break went, and Jacques was in it. In the afternoon there was a 28-kilometre time trial, and he won it by two and a half minutes. That means he beat *everybody* by at least two and a half minutes over 28 kilometres, not just the chaff. Most were losing six or seven minutes, and you had some guys shipping ten or eleven. It almost defies belief that he could be so much better than all the others. When they totted up the day's racing, he led the Tour by almost five minutes. They'd barely got started, but as a sporting contest it was over. I'm wracking my brain to think of a grand tour rider who was better against the watch, but – Induráin aside – nobody has even come close. In that run of four straight Tour wins, Anquetil won nine out of the ten time trials he took part in. The only one he lost was a hill climb to Superbagnères in 1962, when Federico Bahamontes beat him.

Time trialling was much more important during that era, and the make-up of the grand tours reflected the fact. They were about finding the most complete rider, so the time trials tended to be longer and much more frequent. We'll come back to that later . . .

Anyway, the 'Anquetil method' – attack against the watch and defend in the high mountains – pretty much became the blueprint. Others would hone it and refine it, but he built the prototype for guys like Hinault and Induráin, and also for me. He won the Giro twice using it, and in 1963 he helped himself to the Vuelta. Although this one tends to be overlooked, it's worth focusing on for a moment because the race – and the jersey – tells its own story.

That Vuelta took place in the first two weeks in May. Convention had it that you did one or the other – the Vuelta or the Giro – and Jacques had already won the 1960 Giro. He'd ridden the Vuelta the previous year, but he'd fallen ill. He'd been second with two stages to go, but he hadn't wanted to risk making it worse, so he'd abandoned. The organisers hadn't been impressed, and they'd invited Rik Van Looy to be the star rider for 1963. At that time the Vuelta would only invite one big foreign star. They didn't have much money, and setting all the Spaniards against a big champion created intrigue. It made sound commercial sense, but then Van Looy cried off and they were left in a tight spot. Jacques probably felt like he owed them a performance, so when they inserted a second long time trial he agreed to come.

Even though he hadn't raced for nearly two months, he won it comfortably enough. The point, however, is that his winning legitimised a 40-year-old bike race at a stroke. Previously the Vuelta had been regarded as a parochial event in a poor, backward country – the Tour of Switzerland was much more prestigious – but Anquetil put it on the map by winning it. The flip side of that was Franco Balmamion winning a second consecutive Giro. Now, Balmamion was a very good stage racer, probably the second best in the world in 1963, but the gulf between him and Anquetil was vast. He had no

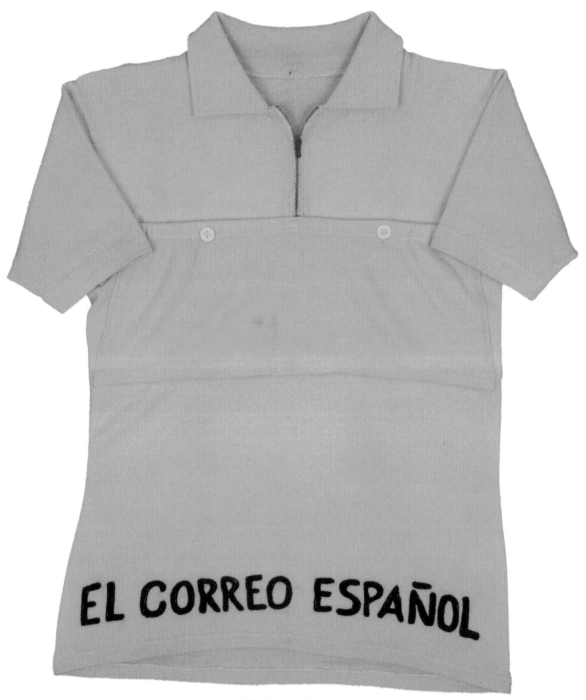

1963 Vuelta leader's jersey

1964 Tour de France *maillot jaune*

particular star quality, he rode defensively and he didn't win a stage. Balmamion was like Anquetil but without the time-trialling ability, the good looks or the intrigue. The prestige of bike races depends on their winners, and in 1963 Anquetil elevated the status of the Vuelta outside of Spain. Nobody else in cycling could have done that.

Anquetil had announced himself in 1953, as a 19-year-old boy. He'd taken part in the Grand Prix des Nations, a 140-kilometre time trial from Versailles to the Parc des Princes. To all intents and purposes, it was an unofficial TT championship of the world (the UCI version wasn't created until 1994), and Jacques won it by six minutes. He'd go on to win every edition he took part in, nine all told, and loads of other *cronos* besides.

During his era you had a dozen or so thoroughbred testers. These days we only see them during stage races, but guys like Ercole Baldini, Rolf Graf and Ferdinand Bracke were so revered that they even had a mini-calendar all to themselves. During the first two weeks of November they did the 'Nations', then two in Switzerland (the Grand Prix Lugano and Martini), and also the mythical Trofeo Baracchi in Italy. That was a two-up time trial between Brescia and Bergamo, and like the 'Nations' it was a major event.

Baldini and Bracke both conquered the Hour Record during their careers, and so did Jacques. In 1956 he broke Coppi's record, which had stood for 14 years. Merckx followed suit in Mexico City, and he told me it was the hardest, most brutal thing he ever did. That's saying something coming from a guy like him, but he understood that his career and legacy would have been incomplete without it. I never truly understood why Bernard Hinault never attempted it. He was one of the greatest who ever lived, and I'm pretty sure he could have broken Merckx's record. He obviously didn't fancy it, which is a shame.

The Hour tends to lie dormant for years on end, then you get a groundswell of interest and a flurry of attempts in a short period of time. It then disappears off the radar for a generation or two, and so it rolls on. Following Merckx's record in 1972 it sat idle for twelve years, before Moser came along and rode 52 kilometres. That sparked a cluster of – unsuccessful – new attempts, and then the dust settled until the last great time-trialling generation came along.

Between 1992 and 1996 there was an immense four-way struggle between Boardman, Obree, Induráin and Tony Rominger, with the second coming of Moser sandwiched among and between them. After that they recalibrated the technical parameters, and in 2000 Boardman broke the record using essentially using the same bike as Eddy had in 1972, but at sea level. Ondrej Sosenka did it in 2005, but then nothing happened for another nine years before I announced that I was going to do it. As usual that created a lot of interest, and quite a few guys broke it in the months preceding my attempt in London. I can't say I blame them for doing it either. They weren't all great testers, but they can say they have something in common with Fausto Coppi, Ercole Baldini, Eddy Merckx and the rest.

A lot of people have said that had I chosen a different track and waited for perfect conditions I could have gone quite a bit further. They're right, but it really didn't matter to me. It was something I wanted to do in my home town, the British public enjoyed it, and – besides – it's 'just' a record. It's going to be broken soon enough, and that's just as it should be.

History suggests it will probably lie dormant for quite a few years now, but I don't think it will ever disappear. That's because in many respects it's the reason you start riding a bike in the first place. One man, one bike, one hour, pure suffering. It's the simplest form of cycling there is, and also the most instinctive. Hopefully I'll be there when it gets broken, and hopefully it will be a rider of stature who does it.

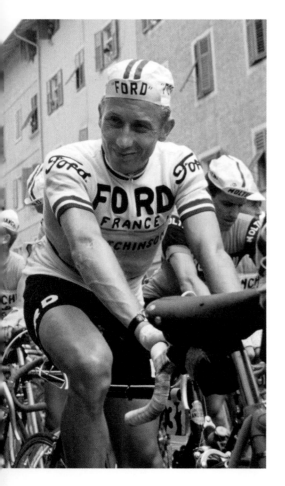

In closing, I'm going to tell you a story from Anquetil's 1965 season. I do so not only because it tells you everything you need to know about his legs, but also a lot about his brain. The previous year he'd emulated Coppi in winning the Giro–Tour double. It was his fourth Tour in succession, but the French public had seen enough. They were tired of watching the same old show, and they were firmly on Poulidor's side. Anquetil found that upsetting – like a lot of athletes he was very sensitive to public opinion.

We've established that the Tour was ... the Tour. It was three weeks of maximum exposure for Ford, his sponsors, three weeks during which they were on the front pages as well as the back. So what Anquetil did was inform them that he wouldn't be present, and that Lucien Aimar, his best *domestique*, would be leading the team instead. They were profoundly upset by that, and demanded to know why.

Left:
Racing for Ford France at the 1966 Giro d'Italia. Anquetil would finish third that year, behind Italians Gianni Motta and Italo Zilioli.

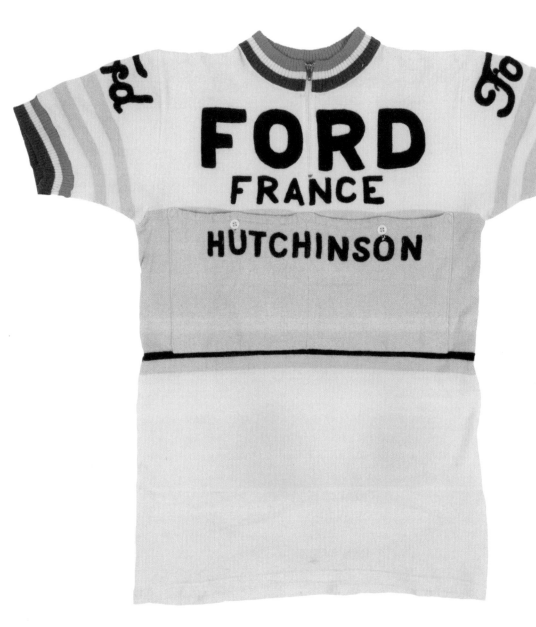

1966 Ford jersey

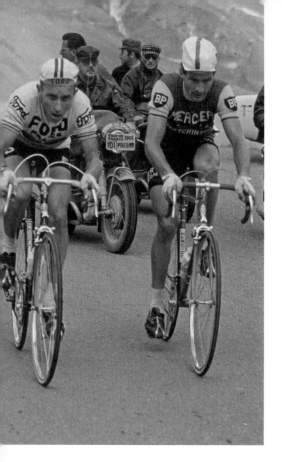

Anquetil's plan was brilliant, simple and daring in equal measure. In relinquishing the Tour he'd be seen to be being magnanimous, to be giving Poulidor a chance. However, he also knew that any Poulidor win would be seriously devalued in his absence, and that if he *failed* to win he'd be exposed as a fraud. One way or another, Poulidor couldn't beat him, because even if he won he'd lose.

The problem was that the suits at Ford still didn't get it. They weren't much interested in mind games, because as sponsors they just wanted their brand exposed. But Jacques told them he had a plan…

The Dauphiné Libéré, eight stages and 1,600 kilometres through the Alps, would finish in Avignon on the afternoon of Saturday 29 May. Poulidor would be racing, because the Dauphiné was a big preparatory race for the Tour. Then in the small hours of the following morning, 600 kilometres west in Bordeaux, cycling's most mythical event would begin. Bordeaux–Paris was an insane single-day endurance test, 15 hours and 557 up-hill-and-down-dale kilometres. The last 150 kilometres took place behind a Derny moped, and the race concluded, like the Tour, at the Parc des Princes. Nobody had even dared to contemplate riding both, because nobody considered it humanly possible. Jacques reasoned that if he could win the Dauphiné he'd put Poulidor firmly in his place. He'd also put Poulidor's Tour – should it materialise – into its rightful context. Then, if he flew to Bordeaux and won Bordeaux–Paris, he'd hand Ford more publicity than they could shake a stick at, while simultaneously performing irrefutably the greatest feat in French cycling history.

He was right. He did – and it was – and Raymond Poulidor finished runner-up (again) at the 1965 Tour de France.

There are some great riders in this book, but only a handful of great men. **Jacques Anquetil was a great man.**

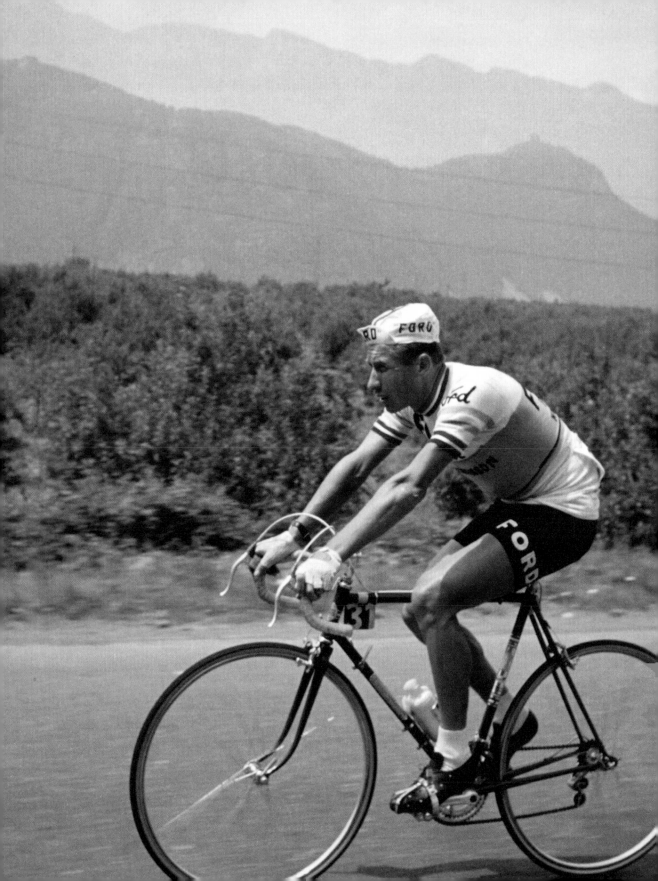

15

Gastone Nencini

1930–1980

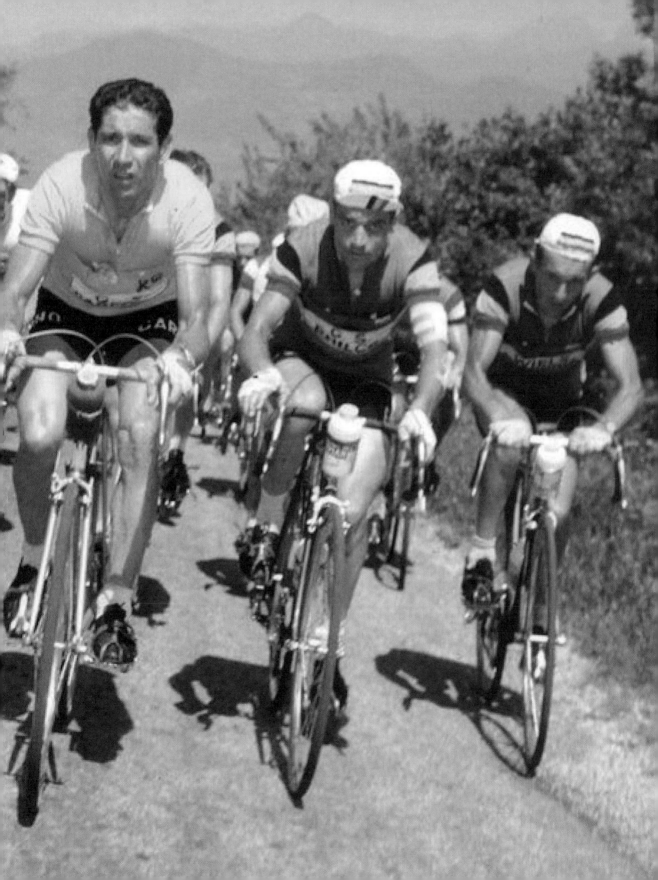

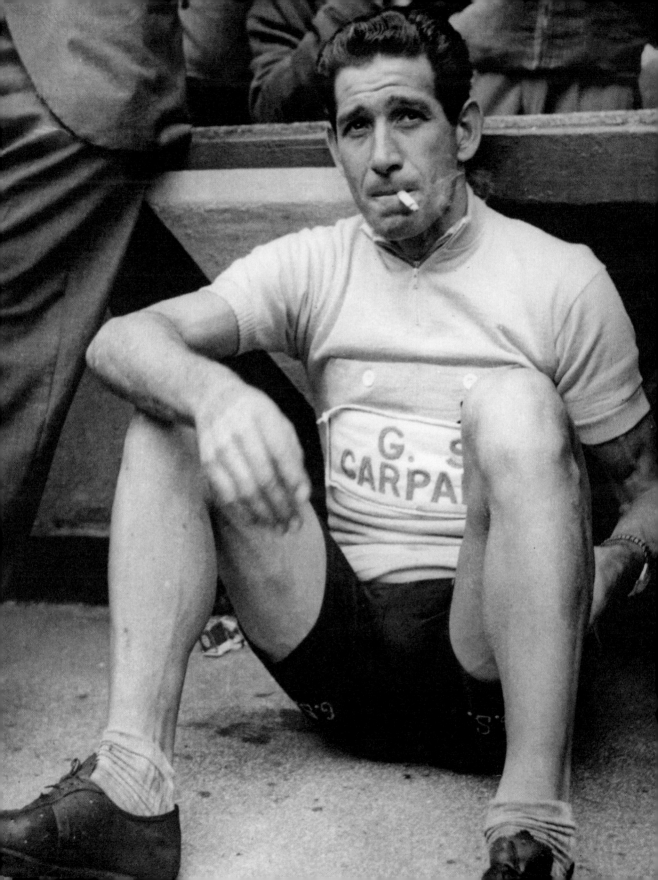

Google almost any Tour de France winner and you'll find a mountain of info. That's because as *maillot jaune* you become, almost by definition, a sporting legend. God knows how many words have been expended on Coppi, on Anquetil, on Pantani and even on me. The Tour has always celebrated itself more than any other great sporting event, and not without reason. It's the most beautiful and the most romantic, and it makes heroes of its competitors. For most people, just taking part in it is a Herculean achievement, let alone winning it.

Gastone Nencini, the 1961 winner, is one of the least famous. That's partly because of his character – he was a bit of a loner, a bit of an introvert and a lot of a rebel – but also because of the circumstances. The Tour was a French race, and he was the third foreigner in a row to win it. The great French hope, Roger Rivière, had been favourite, but he had to be airlifted to hospital with a broken back. He'd been fool enough to try to follow Nencini down the Col de Perjuret, and Gastone was one of the best descenders who ever lived. Following Rivière's crash, nothing much happened. The Italians were easily the strongest, and with no serious challenger the Tour became a bit of a procession.

What you *will* find if you google Nencini – and one of the main reasons I wanted him in the collection – is one of the coolest, most evocative cycling photos I've ever seen. It shows him sitting against a wall at the Parc des Princes. The Tour is won, and they're about to start the ceremony so he looks immaculate. He's a handsome guy anyway, but here his hair is perfectly Brylcreemed, he's not clagged up with road grime and he looks perfectly at peace with the world. He seems completely indifferent to the mayhem around him, and he's enjoying his reward for having beaten the best cyclists in the world over three weeks and 4,200 kilometres. That reward is a fag, and he's taking a long, hard, blissful pull on it.

Sensational.

ECHNICALLY, NENCINI was riding for the Italian national team when he won. In some respects, though, his Tour wasn't so different from my own. It had been years in the making, he was in his thirties by the time it arrived, and he won it with the help of a really strong team. Then, like me, he'd never return to the Tour, let alone win it again.

Unlike me, Gastone won the Giro as well. While his Tour was relatively straightforward (and this is always a relative concept at the Tour), the Giro was anything but. In fact, it was the stuff of cycling legend – and of a kind of cycling that no longer exists.

It was the penultimate Dolomite stage, with a summit finish at Monte Bondone. Charly Gaul, the reigning champion, had the pink jersey, and was easily the best climber in the race. The Giro seemed done and dusted, but as a cyclist Gaul had one major problem – he was friendless. He came across as aloof and a bit big-headed. He'd also upset Louison Bobet, the great French champion.

Bobet had won three Tours, the World Championships and most of the major classics. He had no *maglia rosa*, though, and he understood that without one his palmarès was incomplete. He didn't like Gaul, and the feeling was mutual. Charly was telling anyone who would listen that he was going to humiliate Bobet on the Bondone, and Louison was livid. He ordered his *domestiques* to stay close to Gaul, and to watch him like a hawk.

Early on in the stage, before the racing had really begun in earnest, Gaul stopped for a pee. Barbotin signalled to Bobet, his captain, and then all hell broke loose. It's one of the unwritten rules that you don't attack in these circumstances, but Bobet had had a gutful of Charly Gaul. He went, about 50 others tagged along, and Gaul was left on the roadside looking stupid. Worse still, he had nobody prepared to help him chase – what goes around generally comes around in the peloton – so it was just him and two of his *domestiques* against the best of the rest. For 100 long, hard, miserable kilometres.

Gaul lost eight minutes, and with them the jersey and the Giro. Heading into the final stage, Nencini led Bobet by 19 seconds, so everything was to play for. Nencini had lost the 1955 Giro because he'd punctured at an inopportune moment, and he flatted again here. Punctures were a lot more frequent generally, and he had two of them at the bottom of the final climb, the Brocon. As he and his mechanic struggled with his bike, Bobet (and apparently the *maglia rosa*) floated off into the distance.

Nencini and Charly Gaul on the Rolle Pass during the 1957 Giro d'Italia. Nencini won the GC that year, with Gaul finishing fourth.

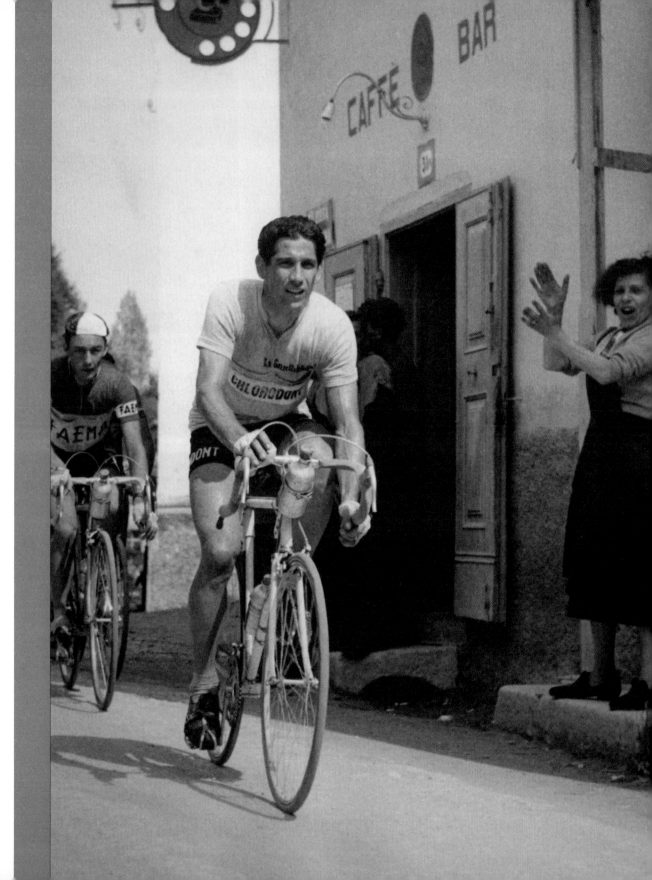

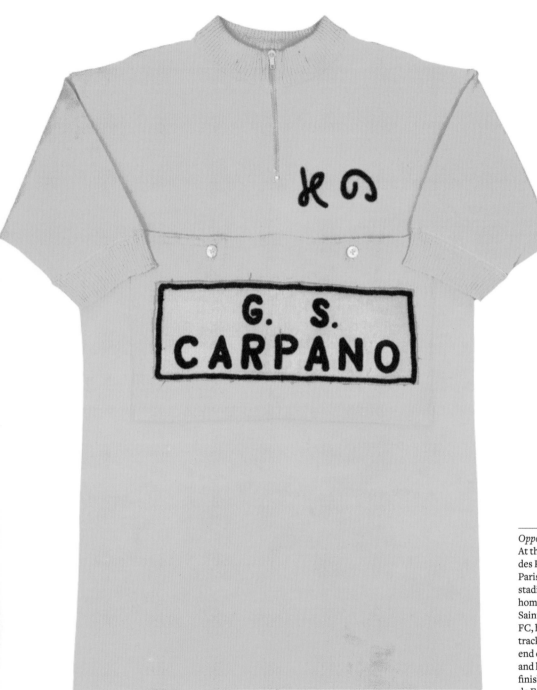

1960 Tour de France *maillot jaune*

Opposite:
At the Parc
des Princes,
Paris, 1955. The
stadium, now
home to Paris
Saint-Germain
FC, had a cycling
track until the
end of the 1960s
and hosted the
finish of the Tour
de France from
1903 to 1967.

Bobet, though, hadn't reckoned on Charly Gaul. He couldn't win the Giro, but he was damned if he was going to sit by and watch his enemy steal it. He first waited for Nencini, and then paced him back up to the Bobet group. Finally, having dropped him off on Bobet's wheel, he danced off into the clouds for the stage win. He had his pound of flesh, Nencini kept the *maglia rosa*, and Bobet left Italy empty-handed.

They reckon it was one of the greatest stage races of all time, and it's not hard to see why.

Nencini won that Giro for a fairly ordinary team, Chlorodont,

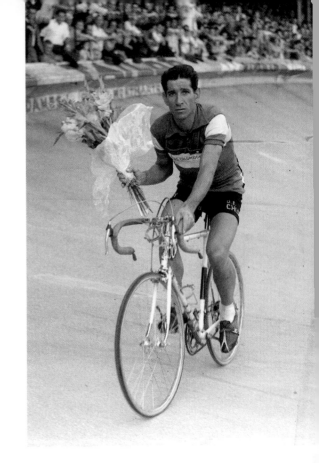

and then signed for an extraordinary one. Carpano were extremely wealthy and extremely ambitious, and they wanted an Italian Tour winner. Nencini was the man most likely, and in that sense our paths cross again because the starting point for the Team Sky project was finding a British Tour de France winner.

I'd been struggling financially before joining Garmin in 2009. One year and one Tour de France later, I was approached by Sky with a generous four-year contract. As well as securing my kids' future, they were offering to build a Tour de France-winning structure around me. As much as I felt I had a moral obligation to honour my contract and as much as I respected Jonathan Vaughters, the Garmin team principal, we both knew I'd have been a fool to turn it down. The respective teams' lawyers battled it out and in December, they had a dramatic, last-ditch meeting in New York. Jonathan's starting position was, 'We'll keep him under contract as a matter of principle. If he doesn't ride, then so be it,' but in reality he knew that Sky needed a British leader. Sky knew that he knew, but they also knew that he was open to some sort of deal. Garmin were a new team, and a good deal would help them secure their medium-term future and improve the overall quality of their roster.

I've an idea that Sky paid quite a substantial amount to buy me out of the contract. I remember Steve Cummings saying, 'Bloody hell – they could have bought Steven Gerrard for that money!'

I like being a Tour de France winner, but I didn't much like winning the Tour de France. What I mean by that is that I didn't much enjoy the three weeks of the actual race, and I *certainly* didn't enjoy the two years preceding it. That doesn't mean I didn't enjoy riding my bike, because for the most part I did. However, where Nencini only decided to take part in the Tour a few weeks beforehand, my winning the race was very much a project. It was quite formulaic and at times repetitive, and there was a lot of number crunching, logistical stuff and general 'management'. In my case, there was also a lot of time away from home on training camps, a hell of a lot of sacrifice and quite a lot of hunger.

I stumbled across the idea that I could be a decent Tour rider, really. By rights I shouldn't have been, because the 21st-century Tour isn't designed for a tester like me. When Coppi won it in 1949 there were time trials of 137 and 92 kilometres, and even in the 1980s they'd ride four or five of them. These days it's geared almost exclusively around the climbers, but I fell on my feet in 2012. Contador wasn't there, and better still they decided to level the playing field by reintroducing a second time trial. At 53 and 41 kilometres they were trifles compared with the ones they used to do, but they gave me a fighting chance.

It might have been different in Nencini's day – though I very much doubt it – but ask any recent Tour winner and they'll tell you that the three weeks themselves are far too pressurised to be fun. They can be a lot of fun for the *domestiques* and the guys hunting for the odd stage win, but not if you're being paid to win it. In my case everyone knew how important it was for Sky and for British Cycling, and because I'd won everything else I started out as the favourite. That was quite stressful, but even with the meticulous preparation and all that 'marginal gains' stuff there were a lot of variables. On the track you can legislate for almost all of these. You can predict them, and as a consequence you can mitigate them. On the road it's not like that at all – just ask Gaul and Nencini – which explains why so many Tour de France favourites fall short. Even guys like Hinault lost Tours they ought to have won, and the list of favourites who never quite made it is as long as your arm. Think Rivière, Poulidor, Hennie Kuiper in 1976, Michel Pollentier in 1978 . . .

The first week of the Tour is dramatic for the fans, but as a rider a lot of what you're doing is avoiding catastrophe. Thankfully we survived it in 2012, and I went

Riding in the Alps in the *maillot jaune* on Stage 18 of the 1960 Tour de France. Nencini won the GC that year, five minutes ahead of Graziano Battistini.

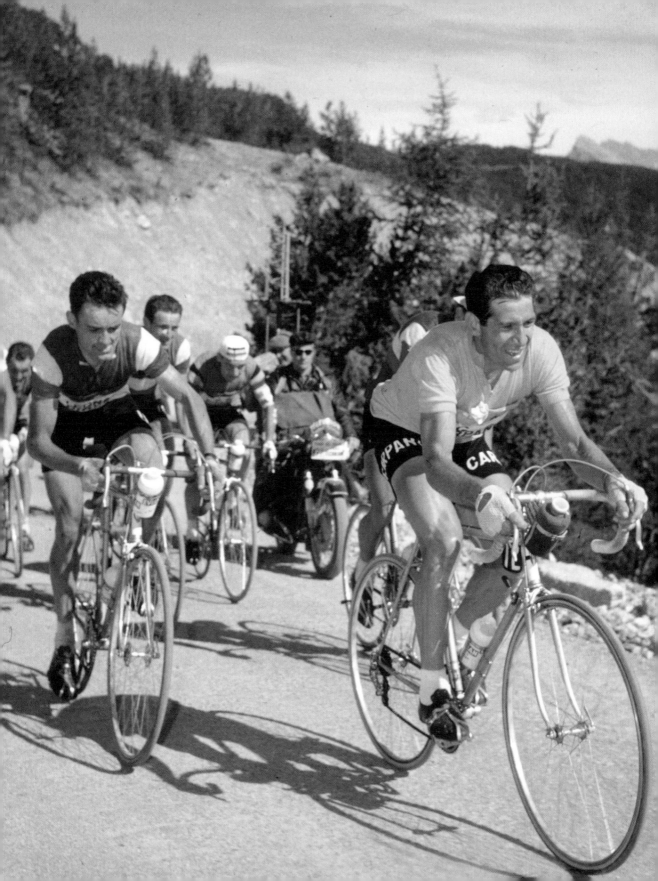

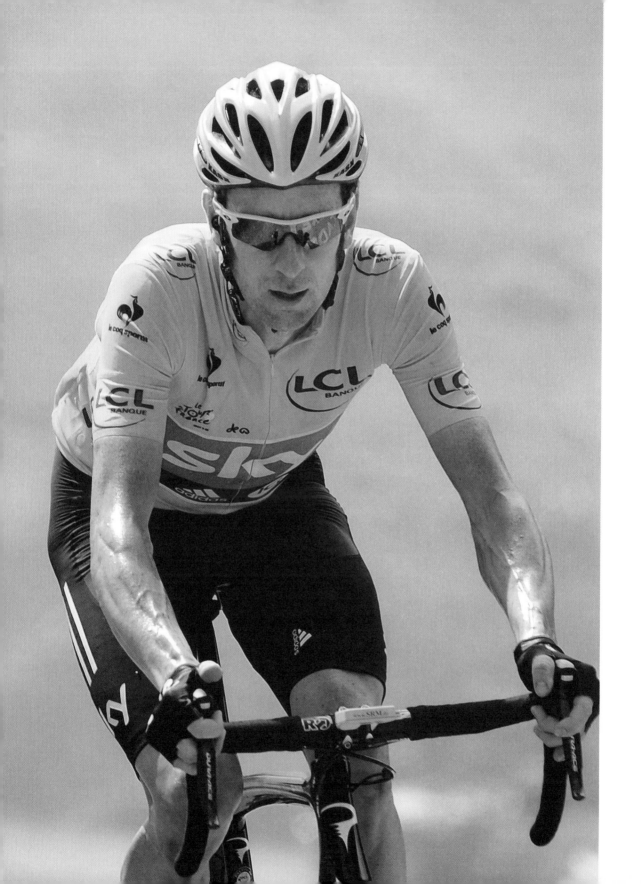

into the time trial in yellow. I came out of it with two minutes on Cadel Evans, with Chris Froome third and Vincenzo Nibali fourth. We were in pretty good shape as a team (though we'd lost Sivtsov), but unbeknownst to me there was trouble ahead.

The second Alpine stage finished with the climb to La Toussuire. Everything was under control, but then Nibali attacked and Evans cracked. That meant that Chris had a job to do, and the job was to ride me across to Vincenzo. For a while that was what he seemed to be doing, but then he drifted off. I assumed he was cooked, so I had to try to get across myself. It amounted to an uphill time trial and, although I wasn't sure I'd make it all the way to Vincenzo, I knew that if I rode sensibly it would be OK. It would only be a matter of seconds, so it would be fine.

So I set off riding tempo, but then at a certain point Chris came flying by me. He started trying to bridge across on his own, riding for himself. As he saw it Evans was in trouble, and Nibali was threatening his GC position. He was absolutely right, but that was of secondary importance. In fact, it was of no importance whatsoever because we had the leadership of the Tour de France to defend. Nobody could understand what Chris was doing, and to cut a long story short he was invited to do his job for the team.

Chris was already a ferocious competitor and one hell of a bike rider, and it was clear to everyone that he was going to become a great champion. That's precisely what he's done and what he is, and in that sense I have a huge amount of respect for him. Despite the narrative created and a few amateur dramatics thrown in, he was never going to win that Tour de France and it wasn't his job to try. There was a financial benefit to his finishing second as opposed to third, and from a structural point of view that's questionable. There's a time and a place for that stuff, however, and this wasn't it.

I'd earned the right to lead the team by winning Paris–Nice, Romandie and the Dauphiné, and if I'd failed in these it would have been me working for Chris. But I had the jersey, there was a long time trial to follow, and we were accomplishing pretty much everything we'd set out to do. I'd thought we were all united. We had world-class guys like Mick Rogers and Richie Porte, and they were sacrificing themselves for the team. We also had Mark Cavendish, the greatest sprinter in the history of the Tour, resplendent in rainbow bands carrying water. That meant the team was winning, not infighting.

As yellow jersey, the further you get into it, the more the pressure ramps up. First you're worried you might crash, then you're worried because the mountains

Wearing the *maillot jaune* on Stage 17 of the 2012 Tour de France.

are coming. Each day ticked off is a day closer to Paris, but the paradox is that with every passing day you have more to lose. In my case I was up against natural climbers, while I was just a time triallist who'd got his weight down. I was as good as I've ever been, but I wasn't deluding myself that they weren't more talented than me in the mountains. By the end I was pretty much just wishing it away, praying that nothing would go wrong.

The release when it's over is incredible. It's not something I'm sure I can really describe, and I think that's one of the reasons I identify with Gastone Nencini smoking his fag at the Parc des Princes.

He's reached Paris and that, for a racing cyclist, is the promised land . . .

At the award ceremony after Stage 10 of the 1960 Tour de France. The stage was won by Roger Rivière, but Nencini took the *maillot jaune* after a lightning-fast descent of the Col d'Aubisque.

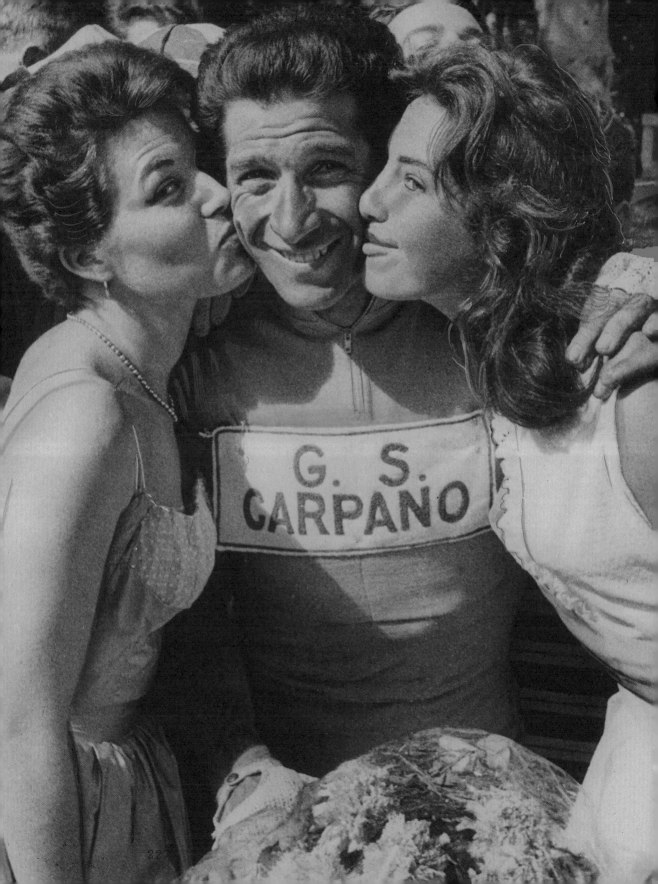

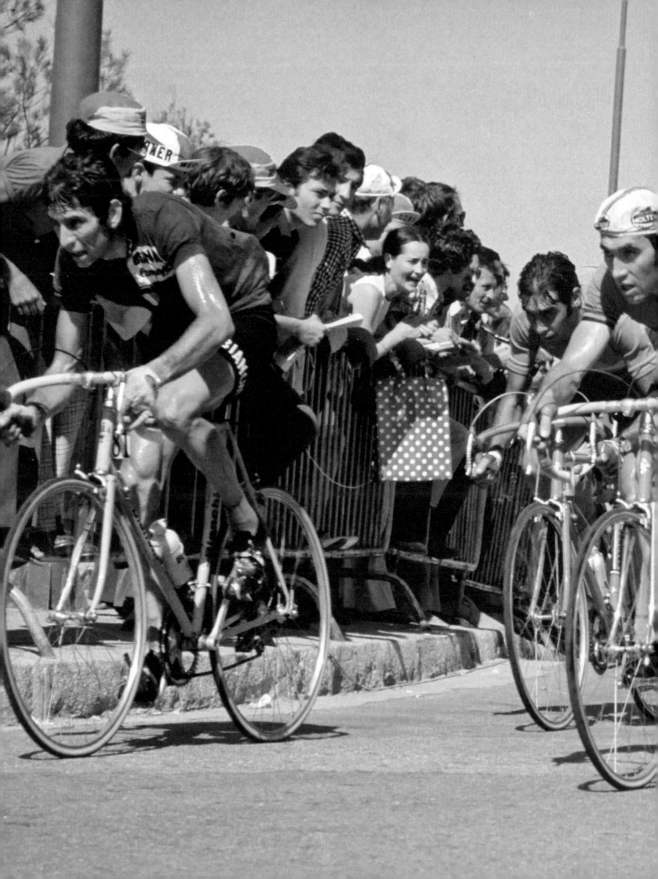

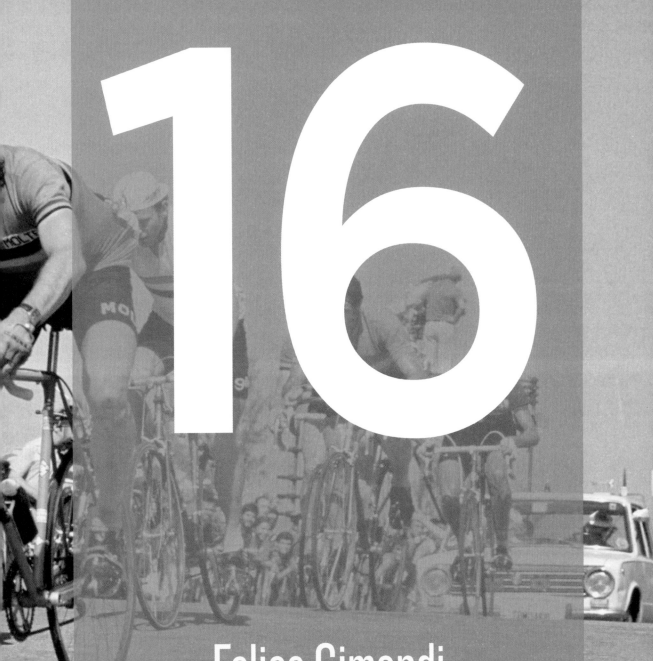

16

Felice Gimondi

1942–

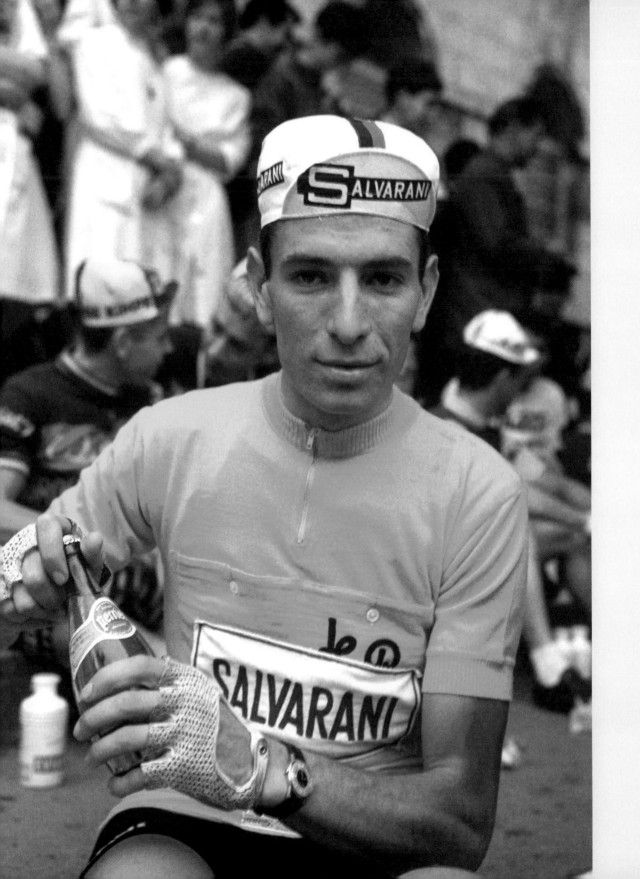

It goes without saying that Merckx was all over those VHS films I watched as a kid. As often as not he won, and as often as not the others seemed beaten before they'd even started. He'd send Deschoenmaecker or Bruyère, his strongest *domestiques*, to the front, and the rest would have this 'here we go again' look about them. They looked like condemned men, because that's precisely what they were.

An exception to this can be seen in a documentary film about Merckx. It's called *La Course en Tête*, it was made in 1976 and it begins with a race Merckx *didn't* win. The 1973 World Championships Road Race in Barcelona is legendary for all sorts of reasons, not least because of the accusations of treachery and skulduggery that have surrounded it ever since. There's enough in that Worlds to warrant a book of its own, but to cut a very long, very complicated story short, it all boils down to a four-man sprint.

Eddy has a team-mate, Freddy Maertens, and in principle his job is to lead out the sprint for his captain. That ought to work, because on paper Eddy is faster than the other two guys, the Spaniard Luis Ocaña and the Italian Felice Gimondi. However, between them Maertens and Merckx make a mess of it – which explains the subsequent rancour – and Eddy finishes fourth. He's convinced that Maertens has double-crossed him and, having lost the Worlds the previous year as well, he's inconsolable.

The winner is Gimondi, Italy's great hero. The *tifosi* worship him because, for all that he's been losing to Merckx for years, he alone has refused to yield. Objectively, Merckx is a much better bike rider than him, but they identify with Gimondi because, like all true cycling champions, he has a limitless depth of resolve. His is to be found in the fact that, although he hasn't often won in the age of Merckx, he has absolutely refused to be beaten.

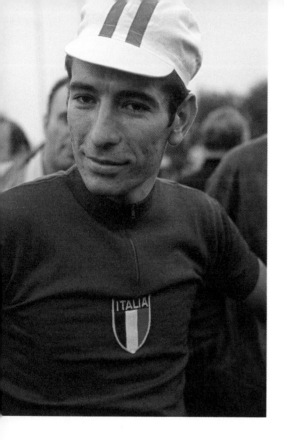

BIKE RACES COME AND GO, and they wax and wane in importance and prestige. Once upon a time the Tour of Switzerland was much more important than, say, the Vuelta, and Flèche Wallonne was more prestigious than Flanders, as were Paris–Brussels, Bordeaux–Paris (now defunct) and even Paris–Tours. But in 1948 things started to change.

The UCI introduced a season-long series called the Challenge Desgrange-Colombo, and it was the first meaningful step towards the 'globalisation' of cycling. In reality, it only included the races run by the big newspapers in France, Italy and Belgium, but Flanders assumed more prestige for being one of them. The great Italian rider Fiorenzo Magni decided to go over there, and he gave it a big boost by winning it. That added to its perceived value, while races like the Tour of Tuscany, which had been left out of the series, suffered as a consequence. In 1959 they revamped the series, since Pernod decided to sponsor it. The Vuelta was included because Pernod wanted to break the Spanish market, and that was why guys like Anquetil rode it. Suddenly the Vuelta started to matter, and ultimately it became the 'third grand tour'. Later, someone – most likely a journalist – decided that Paris–San Remo, Flanders, Liège–Bastogne–Liège, Paris–Roubaix and Lombardy were the five 'Monuments'. In the past they'd always talked about the 'Seven Sisters', but the 'Monuments' idea gained traction, and so it rolled and so it rolls.

I mention all this because it doesn't *really* make sense to compare riders from different eras based on a modern-day perception of their victories. But this doesn't stop us trying, and there's a lot of fun to be had arguing over who was the best. It's human nature, subconsciously or otherwise, and I think most would agree that Merckx and Coppi stand apart from the rest. That probably does a disservice to guys like Alfredo Binda and Costante Girardengo, the *campionissimi* who competed before the Second World War. It's much more difficult to quantify their achievements because there was no globalisation, so they hardly ever rode abroad. They'd also retired long before any of us were born, so they're prehistoric in the same way that Coppi will be fairly soon.

Left:
At the 1968 World Championships at Imola, Italy, where he finished sixth.

Whatever. We're dealing with post-Second World War icons here, and with a half-decent grasp of cycling's evolution we can more or less identify some sort of pecking order. We know that Armstrong was statistically the greatest Tour de France rider ever, at least until they stripped him. We also know that he didn't win the Giro or the Vuelta, because he wasn't interested in them. Everyone knows that Sean Kelly was one of the great classics riders, but that he, like Anquetil and Bartali, failed to win a rainbow jersey. Induráin never won a major classic, Bobet had no *maglia rosa*, and so on and so forth.

We also know that the jerseys speak for themselves, and that there are five meaningful ones. They are the pink and yellow of the Giro and the Tour, and whatever colour the Vuelta winner has happened to wear at any given moment. The other two are – and always were – the rainbow and the national champion's jerseys, and only three cyclists in history have won them all. The first was Merckx. He won five Tours and five Giros between 1967 and 1974, and won the Vuelta in 1973. Hinault did the grand slam before his 26th birthday, and was the second-most successful grand tour rider of all time. He started 13 of them, finished 12 and won 10. He finished second in the other two, and the one DNF, the 1980 Tour, was because his knee failed.

And then there are the five jerseys of Felice Gimondi.

When he won the 1965 Tour de France aged 22, Gimondi became the poster-boy of Italian cycling. That's the power of the Tour, but he confirmed his talent by winning Paris–Roubaix, Paris–Brussels and Lombardy the following year. In 1967 he beat Anquetil to win the 50th-anniversary Giro, and he was still only 25 when he won his third grand tour, the Vuelta, the following spring. The Italians had been searching for the 'new Coppi' for 15 years, and in Gimondi they seemed to have found him. Then, however, Eddy Merckx signed up to ride the Giro.

Day 12 of the race was a Dolomite stage that finished at the Tre Cime di Lavaredo. The Italians had labelled Eddy a classics rider, because at that point he hadn't ridden a grand tour for GC. When he went up the road to the Tre Cime nobody could follow, though, and Gimondi lost over six minutes. The race was blown apart, Gimondi was left in tears, and the face of world cycling was changed forever. Felice Gimondi was still a great bike rider, but he knew his time as the best on the planet was coming to an end.

Gimondi dusted himself down, and that August won the Italian national championship. It was his first professional *maglia tricolore*, and I don't think any other jersey was ever more appropriate. There are all sorts of reasons for that, and I'll try to explain them as best I can.

At the Tre Cime, Merckx's sponsor was Faema, a Milanese coffee company. Italian cycling was the wealthiest and best in the world, so he took part in all of the important races there. Specifically that meant the Giro, Milan–San Remo and Lombardy, and we know that pretty soon he was winning nearly half the races he took part in.

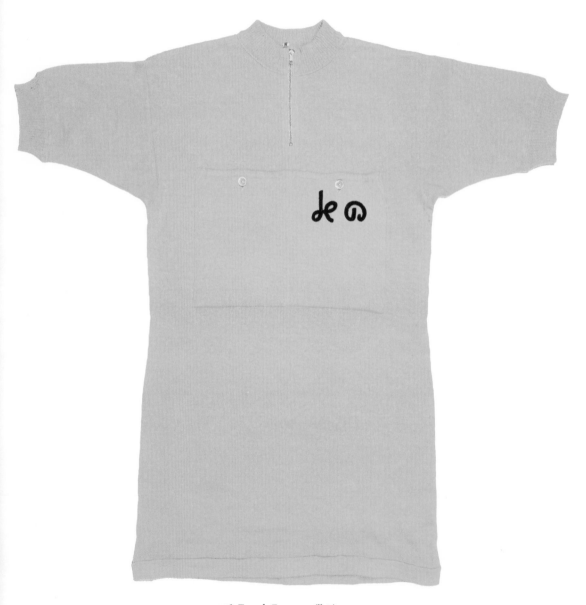

1965 Tour de France *maillot jaune*

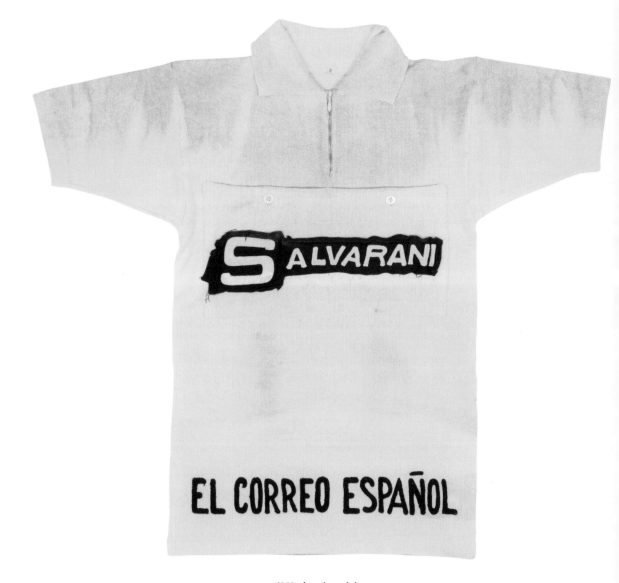

1968 Vuelta winner's jersey

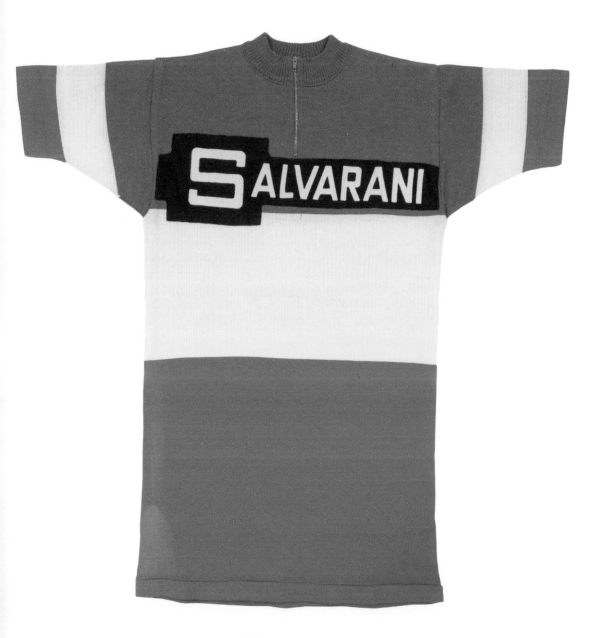

1972 Italian champion's jersey

Merckx couldn't stomach the idea of being beaten by Gimondi. Eddy didn't like losing at the best of times. Between 1968 and 1973 Gimondi never beat him in any of the races that mattered. He won San Remo when Merckx was absent in 1973, and the Giro and Lombardy in 1969 and 1974. He never once beat him on the road, though, because Eddy wouldn't allow it. That's significant, but also paradoxical. That endless losing is the key to understanding just how good Felice Gimondi was, and why having all of his jerseys was so important to me.

Before that fateful day on the Tre Cime, Gimondi had been the best of a brilliant bunch of Italians. Gianni Motta, Franco Bitossi, Vittorio Adorni, Italo Zilioli and Michele Dancelli were fantastic riders. They headed up probably the most talented generation ever produced by any nation at any given time, but when Merckx came along that lot essentially just gave up. They still competed among themselves for the smaller races, but psychologically Merckx had them so broken that they were beaten before they started.

Not so Gimondi. Race after race and year after year he alone carried the fight to Merckx. He couldn't beat him, because Merckx respected him far too much to allow that to happen. He was stronger physically than Gimondi, but Gimondi was stronger mentally than anybody. He was indestructible and so, while the rest capitulated, he just kept going, and going, and going. He was David to Merckx's Goliath, and to the man in the Italian street that was irresistible. He was the symbol of their cycling, and the *maglia tricolore* was the symbol of their journey.

The *maglia tricolore* was the first national champion's jersey, and it was invented by a guy named Giovanni Cuniolo. In 1906 he won the very first Italian road race championship and, because he was a big star, he was invited to Australia to ride some track meets. Evidently he needed something to distinguish him from the locals, so he came up with a brilliant idea. He had a tailor make him a jersey that replicated the Italian flag, and by all accounts it was a big success. He really liked the jersey, so did the fans, and he kept on wearing it when he got home.

I'm not sure that he intended for it to become *the* national champion's jersey, but he won the championship for the next two years so *de facto* it became the champion's jersey. The French often rode in Italy, and obviously someone liked the idea. They adopted it themselves, the rest is history, and as I said before, Italians are *very* keen on their history. They understand that the *maglia tricolore*, perhaps even more than the *maglia rosa*, is the embodiment of their cycling history and culture. The champion keeps it for a full year, and through it he becomes an ambassador for their country. Almost all of the great Italian champions wore it at some point, so it tells a story in its own right.

I know what it means to win a national championship on the road. I managed it in 2011, and it's one of my most important cycling achievements. I loved winning that jersey, and I loved wearing it. I also loved the design of it – whoever came up with it back in the day produced a masterpiece – but most of all I love the *idea* of it.

I guess it all goes back to the Lillywhite thing, to the fact that your heroes remain your heroes regardless of what you accomplish. Yates was winning the British championship when I was a kid, and so were people like Colin Sturgess and John Herety. Further back it was the likes of Les West, Colin Lewis and Phil Edwards. They weren't big international stars like Cavendish, Thomas and Stannard, but for me that's not an issue. They won it because they were the best in Britain, and there are a hell of a lot of fantastic riders who never managed it. Neither Simpson nor Hoban ever won it, nor did Denson, or Graham Jones.

I came up short at the Giro and the Vuelta, but I have a yellow jersey and a rainbow jersey for the time trial. I know that the red, white and blue isn't *considered* as important as either, but to me it means the world.

All of which leads us back, in a roundabout way, to Barcelona and Gimondi. It had been five years and loads of defeats since the Tre Cime, and Merckx had thumped him again at the Giro. By now even the Italians were starting to lose faith. They *wanted* to believe, but wanting to believe and actually believing are completely different things. Gimondi was 31, and his season had amounted to a small stage race in France, a few meaningless criteriums and the Coppa Bernocchi. Time seemed to be running out, and Merckx showed no sign of letting up. He was odds-on when they set off that morning, just as he was odds-on every time he raced.

Gimondi was riding for Italy in Barcelona, which of course is why the race has assumed such historical importance. Had he finally beaten Merckx at the Tre Valli Varesine or the Coppa Agostoni it would have been nice, but not that nice. For the great champions those races are the punctuation marks in the season, but the 1973 World Championships *was* Gimondi's season – and it could be argued it was also the completion of his life's work. Winning the rainbow jersey was one thing, beating Merckx to get it quite another . . .

Gimondi did it again in 1976. By then Merckx was past his best, but old Gim kept on truckin'. They'd written him off once more, but somehow he stormed round Italy to join a very select group. Merckx, Coppi and Binda had each won five *giri*, but they were untouchable. In winning his third, Gimondi joined Magni, Bartali and Giovanni Brunero, three of the greatest of all time. Only Hinault has managed to win three since, which just goes to show how hard it is to win the Giro d'Italia. Three of them – and the yellow, and the rainbow and the *tricolore*. It goes to show you exactly what kind of a bike rider Felice Gimondi was.

An absolute warrior.

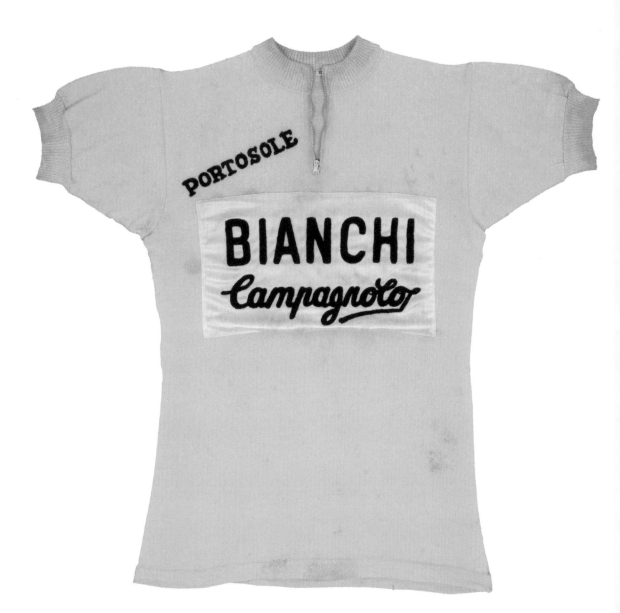

1976 Giro d'Italia *maglia rosa*

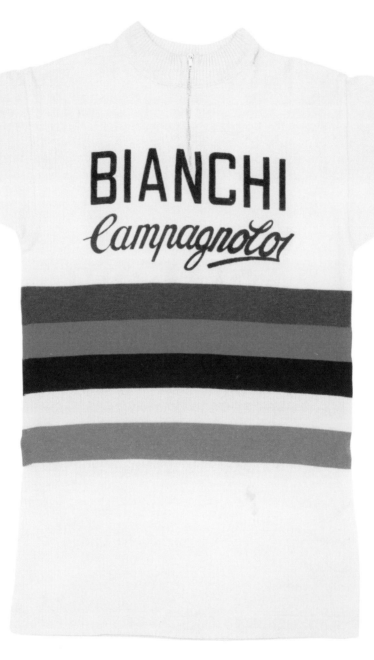

1973 world champion's jersey made by Gianni Vittore,
worn to victory at the Giro del Piemonte, one week after winning the title in Barcelona

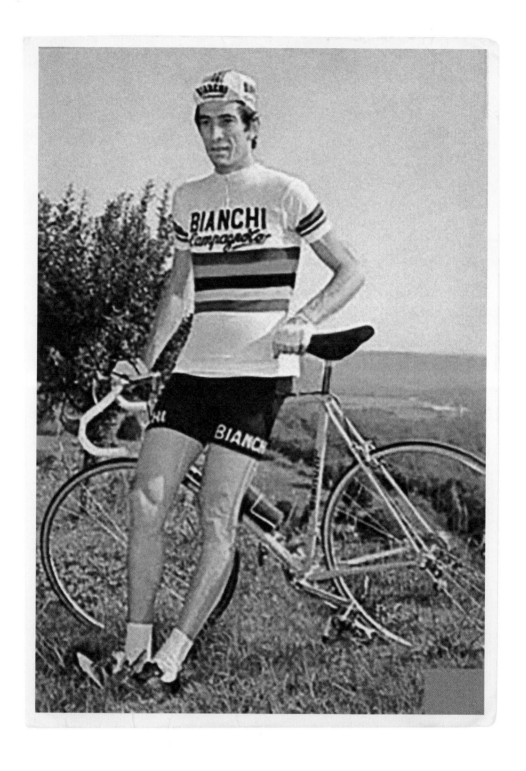

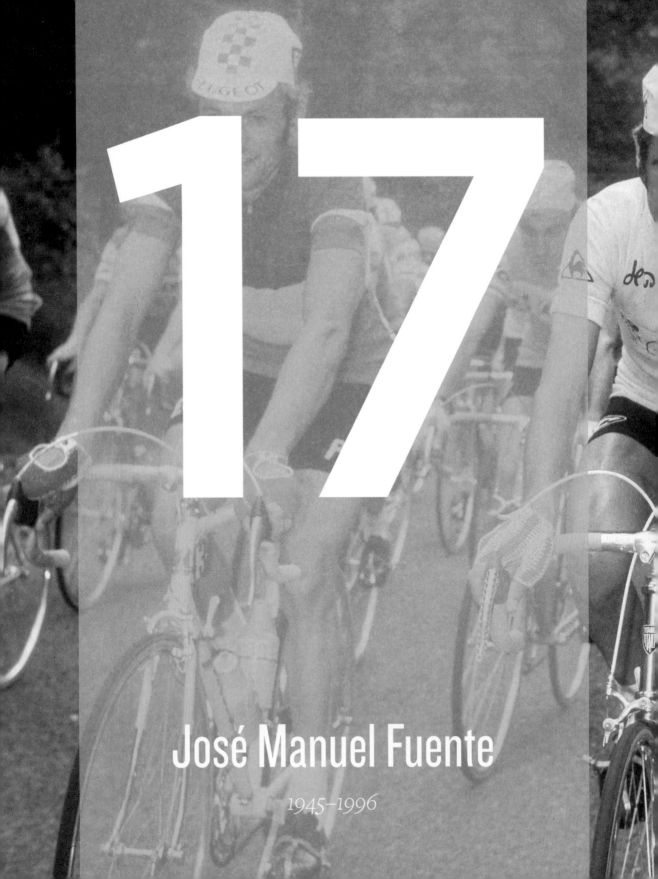

17

José Manuel Fuente

1945–1996

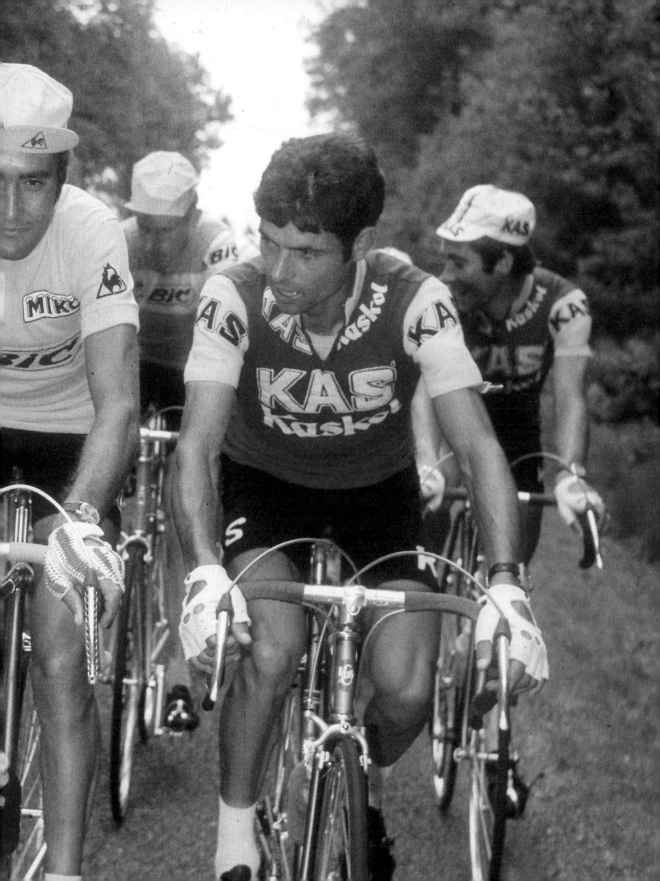

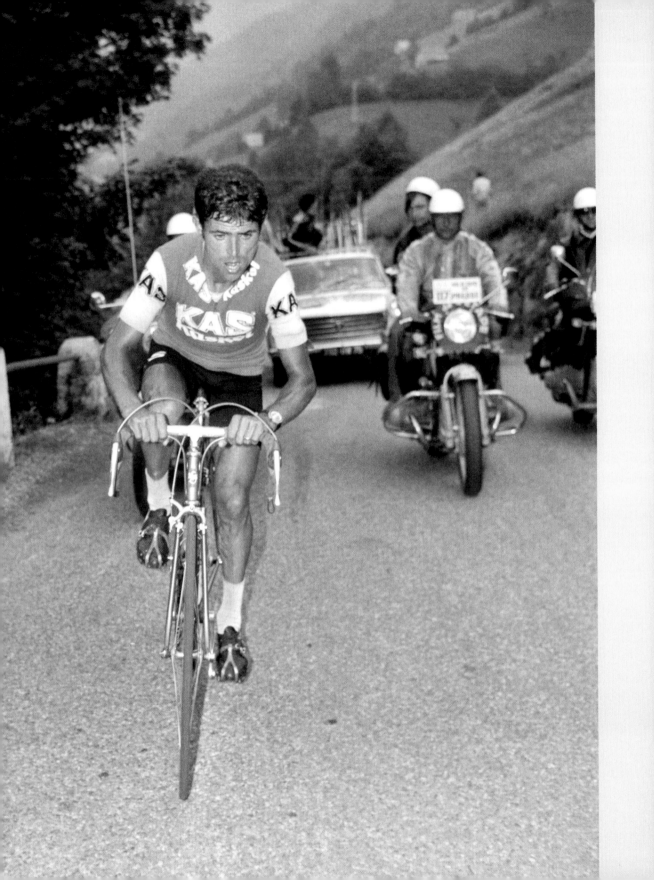

Between 2011 and 2014 I won quite a few stage races, but even before then I'd amassed a small jersey collection of my own. Some of them were nice, but nearly all of them were temporary. From time to time I'd win the prologue or opening time trial, and that would keep me in a job. I didn't tend to keep the jerseys, though, because the minute we hit a climb I'd be out the back. I was too heavy and too focused on the track for it to be any other way.

Even when I was winning big races I wasn't particularly bothered about the jerseys. Like everyone else, I liked winning, but I didn't get precious about my own jerseys in the way that I do about other people's.

There are a couple that I have framed, though, and that I really *do* care about.

You often hear cyclists talk about their 'dream coming true'

when they win a stage or take a jersey. It's a bit of an old cliché, but at the 2010 Giro one of mine genuinely did. Following on from *Stars and Watercarriers*, I'd watched a German documentary about the 1974 Giro. It was called *The Greatest Show on Earth*, and it featured Merckx hammer and tongs with a Spaniard named José Manuel Fuente. He was the best pure climber in the world, he had this beautiful KAS *maglia rosa*, but then he suffered a hunger flat and lost it.

Ultimately Eddy won the Giro, and poor Fuente had to settle for the *maglia verde* of the best climber. Although I'd never even been to Italy when I watched the film, I fell hopelessly in love with its bike race. I wanted a *maglia rosa* of my own, and 15 years later I had my chance.

Stage 13 of the 1973 Tour de France, from Bourg-Madame to Luchon. The stage was won by Luis Ocaña, the overall winner of the Tour that year, in which Fuente took third place, his best result in the race.

THE GIRO STARTED WITH A PROLOGUE IN AMSTERDAM, and I finally got my hands on one. The following day we went to Utrecht, but there was a big crash about 40 kilometres from the finish. I tried to get back into the main group, but it was hopeless. I guess in some ways that sums up the love/hate relationship I've always had with the Giro. What I mean by that is that I've always loved it, but it seemed that, no matter what I did or how hard I tried, it always had it in for me. Problem was that the more it spurned me, the more infatuated I became, and I still love it today. It was a pig's ear pretty much every time I rode it, but I'm still convinced that it's the most beautiful, mystical race on earth. That assertion has no basis whatsoever in fact given my misadventures there, but it doesn't stop me feeling it. I love the Giro much more than I ever loved the Tour, and I love the *maglia rosa* much more than the *maillot jaune*.

The 2003 Giro was my first grand tour. I'd just turned 23, and I remember being really excited because it was another of the races ticked off my mental bucket list. In the two Giro films I'd watched the whole thing had seemed to be total chaos, particularly in the south. I automatically assumed it would have become a lot more orderly and 'civilised' – after all, 30 years had passed – but that wasn't the case at all. It was still the 'old Giro', with 13 Italian teams and all the stages taking place inside the country. They hadn't yet invented the World Tour, and the place still felt like a foreign country and the event like an adventure, because that's what it was. These days the Giro sometimes seems to be a bike race that happens simply to *take place* in Italy, because everyone is speaking English. Back then it was bedlam. Everyone was speaking Italian – and I bloody loved it.

For some reason, FDJ usually sent a team to the race in that era, but we were just a little French outfit. Nominally we had Sandy Casar for the GC, but mostly it was people like me, the third-string. For the Italians it was the be-all and end-all of the season, but most of us were doing our first grand tour. With the exception of Casar, we were the kids who weren't good enough for the Dauphiné – and, by extension, the Tour – so we just tried to stay together and look after one another. We were basically just trying to survive from one day to the next.

Teams didn't have their own chefs then, so the food at the Giro was great. The hotels, on the other hand, were invariably crap, and down in the south they were atrocious. I was rooming with Bernie Eisel, and most of the time we were able to laugh it off. If we hadn't we'd have been distraught, so we lied to ourselves it was all part of the Italian 'charm'. Maybe they gave us the shit hotels because we were a French team, but they seemed to become progressively more bizarre as time went by. We finally cracked when they put us in a room with bunk-beds. Peak Italy!

Riding alongside Merckx in the 1972 Giro d'Italia. Fuente eventually finished second to the Belgian in the race.

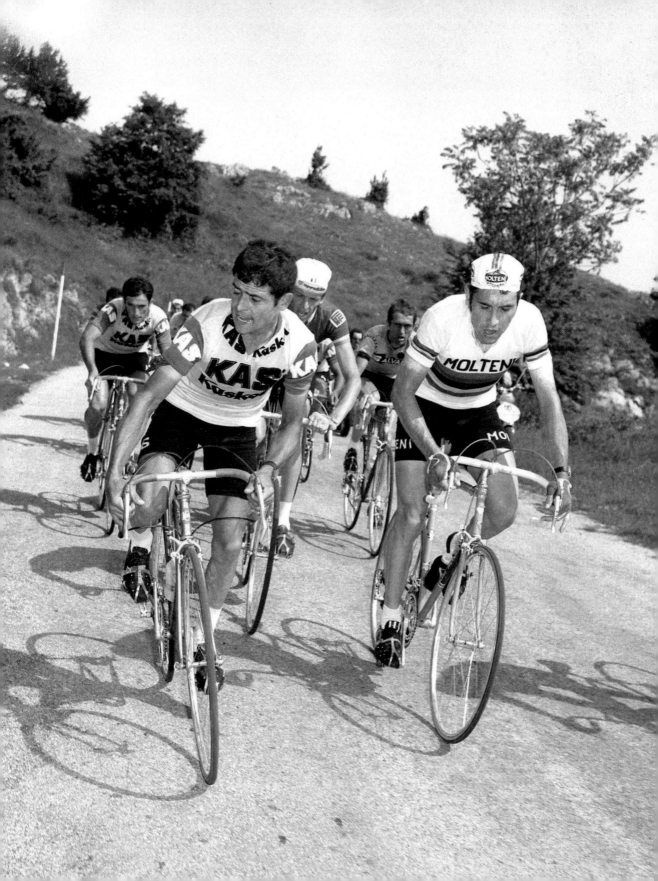

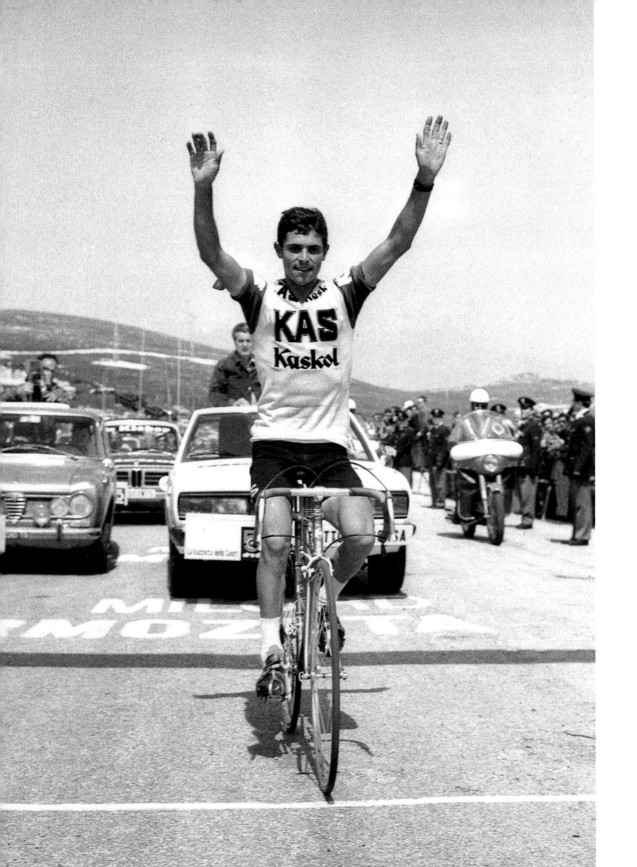

While I was there I had another Cipollini moment. He was going for his 42nd Giro stage win, trying to break Binda's record, but Alessandro Petacchi kept beating him. Cipo was 36, and Petacchi was simply younger and faster. After a week or so we had a stage in central Italy with a big climb, and Cipo's team just went to the front of the peloton. They lined out there and essentially forbade anyone from riding. The whole group twiddled over the climb and back down the other side, and Cipo got his stage win. It was nuts.

Eventually 45 of us were eliminated in the Alps. We were over the time limit, but we all assumed they wouldn't throw us out because there were only three stages left and Petacchi was with us. He'd won six stages and had the points jersey, but they wouldn't budge. So that was it. DNF.

If I were to characterise the difference between the Tour and the Giro I'd say the Tour was quite linear. It was usually quite predictable, whereas with the Giro anything could happen at any time – and it invariably did. You by and large knew what the weather was going to do in France, and how the stages would play out. The first week was about staying out of trouble, but after that you knew what was coming. It was medium mountains, then flat, then big mountains, transition, more big mountains, then time trial, then Paris. The Giro was infinitely more complicated, and the 2010 race was a case in point. You had these insanely hard central Italian stages in apocalyptic weather, then endless transfers, and the only constant was a sort of generalised chaos. I seem to remember Cadel Evans having a punch-up with a guy from Lampre because he was so stressed out by the whole thing.

The problem was that I . . . well, I don't know what the problem was really. Up until July 2012 my whole adult life had been about winning the Tour and the Olympics. I was utterly consumed by it and totally goal-driven. It's difficult to explain how I felt once that goal was achieved. If I'm honest, I'm not sure I've even properly processed it yet. I felt sort of rudderless and a little bit lost. I can count the number of times I went out and got drunk on one hand, although the rhetoric around my behaviour at the time tended to suggest just that. Alongside supporting my kids in their adjustment to all of a sudden having to share their daddy, throw in a court case and I guess you could say I was simply emotionally overwhelmed.

Despite this, I did my best in a physical sense and began training in earnest for the Giro. I started the season tired, but recovered well for Catalunya and Trentino. Heading into the Giro, I think I was walking a tightrope mentally. I fell off it pretty spectacularly.

We started with a team time trial on Ischia. We won it, and I decided to let Salvatore Puccio cross the line first. He was a nice kid from the south, and the *maglia rosa* meant the world to him. There was a long time trial, 55 kilometres I think, and the plan was for me to put three minutes into Nibali and then defend. By rights I should have been

Winning Stage 4a on Blockhaus in the Apennines in the 1972 Giro d'Italia.

able to do that, but I punctured after five kilometres. The problem was I was riding a prototype bike, the Bolide, and the front wheel was held in place by an Allen key. You couldn't just change it as you would normally, so I was given a completely different bike. It was quite wet, the course was rolling and there was a lot of descending, and the long and the short of it was that my head went after the puncture. Alex Dowsett beat me, and I only put a few seconds into Nibali. From there on it was just a downward spiral. I crashed the following day and injured my knee. I wasn't a happy man. In the final analysis I just made a mess of it. The problem with the TT bike wasn't my fault *per se*, but if I'm honest, as well as crashing and getting sick, I didn't have it mentally at that time.

So I never won the Giro. Fuente was a climber and I was a tester, and he was one of the best never to have achieved it. Over the course of his career he spent 15 days in the *maglia rosa*, but he was basically an amateur. Franco Bitossi once said that he raced 'like a maniac', and Bitossi knew a thing or two about racing.

There are pictures of Fuente smoking *during* races, and there were rumours that he was also a big drinker and a womaniser. In terms of climbing ability he was up there with Charly Gaul and Marco Pantani, but just like them he was a bit … *different*. He seemed to treat the Giro as a busman's holiday.

Merckx tells a story about the 1972 Giro, Fuente's second. The previous year Fuente had won two stages and the mountains jersey, and everyone knew he was a GC threat. That was a problem for Eddy, because Fuente came to the Giro having won the Vuelta, and the Giro was very mountainous that year. Then there were only 58 kilometres of TT, although for a climber Fuente wasn't bad against the watch.

Stage 4 was a split stage, and the first part was 48 kilometres. They rolled off the Adriatic coast south of Pescara, did 30 kilometres of false flat, and went straight up the Blockhaus. Fuente not only sent a dozen riders home over the time limit, but he beat Eddy by 2 minutes 35 seconds. He took the jersey, and seemed to have Eddy where he wanted him. They were at anti-doping, and Eddy overheard him telling the journalists that he'd only just got started. In three days' time there was going to be a stage out of Cosenza, starting with a 30-kilometre climb up Monte Scuro. It was one of those murderously hard Calabrese stages, and he said his plan was to attack straight away. He said he'd take Eddy by surprise, and send him home *fuori tempo massimo*.

On the morning of the stage Eddy and the rest of the Moltenis rode for an hour and a half. They were warmed up when the racing started, and Eddy went hard straight away. The peloton shattered, and by the time they reached the summit only four were left: Merckx, Fuente, his KAS *domestique* Lazcano and the Swede Gösta Pettersson. Fuente started sprinting for the mountains prize, but when Eddy came round him he sat up. So Eddy took the points, and Pettersson sprinted over the top in second

Always battling with Merckx. Jos Deschoenmaker and Merckx lead Fuente on Stage 13 of the 1973 Giro d'Italia. Merckx won the GC again that year, with Fuente finishing eighth.

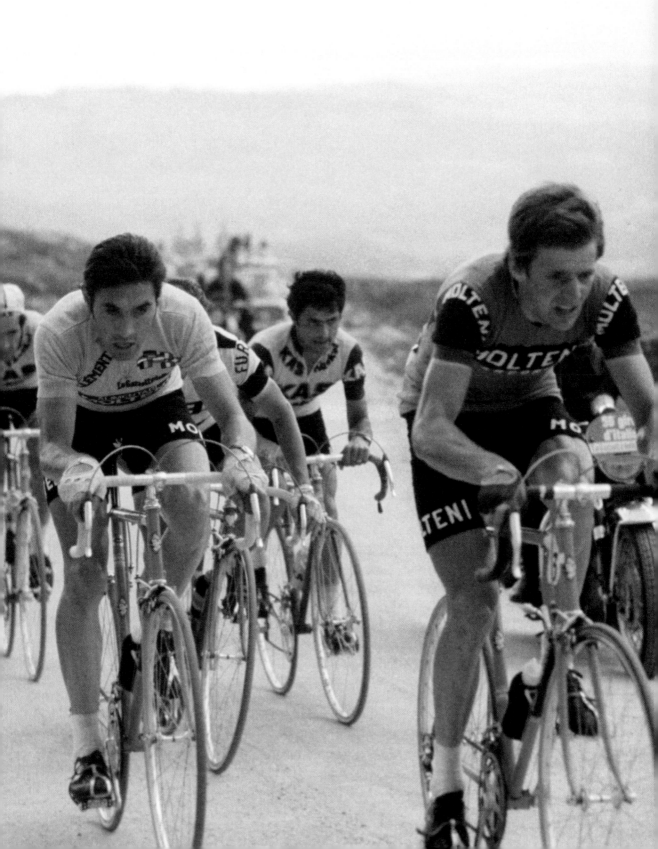

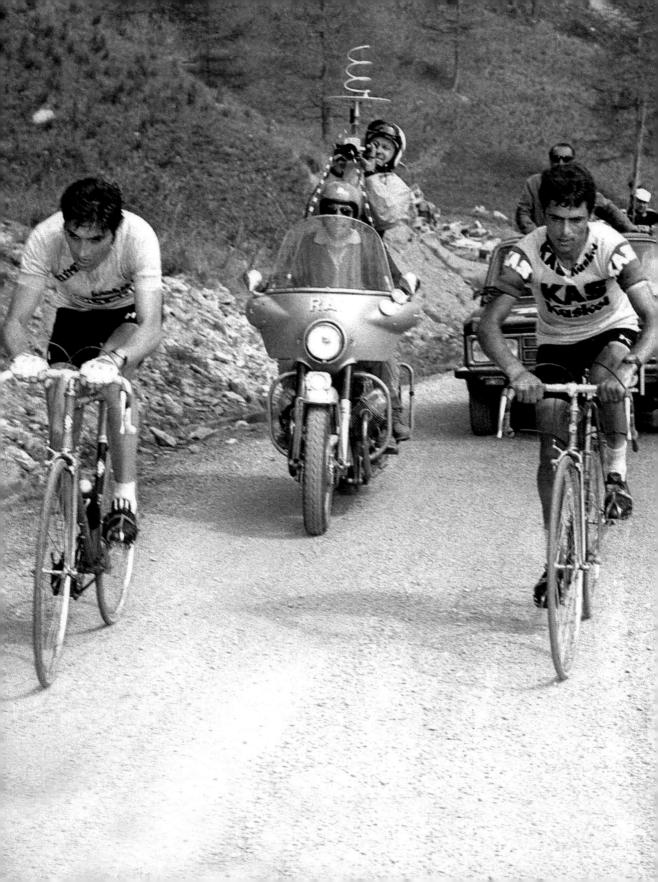

place. Then, while Fuente and Lazcano dithered, the two of them started gunning the descent. By the time Fuente had figured out what was going on it was too late, as Pettersson was both a cracking descender and a great time triallist. He and Eddy rode a 120-kilometre two-up all the way to Catanzaro, and by the time Fuente got there he'd lost over four minutes. Merckx had out-thought him, and the Giro was his.

Two years later Fuente won one of the most dramatic of all Vueltas. He was from Oviedo in Asturias, a poor city in a desperately poor region, and he was its pride and joy. Stage 13 finished at the Santa María del Naranco, the famous church that overlooks the town. The Santa María is the symbol of Oviedo, and so – in a sporting context – was Fuente. He began the stage in the leader's jersey, but KAS, for all that they wore the same jerseys and rode the same bikes, were a motley crew. The company was Basque and most of the riders were Basque, but internally there were all sorts of rivalries. One of the Basques, Miguel María Lasa, attacked the prodigal son on the road to Oviedo. This was diabolical in itself, but worse still he dragged the Portuguese champion Joaquim Agostinho along. Agostinho was a serious GC threat, to a large extent because he was the best time triallist in the race. Fuente produced one of his greatest rides to bring them back, and then clung on in the time trial to beat Agostinho by 11 seconds.

Four days later the Giro started, and Fuente totally dominated Merckx. He won three mountain stages in the south and in the Apennines, and led Merckx before they even *reached* the Dolomites. He looked to have it sewn up, but then he forgot to eat on a rolling stage in Liguria. He famously bonked and lost eight minutes, handing Merckx his fifth Giro on a plate. *The Greatest Show on Earth* doesn't show it, but legend has it all hell broke loose at the hotel that evening. Spain was a much poorer country even than Italy, and his lack of professionalism cost his *domestiques* a fortune in prize money.

The following year he couldn't finish a race. At first nobody understood why, but it transpired he'd developed a kidney complaint. The Spanish Federation refused him a racing licence for 1976, and he had to go cap-in-hand to Felice Gimondi's Bianchi for a ride. It was hopeless, however, and the greatest climber of his generation was finished before his 30th birthday. He opened a bike shop, and later worked for another legendary Spanish team, TEKA, but died aged 50.

José Manuel Fuente's professional career only lasted five years. In that time he won the Vuelta twice and contrived to lose the Giro twice. He remains a romantic, slightly ethereal figure, and he was a very special talent. But you didn't beat Merckx with romance, nor with talent alone. For that you needed discipline, conviction and tactical appreciation, all the things he lacked.

Somehow his *maglia rosa* – damaged, evocative and ultimately lost – is pure José Manuel Fuente . . .

Side by side again with Merckx in the 1972 Giro d'Italia.

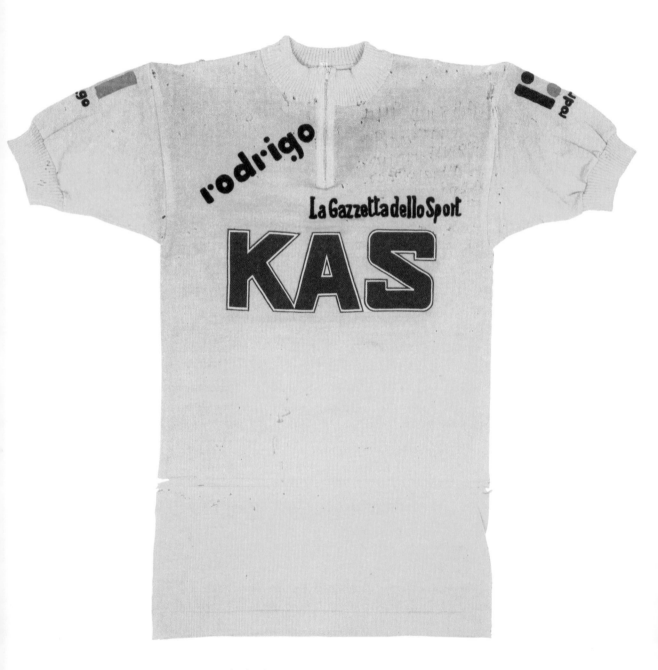

1974 Giro d'Italia *maglia rosa* from Stage 9, Monte Carpegna

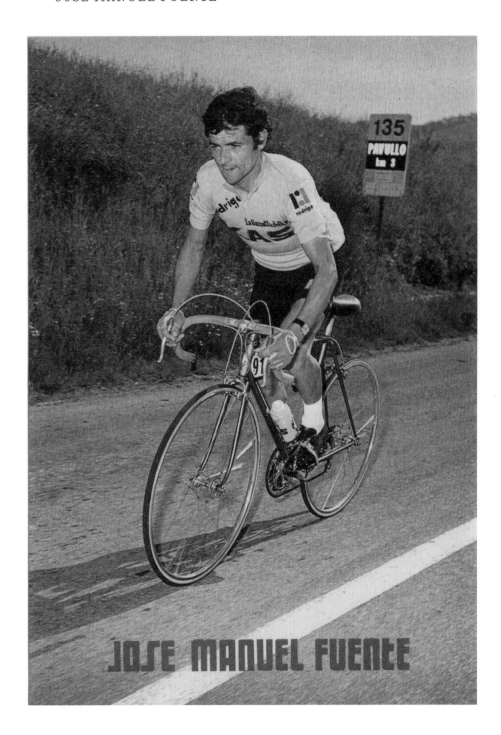

Wearing the *maglia rosa* at the 1974 Giro d'Italia. He'd later bonk and lose eight minutes on the stage to Liguria.

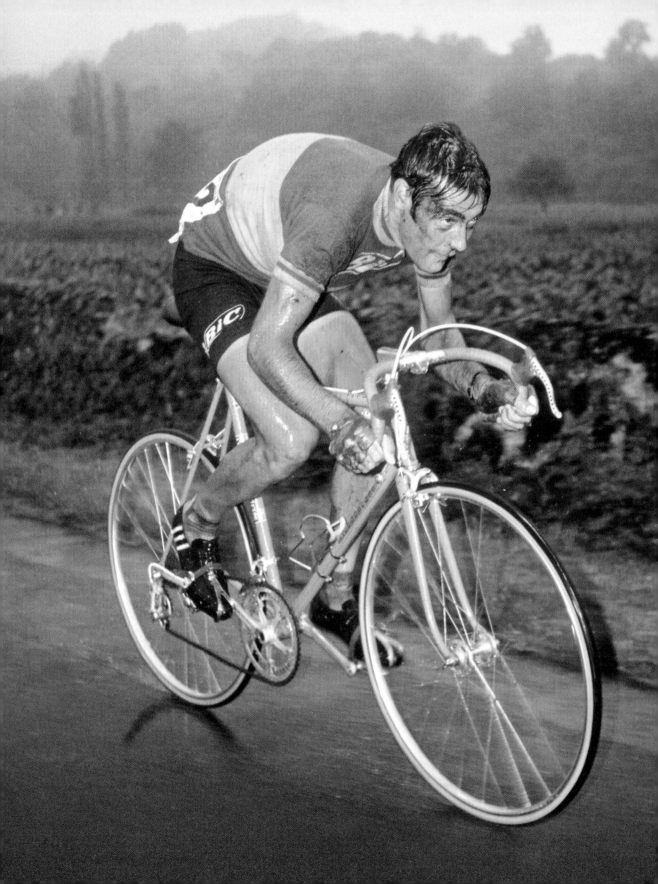

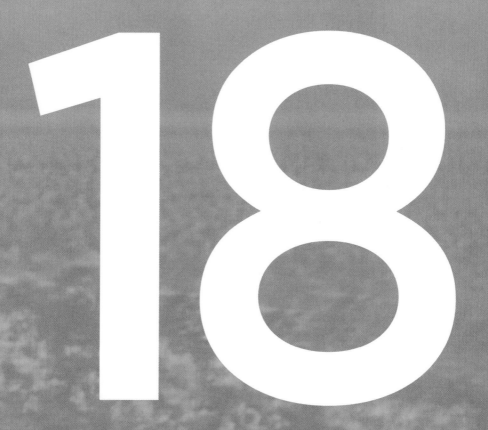

18

Luis Ocaña

1945–1994

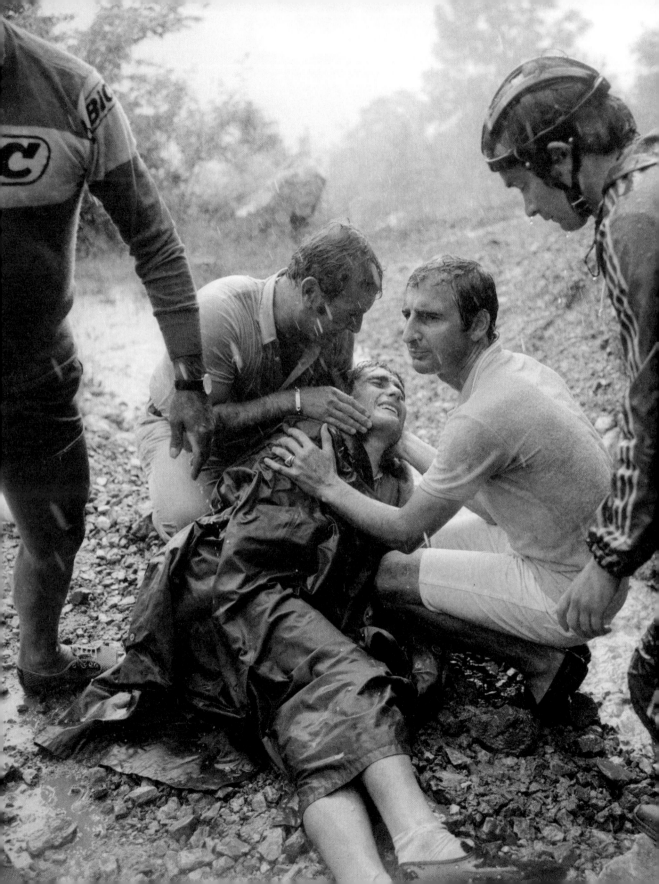

Post-Tour it was just a rollercoaster. I was on every front page, and woke up the following morning to a TV camera pointed at my daughter's bedroom window. Overnight I became much bigger than the sport I was part of, and much bigger than myself. I became a 'celebrity' and I got swept along in it all. Everyone was telling me how great I was and everyone wanted to be my friend.

I was living my childhood dream, but not in some glib, throwaway way. I'd grown up idolising Induráin, and wondering what it must have felt like to win the Tour. Now I was a Tour de France winner and, for all that I was 32, the whole thing felt like make-believe.

The Tour giveth, but the Tour taketh away. I'd been working towards winning it for years. Now I was a bit lost. Nobody from Britain had won the Tour before so there was no trail, no set path, no 'you should do this next'. It was difficult, as well as utterly fantastic (yet at home our daughter, six years old, was struggling to process it all).

The Tour may change your circumstances, but it can't fundamentally change who – and what – you are. Cycling made me famous, but I'm not entirely sure it made me better or more complete. I would never say I wish I hadn't won the Tour, but there have been times, particularly amid the media storm of 2018, when Cath and I have struggled with the *effects* of my having won it.

And I know for a fact that I'm not alone in that . . .

Moments after his crash on the descent of the Col de Menté on Stage 14 of the 1971 Tour de France.

URING MY FIRST GIRO, in 2003, I briefly found myself riding alongside Marco Pantani. By then it was five years on from his Giro–Tour double. They'd excluded him from the 1999 Giro, and since then his life seemed to have spiralled out of control. No matter how many people were around him, he always seemed to be alone. The best way I can describe it is that he seemed to be encircled by some sort of invisible fence, an exclusion zone. I didn't know it at the time, but he was riding a grand tour in the grip of a full-blown cocaine addiction. I have no idea how he managed that, but within nine months he'd commit suicide.

I once sat next to Frank Vandenbroucke on an aeroplane. He was another guy cursed by unimaginable talent who died too soon. A lot of sublimely gifted people – sportsmen or otherwise – are just too magic to fit in this world.

Needless to say I'm no Pantani, but I have a tendency to go off the rails if I don't keep myself in check. I need continuity in my life, and sport is important in that sense. That largely explains my interest in rowing; I took it up when I finished cycling not only because it's healthy for my body, but also for my mind.

There was a time when I thought being famous was great, and I'm thankful for all the opportunities and experiences it's brought me, but you live and learn. I think you mainly learn about yourself, and it's abundantly clear that neither Cath nor I are particularly cut out for it. We're neither of us polished enough – we're both flawed characters – and we have enough on our plates dealing with the day-to-day stuff. The main focus is the kids, who are wonderful, and like most parents our main interest is taking care of them and one another.

We have a place in Mallorca, though, and there's a nice little restaurant on the island that we like to visit. The owner loves cycling, and one day he started telling me about a rider he'd once idolised. This rider was a Tour winner too, but if ever there was a case study in the price of sporting achievement and fame, he was it.

His story is best encapsulated by another of those seminal Tour de France photos, albeit one very different to the image of Nencini at the Parc des Princes. It was taken during the 1971 edition, under a deluge in the Pyrenees, and shows a stricken, tormented bike rider. He's wearing the *maillot jaune*, but his bike is nowhere to be seen. Instead he's on the floor, his body twisted and his face convulsed in agony. He's crashed on the descent of the Col de Menté, near the Spanish border, and his race is over. Where Nencini's photo captures a moment in time, this one captures a life in terrible, tragic microcosm.

Luis Ocaña was born in Cuenca but grew up close to the French border. When he was 12 he and his family crossed the Pyrenees and settled in Aquitaine. He struggled to assimilate and started to have problems with authority, with building and sustaining

With José Manuel Fuente on Stage 17 of the 1973 Tour de France. Ocaña would win the GC that year, with Fuente finishing third.

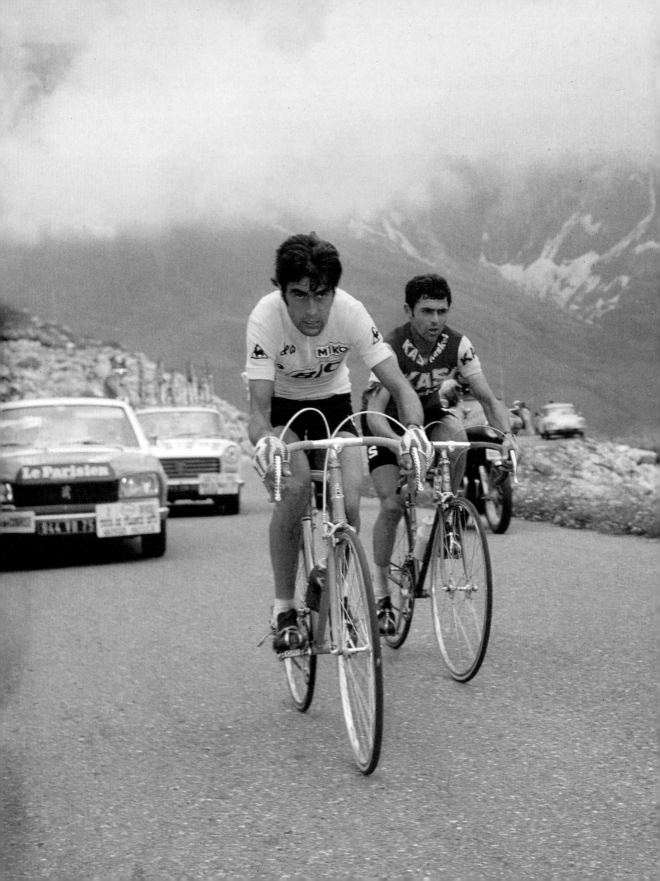

relationships, with intimacy and with his identity. A wilful, fragile and hyper-sensitive character, he seems to have blamed his father for having uprooted him.

He left school at 14, got a job with a local carpenter and borrowed his cousin's bike to get to work. Then, like a lot of conflicted adolescents – yours truly included – he just kept going. It's an old, old story, that of thousands of professional riders over the last hundred years. They start riding for the job, then to escape, then to explore, and finally it becomes their identity and their vocation.

He joined the local club, and it was immediately obvious that he was a natural. Although he instinctively pushed well-wishers away, he developed a close relationship with the club president, Pierre Cescutti, and as his relationship with his father floundered, Cescutti became a sort of surrogate. He would remain a constant throughout Ocaña's life.

By the time he was 21 he was competing as an independent. He won the biggest amateur races in France, and when he rode against the professionals he was among the best of them. As the 1968 season approached he was the hottest property in French cycling, the trade teams queuing up to sign him.

Mercier had been supplying him with bikes and jerseys for two years on the assumption that he'd become naturalised and sign for them. This was Ocaña, however, and he wasn't much for following advice. Instead he turned his back on them, and by extension on French cycling. He chose to assert his Spanish identity by joining Fagor, and that June he became national champion. He took the jersey and offered it, by way of a peace gesture, to his dying father. It was one of the defining moments of Luis's life, but it ended in failure. His father died later that summer, before they were truly reconciled.

The following year he could and should have won the Vuelta. On Stage 12 he looked set to take the jersey on a mountainous stage in Catalonia. He needed only to ride with Roger Pingeon, but instead he decided to go to war with him. Pingeon was too strong and too knowing, and Ocaña blew up. He lost over three minutes and had to settle for second on GC. Following victory at Midi Libre, he began the Tour as Fagor's GC rider but crashed horrifically on a descent in the Vosges. That he finished the stage at all was a miracle, and he insisted that they patch him up for the next day. It was lunacy even to try to ride on but ride on he did, head to toe in bandages. Having proved his bravery, he climbed off the following day.

He made amends by winning the 1970 Vuelta with a blistering final-day time trial, but it didn't endear him to the Spanish public. By then he'd signed for Bic, a French team, and in winning it he overtook the popular climber Agustín Tamames. Whatever he did and whatever he said, he wasn't quite Spanish enough for the Spanish.

Having just signed for Bic, Ocaña rides alongside the master on Stage 4 of the 1970 Tour de France, the second of Merckx's five overall victories at the Tour.

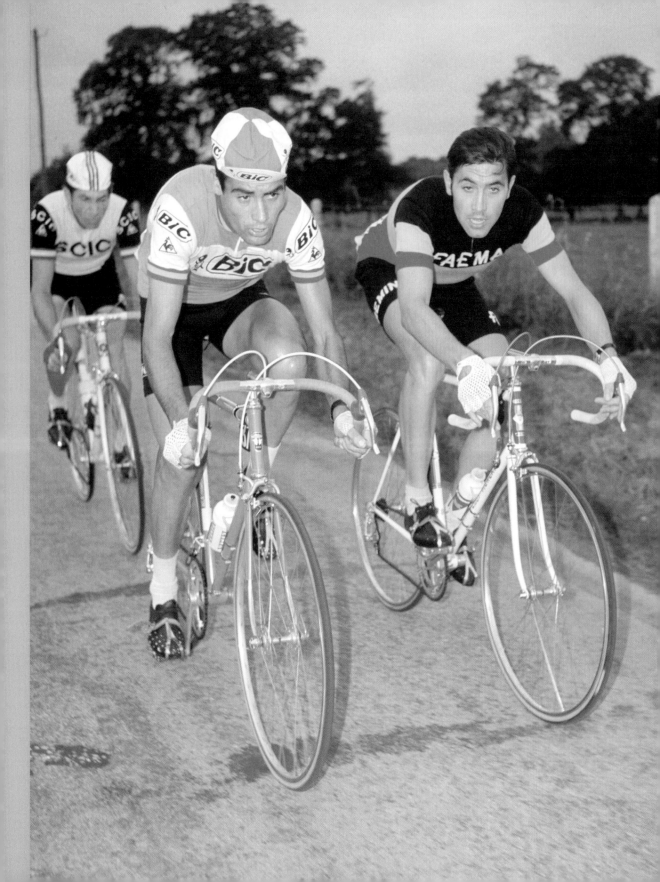

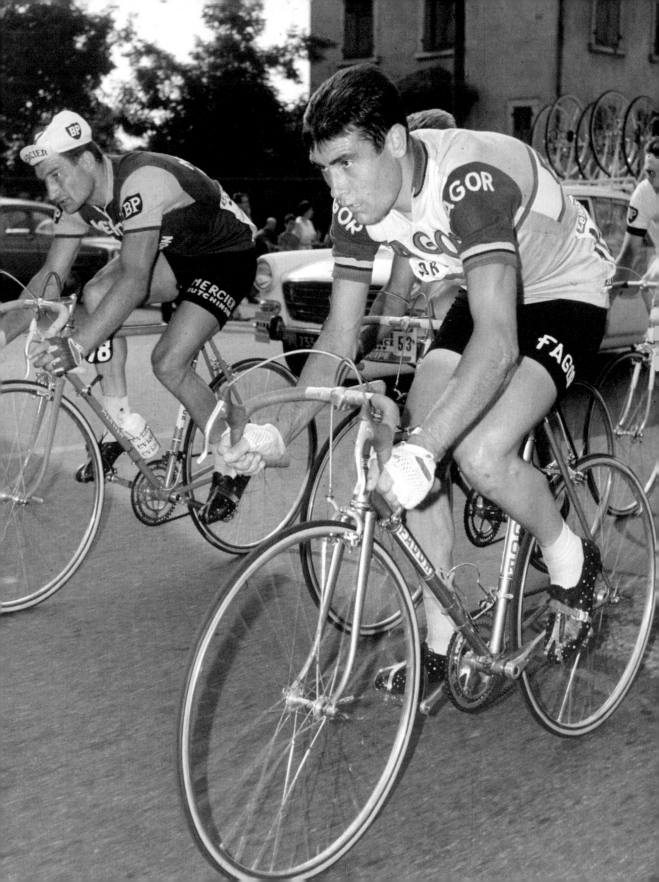

Before that year's Tour he boasted that he'd beat Merckx. It was wishful thinking, and he was naïve to have said it in public. He was off the pace throughout, had to settle for a stage win. What's more, there always seemed to be tension around him. In his personal life he was irascible and unpredictable, and in a cycling context he was virtually unmanageable. Physically he was a tour de force, but psychologically he was completely troubled.

He started to become consumed with beating Merckx, as well as about being beaten by a new star, José Manuel Fuente. People often compare the two of them, as if there were some sort of Spanish anti-Merckx coalition. In fact, there was nothing of the sort and they couldn't have been more different. Where Ocaña was complicated, Fuente was anything but. Where Ocaña needed, absolutely, to be the best, Fuente just needed to ride his bike. Fuente lacked focus, but Ocaña developed tunnel vison. His obsession with proving his strength clouded his judgement, and a cyclist who lacks judgement is a cyclist who crashes. Luis Ocaña crashed. Often.

Fuente was much more popular in Spain. People warmed to his honesty and simplicity, and they very much warmed to his genius as a climber. This was almost unbearable for a soul as hyper-sensitive as Ocaña, and when Fuente won the 1971 Vuelta he became even more desperate. He had to win the Tour, because only by winning the Tour could he win the various arguments raging inside his own head.

He dropped Merckx on the Puy de Dôme, and then put nine minutes into him on an unforgettable stage in the Alps. Heading into the Pyrenees it seemed the Tour would be his, but Merckx was never one for lying down. He reasoned that he probably couldn't beat Ocaña, but he knew that Ocaña was more than capable of beating himself.

As they reached the top of the Col de Menté a storm broke. The descent became treacherous, and for Merckx that meant one thing and one thing only – he attacked. He fell, but then so did the others. When Ocaña came off he was hit first by Agostinho and then by Joop Zoetemelk. He was helicoptered off to hospital as Fuente, of all people, galloped to the stage win, and Merckx to the Tour.

By the time the 1972 Tour came round he could barely bring himself to look at Merckx, let alone talk to him. He was Spanish national champion again, but he was on the edge psychologically and contracted bronchitis during the second week. He climbed off on Stage 14, as Merckx bossed the race again.

The following year Merckx decided not to go to France. He wanted to emulate Anquetil and Gimondi in winning all three grand tours, although the Vuelta was still only 17 stages, so he opted for Spain and Italy instead. In preparation for the Vuelta, he and Ocaña met at Catalan Week. Wearing his silk national champion's jersey, Ocaña thumped Merckx in the time trial to win the GC. They both knew it was the phoney

In Fagor kit at the 1969 Tour de France.

war, but at last he looked back to his pre-Col de Menté best. With Fuente absent at the Tour of Romandie, the scene was set for the mother of all rematches.

But it was no contest. Merckx won six stages, including all the time trials, the 'races of truth'. He dominated the bike race, and he dominated poor, tortured Luis Ocaña.

Ocaña ran away with the Dauphiné, and then with the Tour. He won six stages, wore yellow for eighteen days, and finished 15 minutes in front. It was a stupendous performance, and it settled the argument with Fuente. It settled arguments with Thévenet, Zoetemelk and Van Impe as well, but not the one that mattered. He'd won a Tour without Merckx, and in his gut he knew that a Tour without Merckx was a Tour without anybody.

He'd conquered the Alps and the Pyrenees, but he couldn't and wouldn't conquer his own demons.

From that point on, things pretty much just fell in on themselves. Like so many Tour de France wins (my own included), this was the beginning of the end of his career. In advance of the 1974 Worlds he told the Spanish Federation that if they selected Fuente he wouldn't ride, and to all intents and purposes they told him to take a running jump. He carried on for a few more years, but he never won another grand tour and his performances petered out prematurely.

With his career – and Spain's golden age – over, he worked as a sporting director, but was badly injured in a car crash in 1979. He needed blood transfusions for the rest of his life, and one left him with hepatitis C. When his wine business failed he ran into financial problems, then stood for election with the right-wing Front national.

It didn't work. Nothing did.

By 1994 his will was broken. He'd developed liver cancer and was bankrupt financially, spiritually and mentally.

Aged 48, overwhelmed with the crushing weight of the financial and emotional burden, Ocaña took a gun from the cupboard. An utterly tragic end.

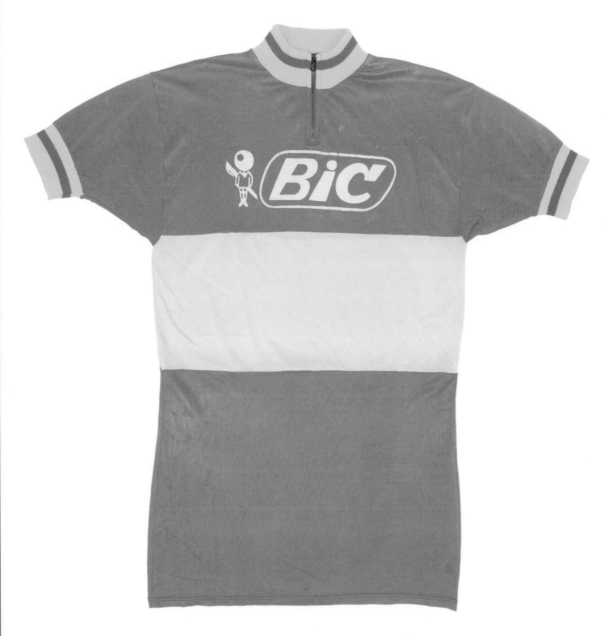

Luis Ocaña's Spanish national champion's jersey worn in the 1973
Vuelta TT

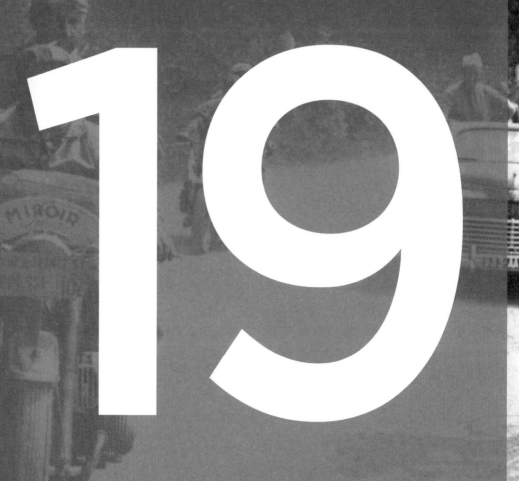

19

Hugo Koblet

1925–1964

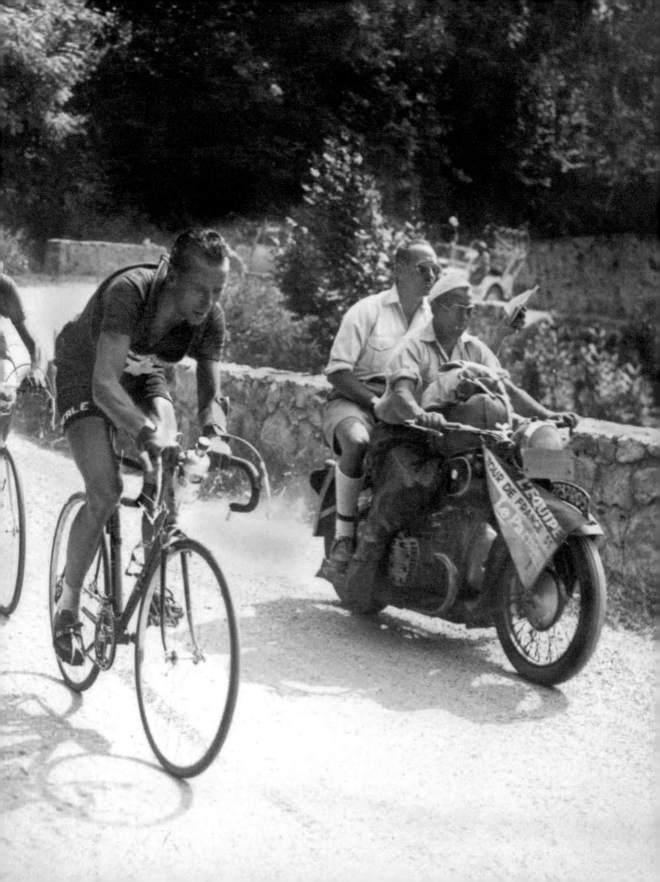

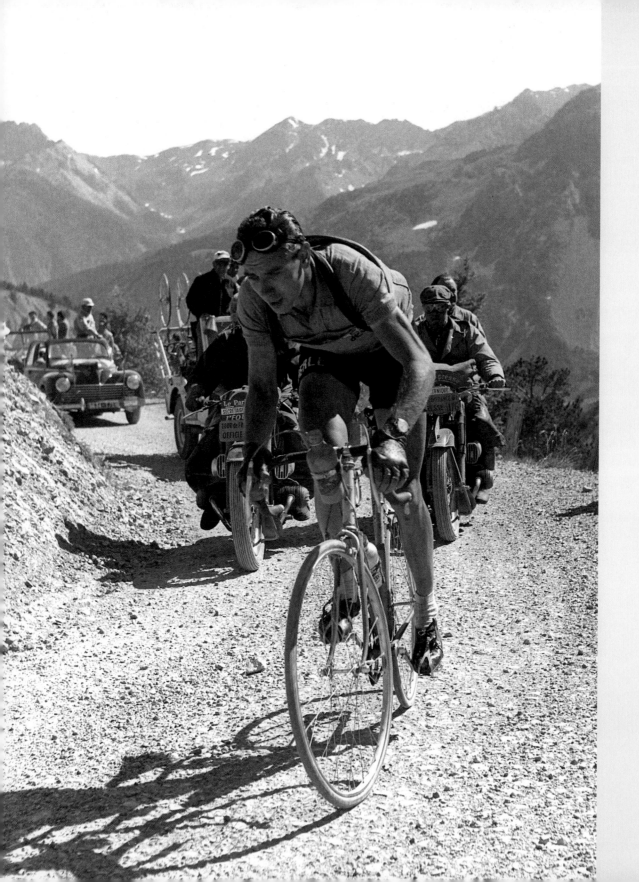

There have been more successful riders than Hugo Koblet, and more enduring riders. I don't think, however, that there's ever been one so mystical, so beautiful or so romantic. It's almost 70 years since he turned Planet Cycling on its axis, but among the *cognoscenti* his star burns just as brightly as it ever did.

Hugo came from Zurich, but in a cycling context he appeared from nowhere. When they announced the start list for the 1950 Giro he wasn't one of the favourites, nor even one of the outsiders. He was a 25-year-old track rider; handy enough as a pursuiter, but with precisely no grand tour experience. His best stage-racing result had been tenth at the Tour de Suisse, and truth be told hardly anyone gave him a second thought.

Having done the Giro–Tour double the previous year, Fausto Coppi was odds-on. Conventional wisdom had it that he'd run away with it, and that Gino Bartali, Fiorenzo Magni and Switzerland's great idol, Ferdi Kübler, would be left to fight over the crumbs. They were

offering 150/1 against Hugo, but it seems that even then they couldn't find any takers. He rolled out of Milan practically unknown, but by the time he arrived in Rome three weeks later he was the talk of the town.

He'd ridden into the pink jersey on the stage to Vicenza, and the following day Coppi had fallen off and hospitalised himself yet again. This time he'd broken his pelvis, and even Fausto couldn't ride a bike in that condition. The Italians threw their lot in with Gino 'The Pious' Bartali – after all, there was to be an audience with the Pope for the winner – but there was nothing to be done. On 13 June 1950 Hugo Koblet became the Giro's first foreign winner and – incredibly – its first *Protestant* winner. He'd won over Italian men with his cycling, and Italian women with his Hollywood good looks. He'd become a household name and, apparently, a bona fide rival to the *campionissimo* Coppi.

And that, by anybody's standard, was a pretty decent return for three weeks of cycling . . .

Racing for the Swiss national team in the 1951 Tour de France, which he won by 22 minutes from Raphaël Géminiani.

WHEN ALBERTO CONTADOR attacked on the climb to Verbier at the 2009 Tour, I was in no position to go with him. He was the best, and I was just happy to be thereabouts. The following year I was useless at the Tour, and in 2011 our paths never crossed. He rode the Giro, and I finished up with a broken collarbone at the Tour. Then Alberto was suspended when I won in 2012, and in 2013 I rode the Giro while he did the Tour. As a latecomer to stage racing that was me pretty much done, and so one way or another I never got to race him on equal terms.

Now Contador was a better stage racer than me – and, for that matter, everyone else of our generation – but I'd have liked to have raced him at least once when I was at my best. I can't say I *regret* his not having been at the 2012 Tour, you can only beat the people you race against. Being on the top step alongside Froome and Nibali is pretty decent by anyone's standards. Contador was one very special bike rider, however, and he was the benchmark by which the rest of us measured ourselves.

I suppose what I'm trying to say, in a roundabout sort of way, is that there are races that happen, and races that don't. There are the races we know about and the races we *think* we know about, because we've read about them in magazines, in books or on the internet. What we think we know often doesn't correspond with the truth, because it's a sequence of events that have been interpreted by journalists who know nothing of what goes on inside the peloton. There's another category to add to that as well. It's what I call the almost-races, the ones that took place in real time, but didn't actually tell us anything.

Hugo Koblet's story is of all of the above. He won one (that 1950 Giro) that we know about, and famously lost another that we *think* we know about. We'll come to that one shortly, but the third, the almost-race – the one that on paper was the greatest Tour de France of all – remains essentially unraced. In practical terms Hugo took part in it and won it, but for reasons that I'll explain it remains a dream unfulfilled . . .

To fully understand all of the above, you need to have a basic grounding in the world as it was back then. We've learned from Coppi's Cuneo-Pinerolo that television existed only as a scientific concept. Sport was consumed via the radio and the newspapers, and the sporting landscape was pretty narrow. Only the super-rich dared even contemplate car ownership, and motor sport's popularity was a reflection of the fact. Golf and skiing weren't so much sports as games played by the ruling classes, and tennis was also the preserve of the wealthy. Rugby was played mainly in Britain, south-western France and a few pockets of the Veneto, and the USA was a long, long way away. Basketball was starting to get a foothold in Europe, but most Europeans were completely ignorant of it. Swimming, athletics and boxing were fairly popular, and in the winter football took centre stage.

We're used to the idea of fooball as a global sport, and as the most popular sport. It's a multi-billion-dollar industry, but it owes its success almost entirely to television.

At the 1954 Giro d'Italia, won by his friend and *gregario* Carlo Clerici.

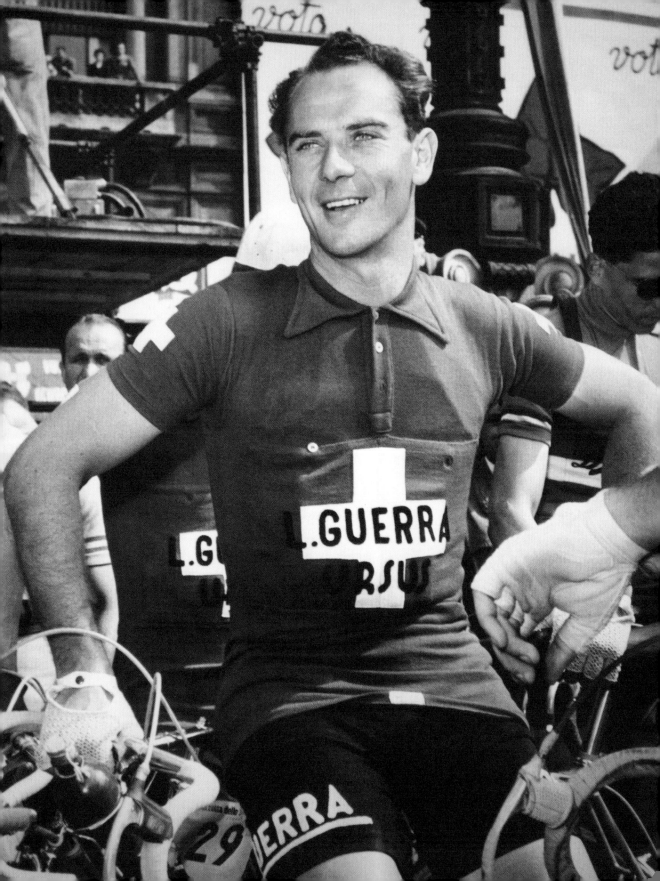

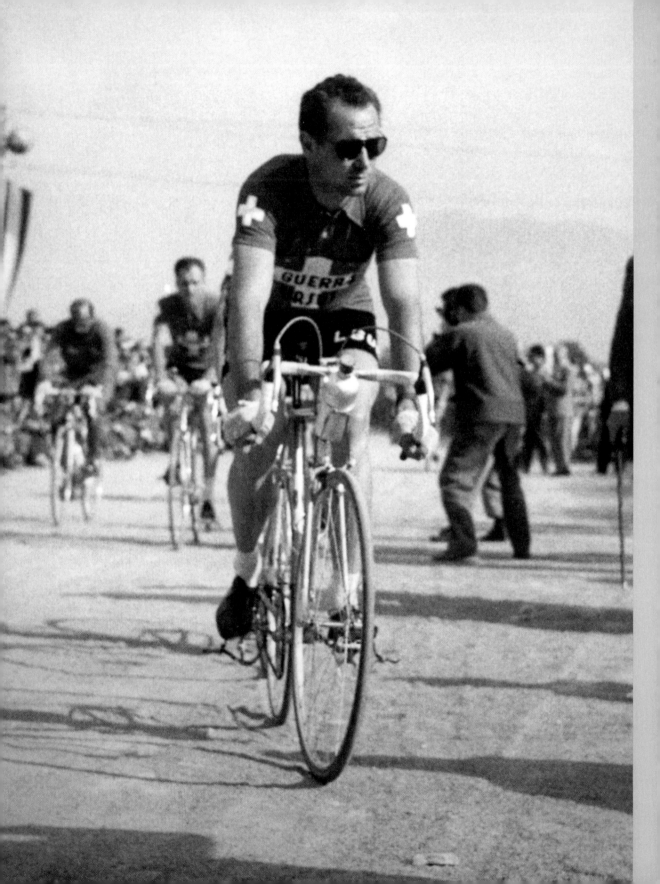

It was – and remains – the perfect TV sport because it was simple and partisan, and because the programmers knew the start, interval and finish times precisely. From a scheduling and advertising point of view, therefore, it was much, much easier than cycling. Our sport was textured and complicated, and it had too many variables for TV. There were no helicopter cameras, and it took place not in a stadium but out on the open road. To make matters worse, the coverage, such as it was in the early days, was lousy. The producers had no idea when the riders would turn up, and when they did they were only able to televise the last couple of minutes. It was basically hopeless, and worse still it played havoc with the schedules.

The so-called 'golden age' of cycling, broadly 1946 to 1953, pre-dated all that. People gathered round the radio to listen to the races, then read about them the following day in sports papers like the *Gazzetta dello Sport*, *L'Équipe* and *Marca*. They watched brief, dramatic newsreel footage of the highlights at the cinema before the main feature, and the racers were portrayed as supermen. Bike ownership was the highest it's ever been (Vespas and Lambrettas were still far too expensive for the majority), and people who ride bikes can easily relate to people who race them. Cycling's champions were household names just as Federer, Hamilton, Neymar and Messi are today. It's no coincidence that the first superstar footballers – the likes of Pelé – didn't emerge until the TV age. As regards post-war fame and public affection, cycling was the only show in town.

Because of all this, Hugo's Giro catapulted him to instant superstardom all across Europe. In addition to his God-given talent he was charming, incredibly handsome and extremely bankable. He confirmed he wasn't a flash-in-the-pan by winning the Tour de Suisse a few weeks later, and suddenly advertisers, manufacturers and sponsors couldn't get enough of him. I know that feeling.

That July his compatriot Kübler concluded a miraculous summer for the Swiss by winning the Tour. They'd been waiting fifty years for a grand tour winner and now, much like me and Froome in modern-day Britain, two had come along all at once. The 'Two Ks' were as different as night and day, a sort of Swiss Coppi and Bartali. A Coppi and a Bartali, a Coe and an Ovett, a Wiggins and a Froome, you name it.

Ferdi Kübler was an old-school, blood-and-thunder sort of a rider. He'd won the Tour in bizarre circumstances – Bartali had forced the entire Italian team to retire while Magni was in yellow – but in truth neither he nor Magni were in Coppi's class over three weeks. Nor, yet, was the young Frenchman Louison Bobet, while 36-year-old Bartali was nearing the end.

Koblet was something else altogether. Like Coppi he was generous and courteous off the bike, and just like Coppi he had immense class on it. He'd so dominated the Giro that many believed he'd have won even if Coppi hadn't fallen off. That was as

Stage 1 of the 1954 Giro d'Italia, the team time trial in Palermo, won by Bianchi.

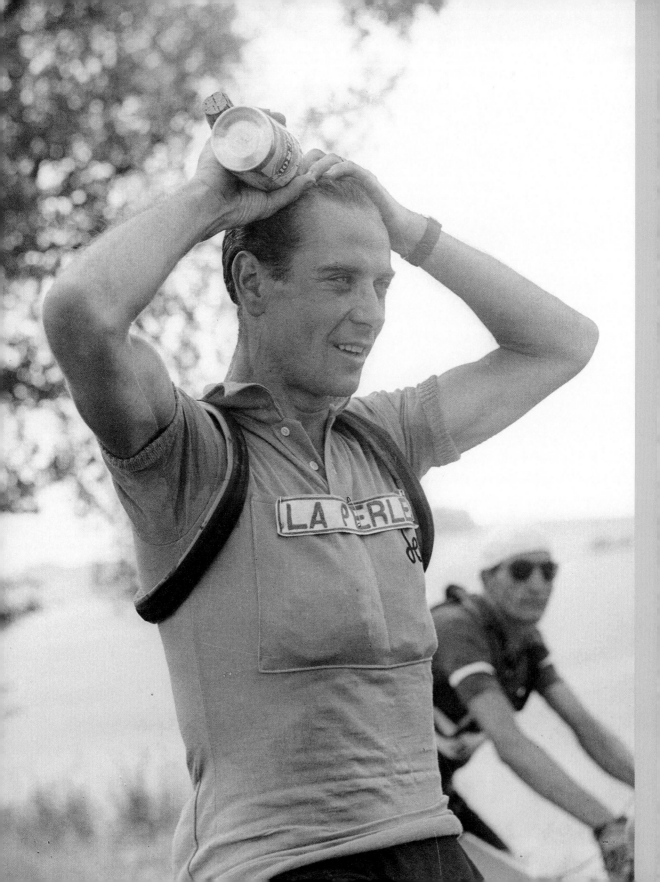

maybe, but when Hugo announced that he was going to ride the 1951 Tour, everyone stood up and took note. Coppi had seen off Bartali, but now he had a new challenger to deal with. He and Koblet, the old *campionissimo* and the new, would be going head to head first at the Giro and then at the Tour. Cycling was in turmoil.

In Italy, the 1951 season opened with Milano–Torino. It took place a week before Milan–San Remo and finished in the velodrome. A group of five broke away from the field, among them Coppi. As they started the sprint, however, Coppi's front wheel collided with Alfredo Martini's back, and (what with him being Coppi and all) he fell and broke his collarbone. He wasn't able to touch his bike for over a month, which meant he arrived at the Giro underdone. Koblet was using the race mainly as training for the Tour, and they both missed the break on the stage to Naples. In the circumstances neither had the form to be able to recover in the mountains, so Fiorenzo Magni won his second Giro. Coppi and Koblet finished fourth and sixth respectively, but everyone had expected the Giro to be the phoney war anyway. They'd reconvene in France on 4 July, for the most eagerly awaited Tour in years.

On 22 June Koblet and Ferdi Kübler fought an immense duel. The penultimate stage of the Tour de Suisse took them over the giant Bernina Pass, and the two of them soon dropped the rest of the field. 'The Dove' Koblet distanced 'The Eagle' Kübler to win the stage, and, although Ferdi held on to win the GC, Hugo's form had arrived just in time. He was ready, while Coppi's final warm-up would be three days later. The Tour of Piedmont promised another finish in Turin's velodrome, a chance to right the wrongs of Milano–Torino and to kick-start the season just in time for the Tour.

Traditionally, many of cycling's great champions have ridden with their brothers as *domestiques*. Juraj Sagan is invaluable to Peter, while the greats Induráin and Louison Bobet were inseparable from Prudencio and Jean respectively. In post-war Italy you had the Maggini brothers, the Zanazzi brothers and the Rossello brothers, but most of all you had the Coppi brothers. Fausto's younger sibling, Serse, was a decent enough rider (he'd been joint winner of the 1949 Paris–Roubaix), but his brain and personality were better than his legs. He was funny, outgoing and popular in the group, and that helped in his role as Fausto's confidant and fixer.

As the peloton charged towards the velodrome, Serse's back wheel got caught in a tramline. He came off, hit his head, and started to complain of a terrible headache shortly afterwards at the hotel. Shortly before midnight, Serse Coppi passed away.

Fausto's wife, Bruna, pleaded with him to stop racing, but the pressure to carry on was overwhelming. People assume that sporting fame and fortune are liberating, but in the main the reverse is true. While you're competing you actually have *less* control, because the amount invested in you grows and grows, and your job is to provide a

Hugo does his hair on the way to Paris in 1951.

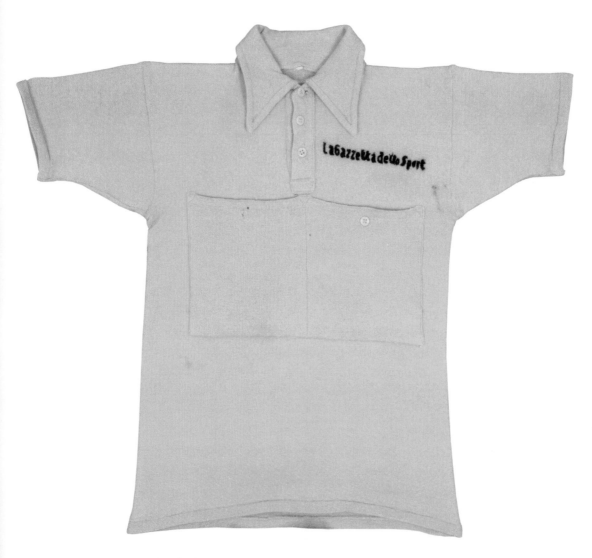

1953 Giro d'Italia *maglia rosa*, in which Koblet finished second to Fausto Coppi

return. Fausto couldn't simply walk away, and for him the bike was existential anyway. Life without Serse didn't bear thinking about, but life without the bike wouldn't be worth living. His morale was on the floor, but he knew that he had no choice either professionally or spiritually but to ride the Tour. He caught the slow train down to Metz.

On Stage 11, Brive to Agen, Hugo produced one of the Tour's most famous exploits. Defying all known cycling logic, he attacked 140 flattish kilometres from the finish. At first the chasers struggled to get organised, but 70 kilometres out they set to reeling him in. They were a 30-man team pursuit and he was one, but he time trialled to the finish to win by 2 minutes and 35 seconds. Afterwards Raphaël Géminiani, the best of the French riders, complained that 'a rider like Koblet isn't possible!', and the following day the French entertainer Jacques Grello famously referred to him as '*le pédaleur de charme*'. The nickname would stick, and sticks to this day. Hugo, they said, was never less than immaculate. He never rode without a comb, and never left home without his eau de Cologne.

The pedaller of charm. Absolutely perfect.

On Stage 16 to Montpellier, Coppi collapsed altogether. Some attributed it to food poisoning, others to stress, but either way he lost 33 minutes. Koblet won the stage, and from there on in the race was a demonstration. Hugo won a 97-kilometre time trial by five minutes and the *maillot jaune* by 22. Poor, wretched, broken Fausto finished tenth, 46 minutes behind.

On paper, the 1951 Tour de France represents Koblet's greatest triumph and Coppi's most appalling tragedy. In point of fact it was both. However, it was also, in some way, the greatest race there never was . . .

Coppi would win the Giro–Tour double for a second time in 1952, but Koblet was never the same rider again. Some said he experimented too much with steroids, some that he overdid it with amphetamines, some that the richer he became, the less he trained. Others said it was wine, women and song, but the chances are it was all of the above and none of the above. What we know for certain is that he contracted a renal complaint. It may or may not have been the consequence of his having 'doped' to satisfy race organisers and sponsors, but it certainly compromised his ability at altitude.

The jersey I have, a beautiful *maglia rosa* from the 1953 Giro, is illustrative. It was another extraordinary, iconic race, one of those we all think we know about but probably don't. The penultimate stage included a new climb, the likes of which had never been seen before. It was called the Passo Stelvio, and its highest point was 2,757 metres above sea level.

Koblet led Coppi by two minutes, and the legend – unsubstantiated – is that the two of them agreed a deal. Giulia Occhini, the *Dama Bianca*, would be at the finish, and Fausto was absolutely smitten. He knew that if they came in together he'd lose, because Hugo was a much better sprinter. As such they're reputed – *reputed*, mind . . . – to have done a deal. Koblet had been the stronger of the two, and now Coppi offered him what amounted to a truce. If Hugo would agree to forgo the stage win, Fausto promised not to attack him on the Stelvio. Instead they'd come in together, Hugo would keep the jersey, and Fausto would get to present the flowers of the stage win to his lover.

In the event Fausto *did* attack on the Stelvio, and *did* drop Hugo to win his fifth and final Giro. In the best cycling tradition there are all sorts of hypotheses as to *why* he did it, but to this day nobody truly knows. What we do know is that neither would win another grand tour, and that both would die prematurely and tragically.

As a sportsman you're driven largely by endorphins, and that's one of the reasons retirement is so difficult. I like to think I've made the transition pretty well, but I'm not going to pretend it's been easy. You can't reproduce the buzz of competition, because it's 100 per cent chemical. A lot of retired cyclists have struggled to come to terms with it, and have become unhealthy psychologically as well as physically. Some just never learned to cope. I think I have the normality of family life with my kids to thank.

Nor, sadly, did poor Hugo. He worked for Alfa Romeo in Caracas for a while, then came home and tried his hand as a radio presenter. He opened petrol stations, but somehow nothing quite worked out. His problem, they said, was that he possessed no business instinct. He spent money he didn't have, he was just too generous, and people took advantage of his kindness. He was also forever in and out of love, and following a string of affairs he found himself alone and in grave financial difficulty. Just past midnight on 2 November 1964, Hugo rammed his car into a sycamore tree on a quiet country road near Zurich. The press release said he'd been avoiding a crossing dog, but it transpired he'd driven up and down that road a few times beforehand. Back and forth, back and forth . . .

Hugo Koblet passed away just after midnight on 6 November. At 39, he was a year younger than Coppi had been when he died, and a year older than me as I write this. My age, more or less, and no age at all. The thought of it breaks my heart.

Hugo Koblet. There but for the grace of God.

Chatting with Fausto Coppi on the penultimate stage of the 1953 Giro d'Italia.

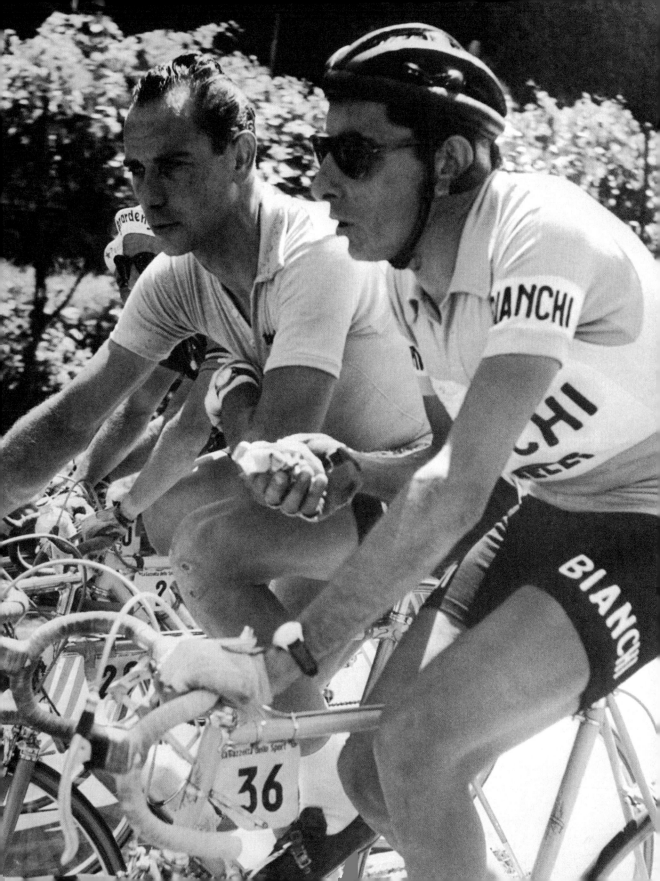

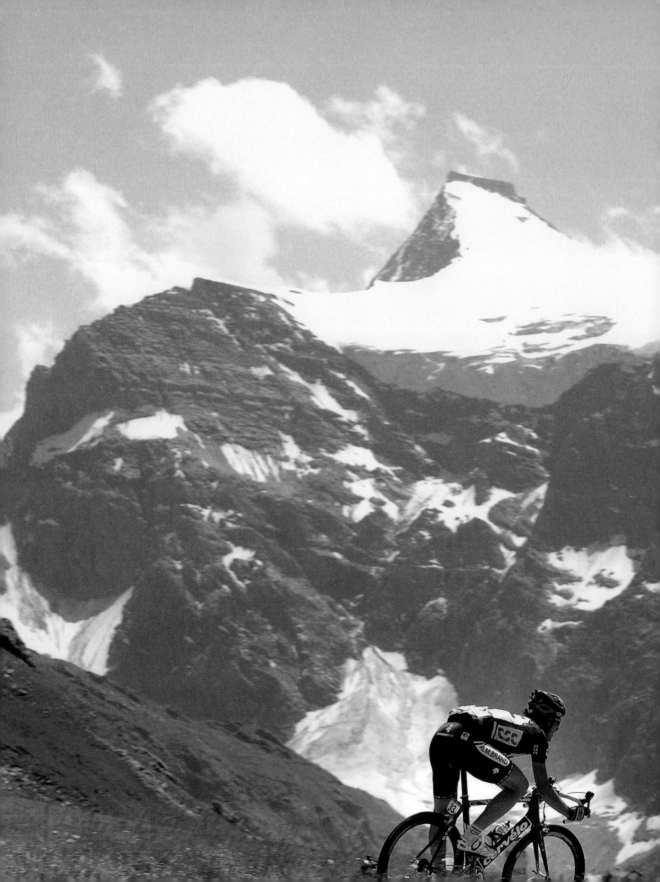

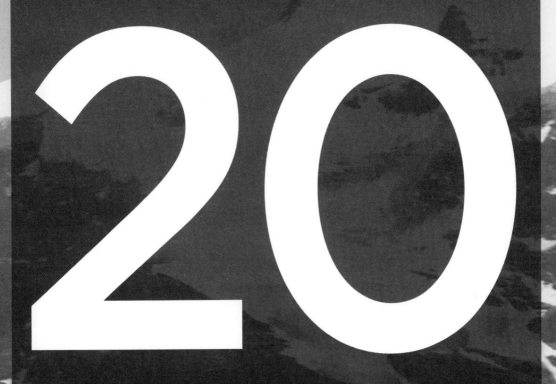

20

Fabian Cancellara

1981–

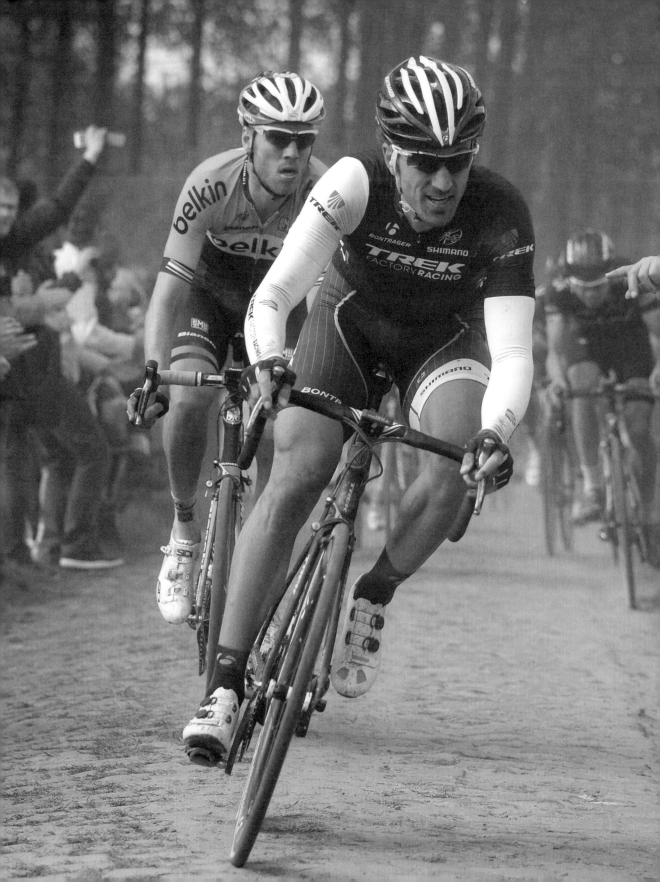

The way you feel on the bike isn't necessarily informed by the talent you have. That's one of the things that makes cycling so compelling for so many people, and one of the things that makes the suffering worthwhile.

There is literally nothing like the feeling you get when you're going well. There are days when you climb effortlessly, and days when the time trial feels like a spiritual experience. Better still, it doesn't actually matter whether you're a champion or not, nor even whether you *win* or not. Of course everyone *wants* to win, but that state of grace can just as easily be granted to a guy in the middle of the peloton. As a matter of fact, it can happen to just about anyone who puts the miles in and gets into shape, because even a club rider can feel like a champion from time to time.

The flip-side is the days when you just know that, irrespective of what you do, how hard you train and how good you thought you were, you're out of your depth.

Mine was the 1998 Junior World Championships time trial in Holland. I was 18, I was winning a lot at home, and like everyone else there I was the best in my country. I was under the impression I was a decent tester, but that day we all ran headlong into an irresistible force.

Fabian Cancellara came from Switzerland. At 17 he was a year younger than most of us, and he looked it until they put him on a bike. Then he started to ride the thing, and it became apparent that he was light years ahead. In terms of strength, speed and straight-up horsepower, he was unlike any junior time trialist I'd ever competed against.

He seemed to be operating at a completely different level to the rest of us, and, for the next 15 years or so, as often as not he pretty much just was . . .

Leading Belgium's Sep Vanmarcke through a cobblestoned sector during the 2014 Paris–Roubaix. Cancellara finished third that year to Vanmarcke's fourth place, with Dutchman Niki Terpstra the winner.

D O YOU REMEMBER THE 2011 TOUR OF BAVARIA? Probably not because . . . well, because it was the Tour of Bavaria! It took place at the end of May, at the same time as the Tour of California, the Tour of Belgium and the final week of the Giro. Commercially they were all much bigger races, but cycling's beauty lies in the fact that it's a broad church. There are three-, four- and five-day stage races, one-week stage races and ten-day stage races. There are fast, flat stage races, mountainous stage races and rolling stage races. There are flat classics, hilly classics and semi-classics, and then there are lots of small, traditional, old, provincial single-day races the wider public never sees.

There are beautiful races that have been running for over 100 years. Because they're not in the World Tour a lot of people don't give them a second thought, but you can bet your life they mean a hell of a lot to the local public and to many of the riders taking part. Not everyone can win the Tour or the Giro, but success in cycling has always been relative. For someone, somewhere, a top-ten finish in the Vuelta a Burgos or the Coppa Bernocchi is a huge result, and that's one of the things I like most about the sport. For all the changes, all the new money and all the re-found popularity, it's still really democratic and it still goes to its public. There are hundreds of professionals who can never dream of riding a grand tour, but it doesn't stop them dreaming, it doesn't preclude them from making a living from riding their bikes, and it doesn't stop them from enjoying a 'day of grace'. There are moments in every cyclist's career when he can't feel the chain, and for the most part they're not at the Giro or the Tour, and nor are they in the Alps or the Dolomites.

On 28 May 2011 Vasily Kiryienka made a long, lone break to win at Sestriere, and he dedicated his stage win to Xavier Tondo. He'd been a team-mate at Movistar who had died in a terrible accident a few days earlier. Alberto Contador came in with the GC group and clinched one of the saddest *maglie rosa* in history. Wouter Weylandt had died during the race. It was a poignant conclusion to a desperate Giro, but as ever Planet Cycling was looking on.

Not me though. I was riding a 30-kilometre time trial in a small German market town called Friedberg. It has a population of around 30,000, many of whom had come out to watch the race. It was a long way from the Giro in every sense, but all the same it's a day I'll never forget.

I was a time trialist. Races against the clock were the bedrock of my professional life, and I won them at the Tour and the Giro, the World Championships and the Olympic Games. Ostensibly that lot were much, much more important than a small stage race in southern Germany, so why the fuss?

Winning Stage 3 of the 2007 Tour de France while wearing the *maillot jaune* that he'd worn since winning the prologue in London.

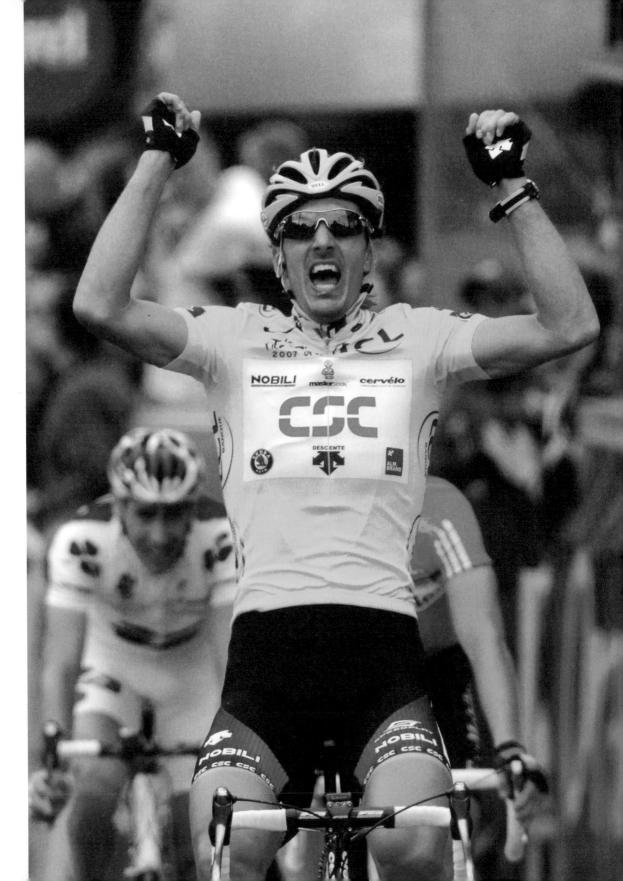

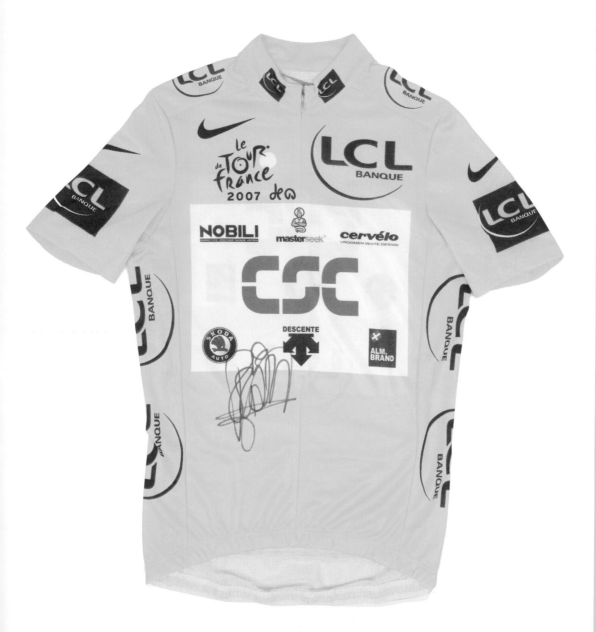

2007 Tour de France *maillot jaune*; my old friend and rival was kind
enough to send me a race-worn *maillot jaune* from each of the Tours
that he spent in yellow

The best way for me to explain is by inviting you to imagine being a sprinter. Imagine winning a stage at the Giro, beating the likes of Sacha Modolo, Davide Appollonio and Giacomo Nizzolo. Now a Giro stage win is a nice thing to have on your CV, but as a pure sporting achievement it's not particularly significant. That lot are fairly ordinary by World Tour standards, so objectively you haven't beaten anybody that *really* matters. Now imagine winning a stage at the Tour of Bavaria, beating guys like Mark Cavendish, André Greipel and Marcel Kittel. There's no comparison. None whatsoever.

On 28 May 2011 I beat Fabian Cancellara in a flat 26-kilometre time trial.

I'm not going to list all of Fabian's achievements here. Most of you will probably be familiar with them, but in essence he won 75 pro races over his career. He won Flanders and Roubaix three times each, and that seems incredible to me. It's incredible not because it's so many but because, for someone like him, it isn't. There were times when it seemed impossible he might lose a race on that sort of terrain, times when you almost had to suspend disbelief because he was so strong. When he was at his best, even Tom Boonen – the great Boonen – had no answer.

Fabian rode away from the entire peloton to win Milan–San Remo, but he didn't do it on the Poggio. He attacked two kilometres from the finish, and they never caught up with him. He also spent 29 days in yellow over six separate Tours de France. (Bear in mind that Fabian wasn't a GC rider and that LeMond, one of the best Tour riders of all time, managed 22.) Throw in two Olympic golds and four rainbow jerseys for the time trial, and you begin to understand why I view Cancellara alongside the all-time greats, the real hard men of the sport, who could do anything. The likes of Van Looy, Freddy Maertens, Sean Kelly . . . and that's before I mention *that* descent on the Tour (look it up on YouTube). There really wasn't anything he wasn't capable of doing on his day, from winning races like Tirreno and Tour de Suisse, bunch sprints, breakaways, as well as being, lest we forget, a pretty awesome teammate to Basso, the Schleks and Sastre.

I beat Fabian again in 2012 – once at the Tour and once more at the Olympics. He wasn't good that day (he'd crashed in the road race), but I was flying so I think I'd have won anyway. It was just about as good as it ever got for me – but it was also, I guess, the beginning of the end for Fabian. If that's not a double-edged sword, then I don't know what is. I remember being told that I'd won. That I was 35 seconds up on Tony Martin with 5km to go. Nobody was giving me references on Cancellara. I refused to believe I'd won until Fabian had crossed the line. I simply couldn't discount him as I knew what he was capable of, and I held him in such high esteem. I think he finished fifth.

You see guys like Cancellara at the Tour because everyone understands that a stage win there is a great shop window. The narrative of a stage win, a super *domestique* or a perfect descent, is something remarkable in itself. As far as my own Tour ambitions after 2012 went, I had a decision to make – my contract with Sky had ended at the end of the 2013 season. I re-signed and made it clear that I was happy to work for Chris the following year. I'd have made it my business to be a good *domestique*, and still more so in light of what happened at the 2012 Tour. My pride wouldn't have allowed me to be anything but, and I wanted to ride it one more time without the pressure of trying to win it. I felt that I'd earned that, but Chris really didn't want me there. That was his prerogative – like a lot of champions he was fairly ruthless in bending things to his will, and the upshot was a 'him or me' situation. It fell upon Dave Brailsford to decide, and he decided he wanted Froome.

People often ask me about Sky in general, and Brailsford in particular. My answer is that he's not someone I would call a friend. I simply can't put my finger on it with him. His words don't always follow his actions and vice versa. Sky have developed proven working practices, and they turn talented riders into excellent ones. Whether you like it or not, they're easily the best grand tour team out there right now.

Some of what Sky do is genuinely new and revolutionary, but some is just standard stuff with a new spin on it. I think that partly explains why there are people who still see them as intruders, but the fans seem to be more strident than ever. They were always very passionate and ruled by their hearts – nothing wrong with that. Some are better informed than others, but they're predictable, if nothing else . . .

Comparing Team Sky to Lance's US Postal/Discovery Channel seems to have become a bit of a sport recently, and there probably are some similarities in terms of human behaviour. There's no vertical doping anymore, but the teams are not so very different because they're not far removed from each other in the evolutionary curve. Discovery closed down in 2007 and Sky started three years later, so it's hardly a surprise that there are similarities in the way they operate and ride. That said, anybody who really understands cycling history can draw parallels with Merckx's Molteni, and even Coppi's Bianchi. They each had *domestiques* with big, powerful engines, and neither team was in the business of allowing bike races to become a free-for-all.

Before Geraint Thomas became a deserved and popular winner this summer, it had seemed that Sky had long-since given up trying to ingratiate themselves with the fans. But that's nothing new. Anquetil's team was the same, and Molteni were French public enemy number one by the time Bernard Thévenet beat Merckx at the 1975 Tour. So while Sky haven't necessarily helped themselves with the die-hards in the past, theirs is a path well-trodden. They win the Tour de France, and to the casual observer the Tour de France is cycling.

But it's easy to get side-tracked when talking about the Tour with respect to its teams. For me, the beauty of cycling is in the talent of the individual cyclists it showcases,

In the Swiss champion's jersey during Stage 3 of the 2011 Tour de France.

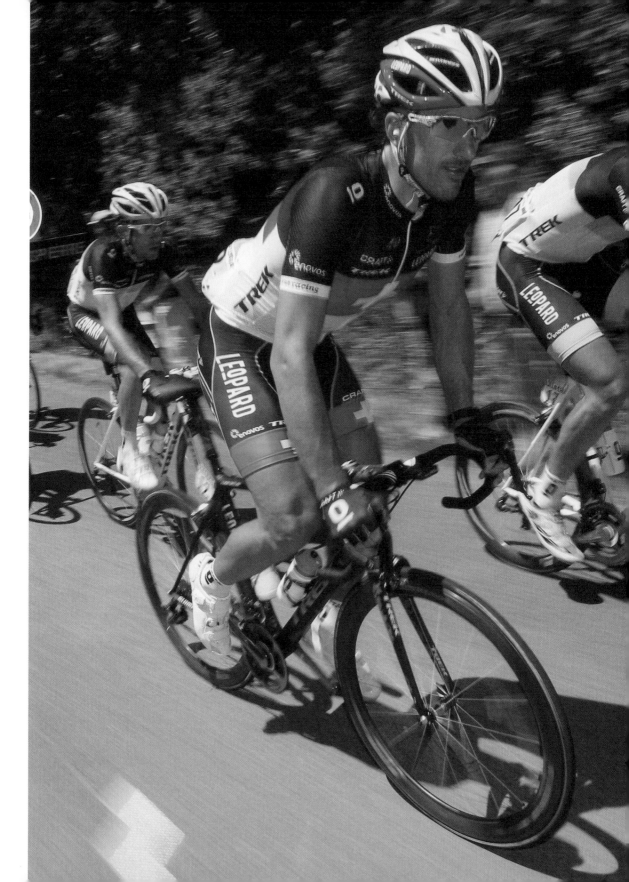

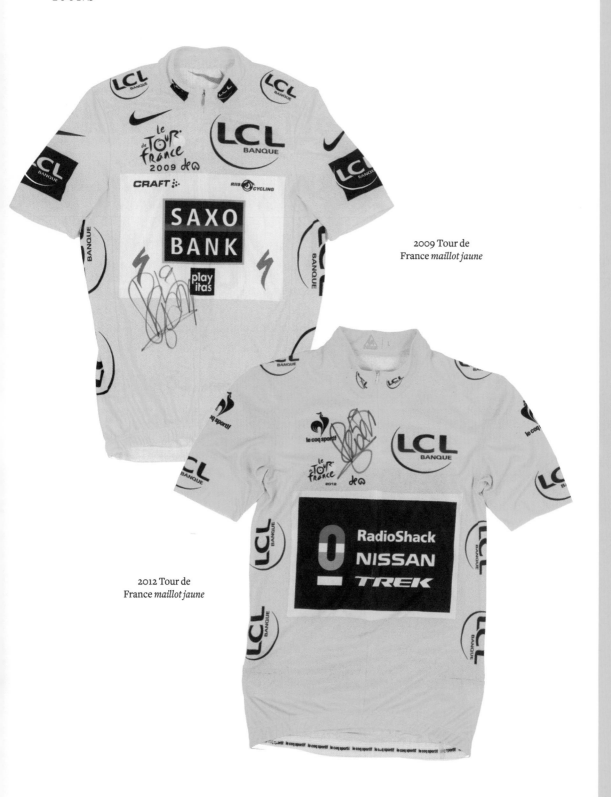

2009 Tour de
France *maillot jaune*

2012 Tour de
France *maillot jaune*

of whom Cancellara (in my mind) is one of the greatest. What a bike rider he was – to have really appreciated it, you needed to see him up close: his position on the bike, low down to the handlebars, sleek and smooth into the wind. He had, as much as any rider I've written about here, perfect form. For me, cycling is as much about competition and endurance as it is about beauty – of the body in harmony with the bike, of the postcard-perfect imagery of Alpine scenery and the vibrant colours of the peloton as it passes through the countryside. Cancellara is the kind of rider who makes me appreciate the joys not just of being a competitor, but also of being a fan.

As I mentioned earlier, cyclists have always made up fancy nicknames for themselves. It's their stock-in-trade, but I'm not sure anyone has had a better, more appropriate one.

Spartacus.

Absolutely brilliant.

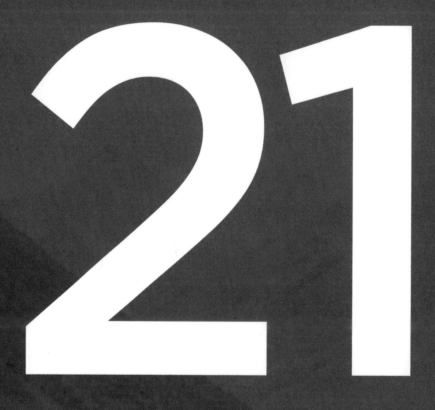

21

Fausto Coppi

1919–1960

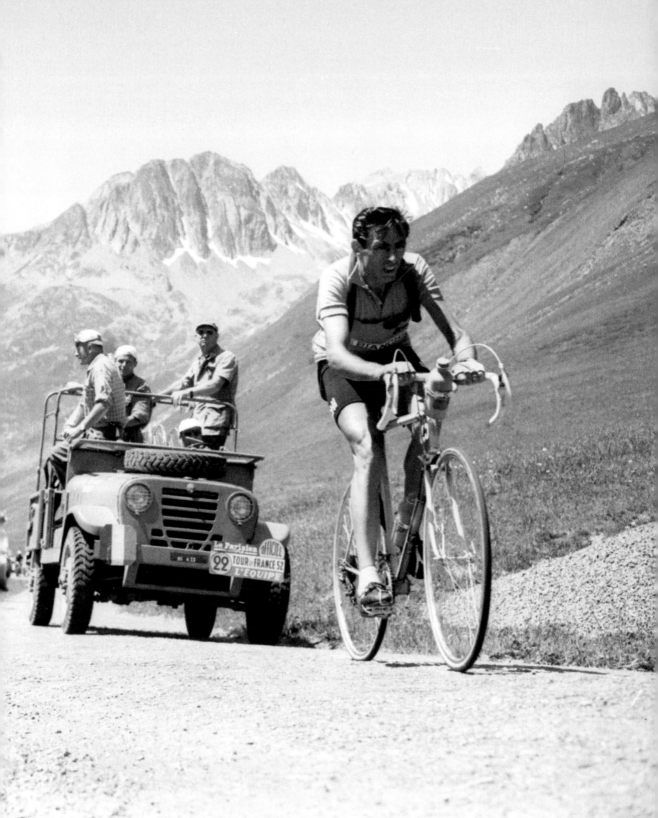

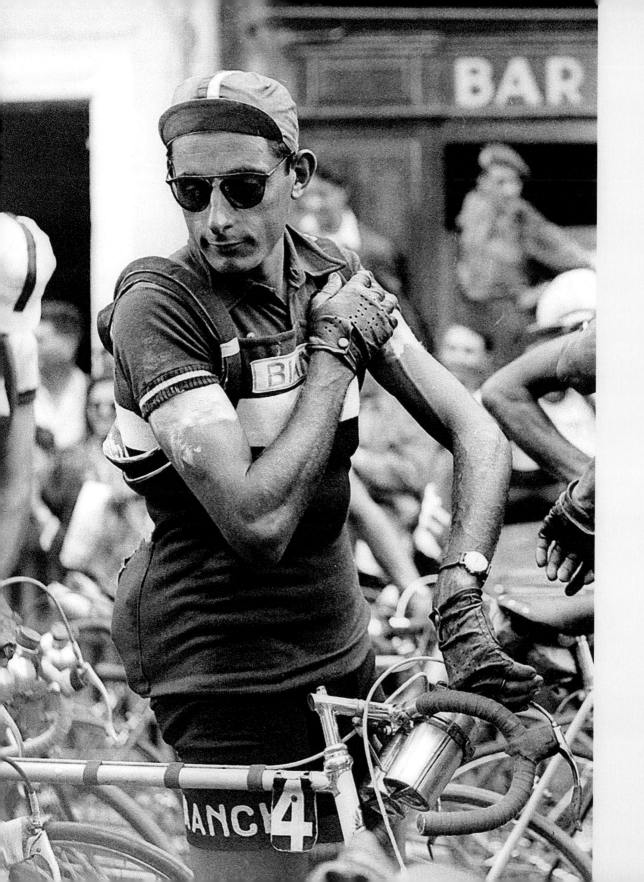

And so to cycling's eternal question...

Coppi or Merckx?

Or – depending on which side of the fence you sit – Merckx or Coppi?

We touched on the 'greatest of all time' argument in the Anquetil chapter. I think I've already declared for Eddy, but as always with sports it's personal. I discovered Eddy as I was falling in love with cycling, when I was a dreamer. As such he's synonymous – for me, at least – with a time of hope, optimism and discovery.

However, cycling is different things to different people. Although Eddy won the most, cycling is about much more than dry numbers. They are indicative and important, but they're not the only barometer because there are so many variables at play. The most interesting are the contextual forces that influence the way cycling has evolved. We don't always take the time to understand them fully, but we do know that they have a significant bearing on both performance and results.

I guess that in the final analysis, real greatness is made up of three elements: performance, impact and legacy. Or, to put it another way, it's about what sporting icons do, what their achievements mean when they do them, and whether or not they stand the test of time.

I think that in this sense Fausto Coppi is unique not only in cycling, but probably in the history of sport. I say that because, for all that he was an incomparable bike rider, he was much, much more than the races he won and lost. There was nobody even remotely like him, and the evolution of the sport suggests that there never will be.

In Italy they say that while Eddy is the best of all time, Fausto is the *greatest* of all time. Of course, they *would* say that, and who am I to disagree?

Turning out for the Italian national team on Stage 11 of the 1949 Tour de France. Coppi went on to win the GC, but there was controversy from the start as to whether he or Gino Bartali should be team leader.

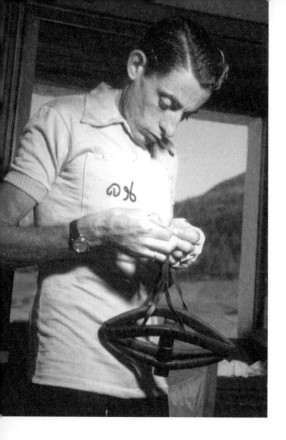

WHEN I WON THE TOUR IN 2012 there was a media feeding frenzy. So-called 'Wiggomania' took hold, and suddenly everything I did was news. I was a racing cyclist, but overnight my public persona grew bigger than what I actually did. It was, however, a massive change for me and my family, and it took a lot of getting used to.

Long before TV revolutionised sport in football's favour, Fausto Coppi was the first true sporting superstar. He was the first athlete whose professional and private lives became intertwined in the public consciousness, and the first to be subjected to intense media scrutiny. Or, to put it another way, Fausto Coppi was the first sportsman to occupy both the front *and* back pages.

During the years following the Second World War, Fausto Coppi's life on and off the bike was incredible. When I use the word 'incredible' I don't mean it in some lazy, throwaway sense; I mean it quite literally. As a racing cyclist he did things that nobody had previously conceived of. The impact his career had on everyday life – his own and those of his countrymen – was unprecedented and, I think, unique. He lived during a time of great social and cultural upheaval. Italy was becoming less agrarian and less Catholic, more industrial and more secular. Coppi and Gino Bartali were the perfect symbols of that, and they came to the fore at a time when Italy, crippled by the war, had genuine need of heroes. Post-war, cycling was still *the* sport in Europe and, as Tour de France winners and perennial rivals, the pair were idolised by millions. It's no exaggeration to state that they were the most famous people in Italy, and in all probability the most important. Rivalry is the heart and soul of sport, but I'm not sure there's been any other that has simultaneously enveloped and divided a country to such an extent.

We've established that cycling, with its up-hill and down-dale storyline, is the great sporting metaphor. Every long, endless climb has a descent, for every headwind there's a tailwind, and sooner or later all the wet, miserable, grovelling afternoons are

Left:
Inspecting his helmet strap, Stage 11 of the 1952 Tour de France.

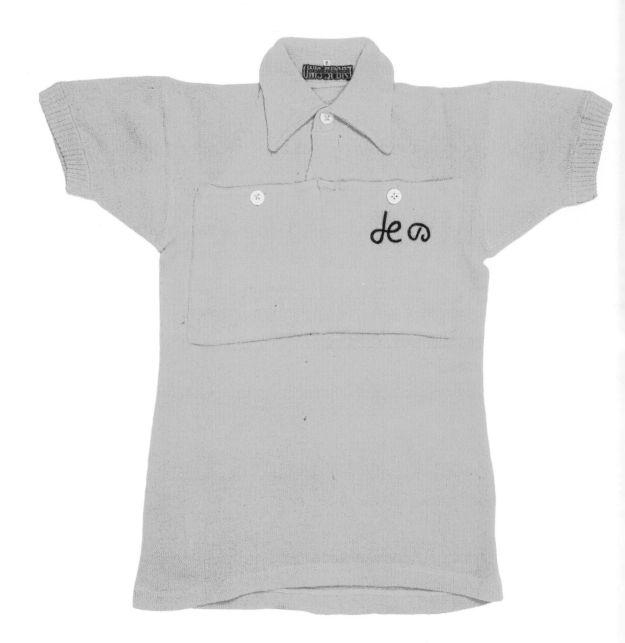

Fausto Coppi's 1949 *maillot jaune*, the oldest jersey in my collection

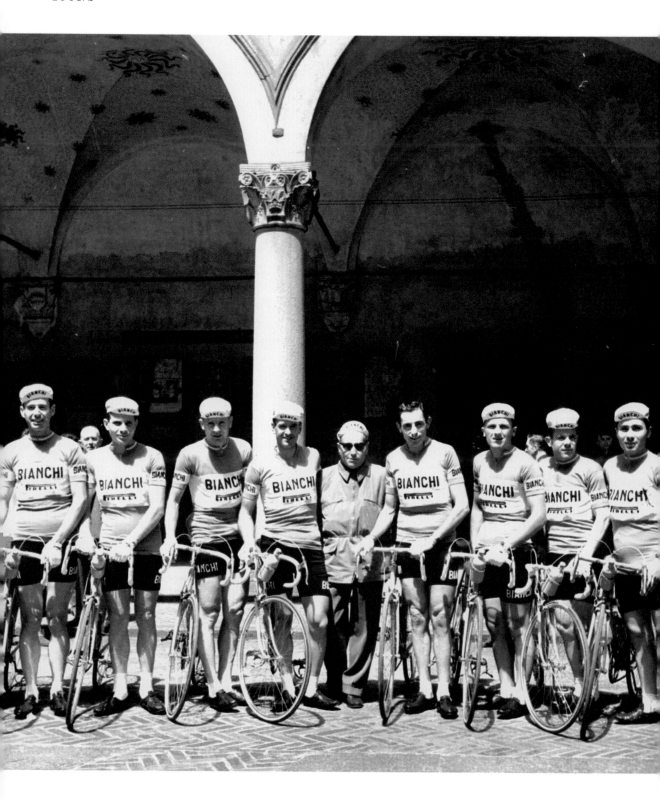

going to be rewarded with a day in the sun. Coppi personified that vision of the sport better than anyone – and more than anyone. He did things on a bike that were hitherto considered impossible, but he paid the heaviest price of anyone for his genius as a rider. He was a simple, humble, kindly man, and yet his was a life marked by tragedy and farce, and ultimately by a profound sadness.

In 1951 he lost his brother in a terrible racing accident, and he never truly recovered his equilibrium. His life became a soap opera, and in 1954 news broke that he'd left his wife and daughter for a married woman. It represented a watershed moment in Italy, because previously there'd been a tacit agreement that publishing the intimate secrets of high-profile public figures was off-limits.

Coppi's affair with Giulia Occhini, the '*Dama Biancha*', polarised and scandalised in equal measure. She actually went to prison for adultery, and the birth of their son, conceived out of wedlock and born in Argentina so as to assume his father's surname, was a seismic event in Catholic Italy. Everyone knew about it, everyone had an opinion on it, and it cut to the heart of the debate about liberal morality and the power of the Church. So when today's 'celebrities' complain about being in the public eye, perhaps we should try to be a little more objective about it. The eye of the public is one thing, but the eye of a public hurricane is something else entirely.

When Fausto died suddenly and (it must be said) dramatically of malaria in 1960, an entire country mourned. For Italians it was one of those 'Where were you?' moments, like when JFK was shot or Princess Diana died. That was Fausto Coppi, that was what he meant, and, regardless of performance, no cyclist has ever meant so much to so many since. They did a poll in Italy a few years ago, and it concluded that he was their greatest-ever sportsman. That's instructive, because he'd stopped winning by 1955 and there aren't many Italians left who saw him at his best. Most tellingly of all, though, he pre-dated TV. They didn't see him ride, but they understand what he was, what he represented, and the depth of influence his story has on their own.

What, though, of Coppi the cyclist? It's not easy to articulate just how good he was, but I'll try, as best I can, to explain . . .

To win the Giro–Tour double is the Holy Grail for stage racers. Very few achieve it, and it goes without saying that those who do are freakishly talented. To fully appreciate just how hard it is, keep in mind that it was beyond champions like Lance Armstrong, Greg LeMond and Alberto Contador. It's been 20 years since Marco Pantani did it, but we're used to the idea that, from time to time, a great champion emerges to have a crack at it. Anquetil and Merckx did it, so did Hinault and Induráin, and Stephen Roche did it in 1987, his year of grace. As I write this, Chris Froome just failed to add his name to the list, having already landed a bruising Giro.

The Bianchi team presentation in Milan in 1959.

To put all of the above into some sort of context I want to rewind to 1949. By then Coppi was 29, and approaching his peak as a bike rider. Nine years earlier he'd begun the Giro as a scrawny *gregario* for Bartali, and finished up running away with the *maglia rosa*. Italy had declared war the following week and, save for the odd semi-classic and the Hour Record in 1942, Fausto's career had been placed on hold for five years.

The first big race back had been the 1946 Milan–San Remo. He'd won it by 15 minutes (the radio broadcaster had played 'dance music' while they waited for the rest of the field to arrive), but then he'd been beaten by Bartali at the Giro. From there on in, their rivalry had gripped Italy, and the odd race in Switzerland aside it had been played out almost exclusively at home. It was tit-for-tat, and at times really caustic. However, at San Remo and Lombardy, the two great Italian classics, Fausto had ridden away pretty much as he'd pleased. Put simply, he couldn't be beaten.

In winning the 1938 Tour, Gino Bartali had become a national hero. He'd been a Christian Democrat at a time when Italy was rapidly falling out of love with Mussolini's fascism, and the symbolism of that had been very important. In Coppi's absence he'd done it again ten years later, at the ripe old age of 34. Now Italians, particularly traditionalists and folks in the centre and south, couldn't get enough of 'Gino the Pious'. Suddenly there were Bartali-branded razors, Bartali raincoats and Bartali Chianti, Bartali bikes and even Bartali scooters. Objectively, Coppi was younger and better, but whether he liked it or not the Tour was the Tour. Italians, millions of them, lined up behind the old lion Bartali.

Upon Bartali's triumphant return from France, the two of them were selected to ride for Italy at the 1948 World Championships in Holland. When the decisive break went, they chose not to go with it, but instead to sit and mark one another. With the race disappearing up the road they remained passive because neither dared contemplate the idea that the other might win. For Coppi – and for Bianchi, his sponsor – another big Bartali victory would have been catastrophic. For Bartali, just then in the ascendency, it was a no-brainer. Anybody, he reasoned, but Coppi. In the end, the Belgian Briek Schotte won the race.

Coppi and Bartali had averted disaster, but for Italian cycling the stalemate was a calamity. Both were fined and banned by the federation, but when the dust settled most of the *tifosi* sided with Bartali. Coppi was losing the battle for hearts and minds, it was costing him millions of lire, and worst of all it was costing him his psychological well-being. Heading into that 1949 season, he needed to find a solution and to prove that there was an abyss between him and Bartali.

Most reasoned cycling people believed the Giro–Tour double to be impossible. The combined distance of the 1949 editions was 8,800 kilometres, and the Tour started

With team-mate Adolfo Leoni after Stage 20 of the 1947 Giro d'Italia, the third of Coppi's five Giro victories.

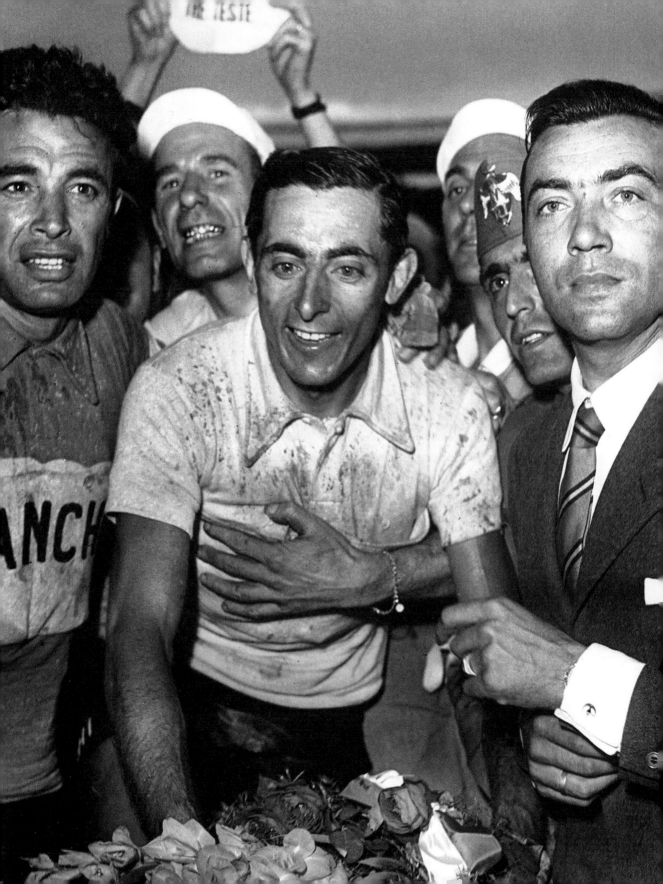

just 18 days after the Giro – not long enough to recover, but too long to hold form. (By comparison, the 2017 distance was 7,100 kilometres, with 34 days in between.) Coppi, though, had had a gutful of Bartali, and a gutful of the tittle-tattle that always seemed to surround him. He decided to risk everything, to settle the argument once and for all.

Every sport has its high watermark, and everyone can point to a 'golden age' of cycling. It's open to debate, but what's not in question is the events of 10 June 1949. That was the day of Cuneo-Pinerolo, the hardest mountain stage ever conceived. Over 254 kilometres they would scale the great cols – Vars, Izoard, Maddalena, Montgenèvre and Sestriere. When Fausto Coppi attacked 192 kilometres (that's *one hundred and ninety-two*) kilometres from home, the mortals of the peloton were incredulous. Bartali was still incredulous when he finished second, almost twelve minutes in arrears and utterly broken.

Cuneo-Pinerolo is worthy of a book in its own right, but most cycling historians agree that it was as good as it ever got, the apogee both of cycling's popularity and Coppi's greatness. That's a bold claim, and as such it begs one simple, obvious question – why?

Everyone in England is familiar with Kenneth Wolstenholme's 'Some people are on the pitch . . .' For millions it's intrinsic to and indivisible from the 1966 World Cup Final, the greatest moment in English sporting history. In pre-TV Italy, cycling was consumed via the radio, and the commentator that day was a certain Mario Ferretti. He began his broadcast by exclaiming, breathlessly, that '*Un uomo solo è al comando, la sua maglia è bianco-celeste, il suo nome è Fausto Coppi!*'.

It means, 'One man alone is leading, his jersey is sky blue and his name is Fausto Coppi.' It's a perfect distillation of cycling in the age of Coppi, and it encapsulates an era not only of Italian sport, but of Italian social history.

Coppi would win the Giro by 23 minutes and – part one of the impossible double complete – made for Paris. With the Tour organised along national lines as distinct to trade teams, he was compelled to share leadership of the Italian team with Bartali. He found the stress of that almost impossible to cope with and, his nerves shredded, he lost 18 minutes on the stage in Brittany. After a week's racing he trailed the great Swiss champion Ferdi Kübler by 22 minutes, Bartali by 13. Worse still, he fell victim to a profound moral and physical crisis. He told Alfredo Binda, the team manager, that he could no longer ride with Bartali, and had to be persuaded to carry on *in extremis*.

Then, what with being Fausto Coppi and all, he went and produced the most astonishing comeback in the history of the sport.

On 24 July he rolled into Paris in yellow, with Bartali conclusively defeated and the argument finally settled. It was perhaps the greatest of all the Tours de France, and

In front of the Castello Sforzesco in Milan with his Bianchi team-mates.

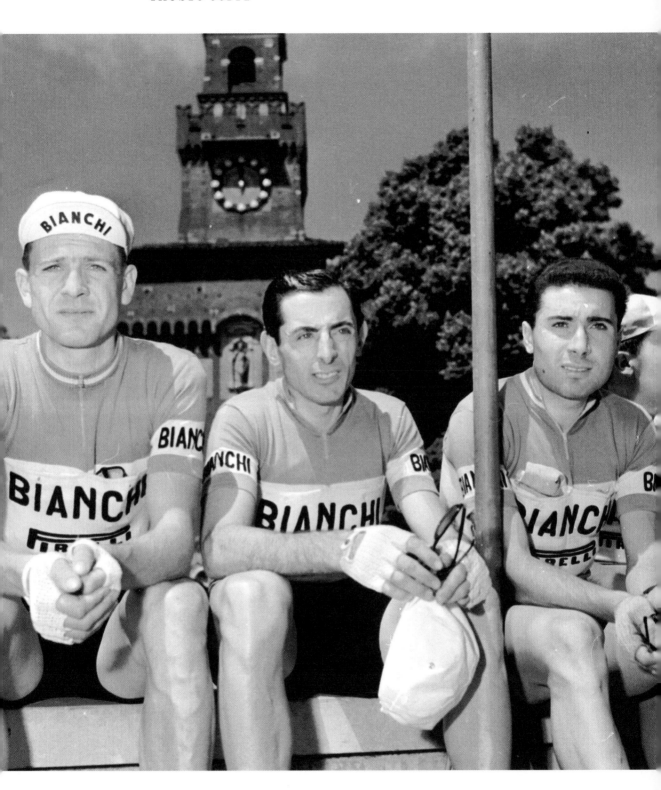

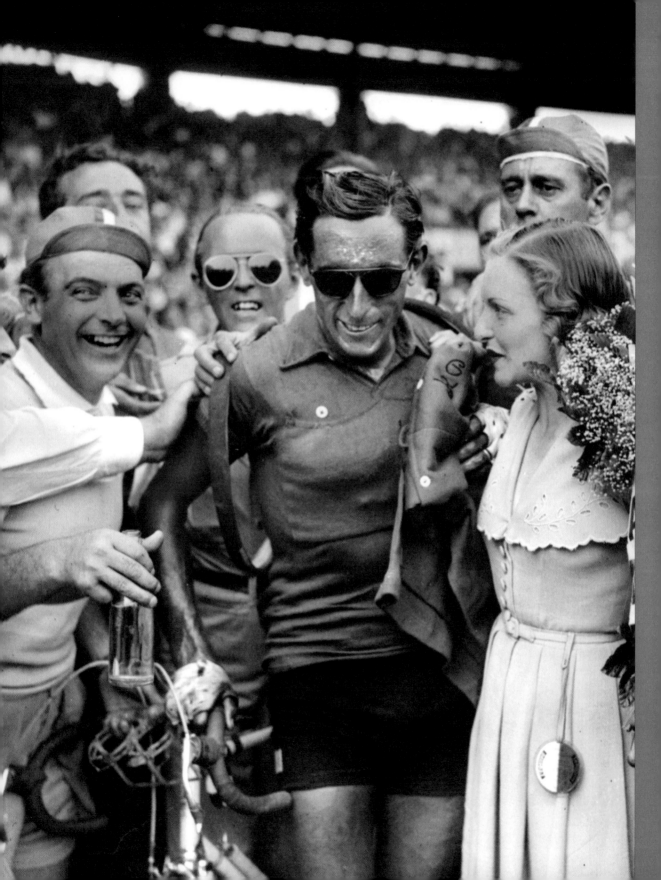

irrefutably the greatest stage-racing feat in history. Fausto would repeat the double in 1952, and those who witnessed it say that nobody – Eddy included – would ever replicate that level of performance.

They called him 'The Heron', and never was a cycling nickname more fitting. Off the bike he was shy, unremarkable and physically somewhat awkward. He had a distended chest cavity and skinny legs, but in flight they transformed him into a thing of wonder; elegant, graceful, absolutely sublime.

And yet . . . And yet through it all he was blighted by bad luck, illness and injury. There was always tension around him, and always the feeling that what could go wrong inevitably would. They said he had 'light bones', because when he crashed something always seemed to break. Somehow the injuries, the war, the tragedies, the scandals and the vagaries of post-war racing saw to it that he won 'only' five editions of the Giro, only two of the three Tours de France in which he competed and, in 1953, his one and only road rainbow jersey.

Of course there were countless others as well (Paris–Roubaix, Flèche Wallonne, World Pursuit Championships, the Grand Prix des Nations), but in some respects even the results aren't the issue. The issue with Coppi is who he was and what he represents, and the profound impact he had on those who knew him and those who didn't. He rode in cycling's age of plenty, when its popularity seemed boundless. It was an era of true greats, the era of Bartali and Fiorenzo Magni, Rik Van Steenbergen and Stan Ockers, of Ferdi Kübler, Hugo Koblet and Louison Bobet.

These were immense bike riders but, by their own admission, 'The Heron' was something else.

Coppi is congratulated upon his arrival, 24 July 1949 at the Parc des Princes in Paris, after winning the Tour de France.

AFTERWORD

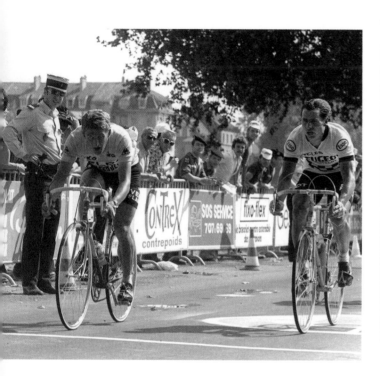

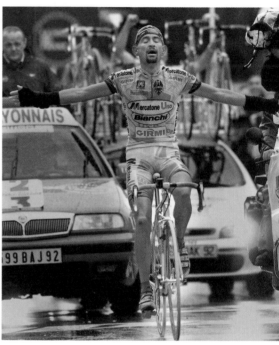

I think it's fair to say that 2018 hasn't exactly been my favourite year on record, but writing this book has been hugely motivating and a welcome distraction. I have been given the opportunity to reflect on and remember all those cyclists who've genuinely inspired me over the years. It's a bit of a cliché, but I have no doubt that these men not only helped shape me as a rider, but also as an individual.

I think one of the best things about putting the book together and immersing myself in my collection is that it has reminded me why I fell in love with this sport in the first place. I am no spring chicken these days, but cycling can still make me feel like that giddy young boy watching Johan Museeuw winning the Worlds in 1993 in his beautiful tricolour jersey.

That said, having to select only 21 riders has been a hell of a job. I would have loved to have written about Matt Illingworth, Colin Sturgess, and Malcolm Eliott but sadly, you have to draw the line somewhere. At the very least, I wanted to mention a few more here:

Left to right: Champions past and present: Freddy Maertens, Marco Pantani, Geraint Thomas and Peter Sagan.

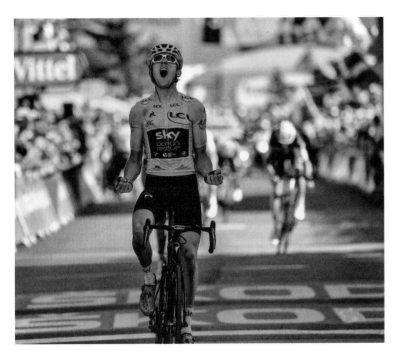

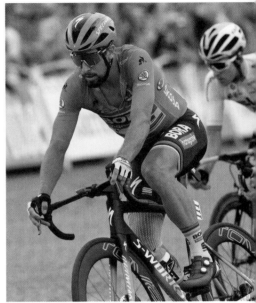

The great Freddy Maertens – two-time champion at the Worlds – had a turbulent but often astonishing career. He pushed Eddy all the way and it made him a better rider for it. His comeback in 1981, after years in the wilderness, should be recognised as one of the most iconic redemptions in the history of the sport. I've referenced him before in this book and it goes without saying, the 'pirate' Marco Pantani was a similarly combustible and utterly amazing rider. He was an outrageous climbing machine, but it was his innate charisma that gave him genuinely iconic status amongst his fan base. Last but certainly not least, Philippa York is one of the UK's most important riders of all time – the first Brit to win a major Tour classification and someone who massively raised the bar for British cycling.

I guess I might also get a bit of a shoeing for not including any current riders in my line up. So I have to say that it's been an absolute pleasure to witness the rise and rise of Peter Sagan. Characters like him are exactly what this sport needs and such a potent mixture of personality and ability keeps cycling relevant and enjoyable. And

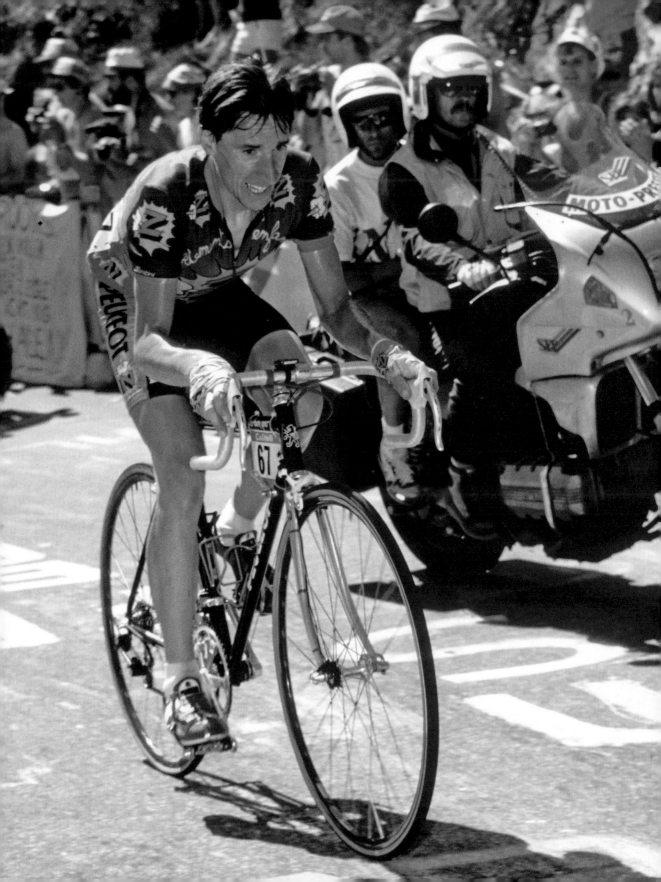

I obviously can't write this afterword without mentioning 'G'! What a fantastically dominant performance and I am incredibly proud of him, knowing just how much hard work was put into that. I am banging on but I must add that I have complete faith that the sport is in great hands. These guys will undoubtedly inspire others in the same way that the 21 icons in this book inspired me.

What else is there to say? Cycling is incredibly demanding, both physically and mentally, and as a professional sport it attracts a certain kind of individual. I hope I've managed to capture something of this mindset in the book – the unique psychology, character trait or obsession that allows or even propels someone to succeed. I feel privileged to be a member of this group of nutters; we are not what you might call 'normal' people, but 'normal' certainly doesn't win you a Tour!

The final – and perhaps most important – point of this book is to say that while cycling is clearly an exhilarating and physical sport to watch or compete in, it's just so vital for us all to appreciate its history and culture. I have nothing against the celebration of modern tactics and the incredible leaps in data analytics, but I am a romantic and don't want to see the pursuit of precision come at the expense of cycling's soul. Cycling is not simply a sport but an art: this is what makes it exceptional.

Anyway, to sign off I will paraphrase the great Maya Angelou: you can forget what they said, you can forget what they did, but you can't forget how they made you feel. This has been a blast and I have no regrets. I fulfilled my dream, riding in the slipstream of the greats.

Sir Bradley Wiggins

Opposite: Robert Millar, now Philippa York, on a gruelling stage with the Z team.

#icons21

311

GLOSSARY OF CYCLING TERMS

bidon – water bottle carried in cage on bike

....

bit-and-bit riding – alternating riding at front to share aerodynamic benefit of slipstream when riding behind

....

bonk/hitting the wall – complete loss of energy while riding

....

broomwagon – support vehicle that collects riders who cannot continue in race

....

classics – one-day races with historic status; *see also* northern classics

....

criterium – multiple-lap race

....

crono – time trial

....

directeur sportif (**DS**) – manager of cycling team, also known as sporting director

....

disc wheel – aerodynamic back wheel used in time trial

....

domestique – rider who supports team or team leader; *see also gregario*

....

GC (**general classification**) – ordering of stage race based on cumulative riding time

....

grand tour – three-week stage races: Giro d'Italia, Tour de France, Vuelta a España

....

gregario – Italian for *domestique*

....

Hour Record – furthest distance ridden over one hour, usually in indoor velodrome

....

kermesse – multiple-lap race, usually staged in Belgium or Holland

....

madison – team track race, where members of team replace each other on track, often by using slingshot

....

maglia rosa – jersey worn by GC leader in Giro d'Italia

....

maglia verde – jersey worn by points leader for sprinting in Giro d'Italia

....

maillot blanc – jersey worn by leader of young riders' competition in Tour de France

....

maillot jaune – jersey worn by GC leader in Tour de France

Monuments – five ultra-classic one-day races: Liège–Bastogne–Liège, Milan–San Remo, Paris–Roubaix, Tour of Flanders, Tour of Lombardy

musette – bag containing food given to a rider while riding

northern classics – one-day races held in France and Belgium in spring, often on cobbles (*pavé*)

omnium – multi-event track race

palmarès – list of rider's major wins and placings

passista – rider who can do long turn at front, particularly in northern classics

patron – boss of peloton

pavé – cobbles

percorso (**French:** *parcours*) – route taken by race

prologue – short time-trial before first stage of stage race

pursuit – individual or team event in velodrome with aim of catching opponents starting at opposite side of track

rainbow jersey – world champion's jersey

rouleur – rider excelling on flat or gently undulating terrain

sagwagon *see* **broomwagon**

six-day race – race at velodrome, usually involving teams of two

soigneur – team support worker who also gives massages

sporting director *see directeur sportif*

tempo, riding at – fastest sustainable pace

tester – rider specialising in time trials

tifosi – Italian cycling fans

time trial – form of racing where riders start one by one and race against clock

yellow jersey *see maillot jaune*

INDEX

PICTURE CREDITS

Photos of memorabilia © Andrew Brown

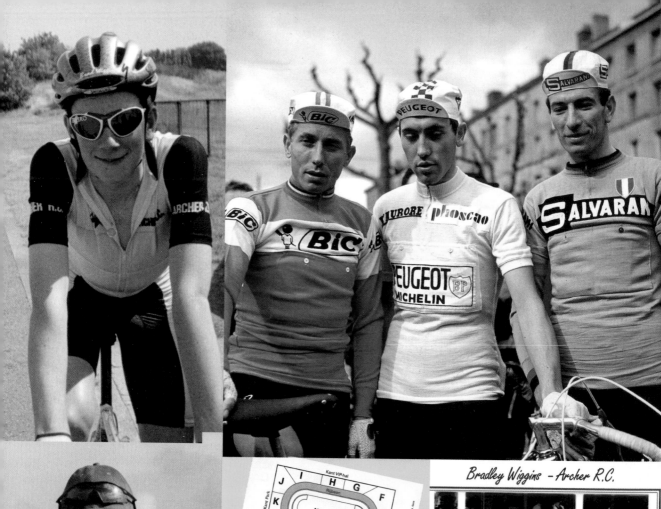

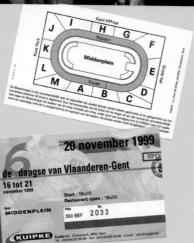

Bradley Wiggins - Archer R.C.

20 november 1999
de daagse van Vlaanderen-Gent
16 tot 21
november 1999

Start : 19u00
Restaurant open : 18u00

Middenplein

Prijs   Nr
350 BEF   2033

KUIPKE   Kuipke nv - Citadelpark, 9000 Gent
Tel +32(0)9/222.06.36 - Fax +32(0)9/220.54.94 - e-mail : info@kuipke.be

Wiggins — how he won

WHEN Bradley Wiggins became Britain's first-ever junior world track champion in Cuba recently — winning the pursuit title — he felt no great surge of excitement at his achievement. He simply couldn't take it in, which may well turn out be a portent for his future, for that is exactly how Chris Boardman felt when he won the Olympic pursuit title in Barcelona six years before.

"It was weird. I thought I'd be ecstatic winning, but I wasn't," recalled Wiggins upon returning home to London last week.

By then, however, the significance of his achievement had def-

national track titles last year — in the pursuit, kilo, points and scratch — and was not alone in believing that the youngster was destined for greater things. His world title now confirms that feeling. Strange as it may seem, it was the World points title he had trained for, though, not the pursuit.

"I'd planned everything around winning the points," he said. "I'd had this big build-up through the winter and I decided to put a lot into it and built my whole season around the points race." He had plenty of incentive after finishing fourth in the race last year, missing a medal by one point.

"Al... for the ... "Then ... at the ... for the ...

Tha... Brite p... super t...

"I c... 3.24 3... the nati... said W... the Li... right. "... can wi...

est London Juvenile Divisional Road Champion 1994
CA London & Home Counties Criterium Champion 1993/4
out the Hill Monday Competition Juvenile Track Champion 1994